METHODS IN MOLECULAR BIOLOGY

Series Editor
John M. Walker
University of Hertfordshire
School of Life and Medical Sciences
Hatfield, Hertfordshire, UK

For further volumes:
http://www.springer.com/series/7651

Cancer Nanotechnology

Methods and Protocols

Edited by

Reema Zeineldin

School of Applied Sciences
Mount Ida College
Newton, MA, USA

Humana Press

Editor
Reema Zeineldin
School of Applied Sciences
Mount Ida College
Newton, MA, USA

ISSN 1064-3745 ISSN 1940-6029 (electronic)
Methods in Molecular Biology
ISBN 978-1-4939-6644-8 ISBN 978-1-4939-6646-2 (eBook)
DOI 10.1007/978-1-4939-6646-2

Library of Congress Control Number: 2017932075

Printed on acid-free paper

This Humana Press imprint is published by Springer Nature
The registered company is Springer Science+Business Media LLC
The registered company address is: 233 Spring Street, New York, NY 10013, U.S.A.

Preface

This volume presents protocols for advancing the utility of nanotechnology in cancer research toward improving our understanding of cancer biology, prevention, diagnosis, and therapy. There are continuously new discoveries in the field of nanotechnology, thus creating new imaging systems or therapies. This volume does not aim at covering those expansive discoveries; instead, it focuses on how to employ certain discoveries for studying cancer by presenting principles along with techniques to allow for the transformation of any new discoveries in the field into cancer-studying tools. The audience for the field of nanotechnology in cancer is diverse and includes physical scientists, engineers, and biomedical scientists. A major deficiency in the field of cancer nanotechnology has been the limited involvement of biomedical scientists who can enhance the speed of discoveries toward cancer diagnosis and therapy. This volume of the *Methods in Molecular Biology* series in cancer nanotechnology may help focus the biomedical scientists on the potential in this field and improve their understanding of the utility of this field for conquering cancer. This volume also serves as a resource for physical scientists and engineers interested in employing nanotechnology in cancer diagnosis and therapy.

Newton, MA *Reema Zeineldin*

Contents

Part III Nanotechnology to Study Cancer

Part IV Nanotechnology for Prevention and Detection/Imaging of Cancer

Part V Nanotechnology-Based Therapies

Contributors

W. Russ Algar • *Department of Chemistry, University of British Columbia, Vancouver, BC, Canada*

Aws Alshamsan • *Nanomedicine Research Unit, Department of Pharmaceutics, College of Pharmacy, King Saud University, Riyadh, Saudi Arabia; King Abdullah Institute for Nanotechnology, King Saud University, Riyadh, Saudi Arabia*

Bhawani Aryasomayajula • *Center for Pharmaceutical Biotechnology and Nanomedicine, Northeastern University, Boston, MA, USA*

Paige Baldwin • *Department of Bioengineering, Northeastern University, Boston, MA, USA; Nanomedicine Science and Technology Center, Northeastern University, Boston, MA, USA*

Shashwat S. Banerjee • *Maharashtra Institute of Medical Education and Research Medical College, Talegaon Dabhade, Pune, India*

Pedro V. Baptista • *UCIBIO, Departamento de Ciências da Vida, Faculdade de Ciências e Tecnologia, Universidade NOVA de Lisboa, Caparica, Portugal*

Jodi Belz • *Department of Bioengineering, Northeastern University, Boston, MA, USA; Nanomedicine Science and Technology Center, Northeastern University, Boston, MA, USA*

Sandra W. Bishnoi • *Rice 360 Institute for Global Health, Rice University, Houston, TX, USA*

Ann-Marie Broome • *Department of Radiology and Radiological Science, Medical University of South Carolina, Charleston, SC, USA; Center of Biomedical Imaging, Medical University of South Carolina, Charleston, SC, USA; Department of Cell and Molecular Pharmacology & Experimental Therapeutics, Medical University of South Carolina, Charleston, SC, USA*

Robert B. Campbell • *Department of Pharmaceutical Sciences, MCPHS University, Worcester, MA, USA*

Noelle Castilla-Ojo • *Nanomedicine Science and Technology Center, Northeastern University, Boston, MA, USA*

Xiaoyuan Chen • *Laboratory of Molecular Imaging and Nanomedicine (LOMIN), National Institute of Biomedical Imaging and Bioengineering (NIBIB), National Institutes of Health (NIH), Bethesda, MD, USA*

Bei Cheng • *Department of Drug Discovery and Biomedical Sciences, University of South Carolina, Columbia, SC, USA*

Charlene M. Dawidczyk • *Department of Materials Science and Engineering, Johns Hopkins University, Baltimore, MD, USA; Institute for NanoBioTechnology, Johns Hopkins University, Baltimore, MD, USA*

Suraj Dixit • *Department of Radiology and Radiological Science, Medical University of South Carolina, Charleston, SC, USA*

Maxim E. Dokukin • *Department of Mechanical Engineering, Tufts University, Medford, MA, USA*

Rockford Draper • *Department of Biological Sciences, The University of Texas at Dallas, Richardson, TX, USA; Department of Chemistry and Biochemistry, The University of Texas at Dallas, Richardson, TX, USA*

Tarek M. Fahmy • *Department of Biomedical Engineering, Yale University, New Haven, CT, USA*
Brenda Farrell • *Department of Otolaryngology – Head and Neck Surgery, Baylor College of Medicine, Houston, TX, USA*
Alexandra R. Fernandes • *UCIBIO, Departamento de Ciências da Vida, Faculdade de Ciências e Tecnologia, Universidade NOVA de Lisboa, Caparica, Portugal*
Steven Fiering • *Department of Microbiology and Immunology, Geisel School of Medicine at Dartmouth University, Hanover, NH, USA; Department of Genetics, Geisel School of Medicine at Dartmouth University, Hanover, NH, USA; Norris Cotton Cancer Center, Dartmouth Hitchcock Medical Center, Lebanon, NH, USA*
Christian Foster • *Ligandal Inc., Berkeley, CA, USA*
Derek Hargrove • *Department of Pharmaceutical Sciences, University of Connecticut, Storrs, CT, USA*
Nazila Kamaly • *Department of Micro and Nanotechnology, DTU Nanotech, Technical University of Denmark, Kongens Lyngby, Denmark*
Joseph Kaplinsky • *Department of Micro and Nanotechnology, DTU Nanotech, Technical University of Denmark, Kongens Lyngby, Denmark*
Jayant Khandare • *MAEER's Maharashtra Institute of Pharmacy, Pune, India*
Vrushali Khobragade • *Actorius Innovations and Research, Pune, India*
Dongin Kim • *Department of Biomedical Engineering, Yale University, New Haven, CT, USA; Department of Pharmaceutical Sciences, Irma Lerma Rangel College of Pharmacy, Texas A&M HSC, College Station, TX, USA*
Rajiv Kumar • *Department of Physics, Northeastern University, Boston, MA, USA; Nanomedicine Science and Technology Center, Northeastern University, Boston, MA, USA*
Samuel K. Lai • *Division of Molecular Pharmaceutics, University of North Carolina at Chapel Hill, Chapel Hill, NC, USA*
Dmitri O. Lapotko • *Department of BioSciences, Rice University, Houston, TX, USA*
Jia Jun Li • *Department of Chemistry, University of British Columbia, Vancouver, BC, Canada*
Yujen Lin • *Institute of Chemistry, Academia Sinica, Taipei, Taiwan, China*
Dingbin Liu • *College of Chemistry, Research Center for Analytical Sciences, State Key Laboratory of Medicinal Chemical Biology, Tianjin Key Laboratory of Molecular Recognition and Biosensing, and Collaborative Innovation Center of Chemical Science and Engineering, Nankai University, Tianjin, China*
Xiuling Lu • *Department of Pharmaceutical Sciences, University of Connecticut, Storrs, CT, USA*
Ekaterina Y. Lukianova-Hleb • *Department of BioSciences, Rice University, Houston, TX, USA*
Melissa Massey • *Department of Chemistry, University of British Columbia, Vancouver, BC, Canada*
Amber A. McBride • *Sandia National Laboratories, Albuquerque, NM, USA*
Emilie McKinnon • *Department of Radiology and Radiological Science, Medical University of South Carolina, Charleston, SC, USA*
Alfred Moore • *Department of Radiology and Radiological Science, Medical University of South Carolina, Charleston, SC, USA; Center of Biomedical Imaging, Medical University of South Carolina, Charleston, SC, USA*
Vasanth S. Murali • *Department of Biological Sciences, The University of Texas at Dallas, Richardson, TX, USA*

PAVAN MUTTIL • *Department of Pharmaceutical Sciences, College of Pharmacy, University of New Mexico, Albuquerque, NM, USA*
AUTUMN D. PARO • *Department of Chemical Engineering, Northeastern University, Boston, MA, USA; Nanomedicine Science and Technology Center, Northeastern University, Boston, MA, USA*
DOMINIQUE N. PRICE • *Department of Pharmaceutical Sciences, College of Pharmacy, University of New Mexico, Albuquerque, NM, USA*
VIVEK RAJASEKHARAN • *Department of Otolaryngology – Head and Neck Surgery, Baylor College of Medicine, Houston, TX, USA; Department of Molecular and Cellular Biology, Baylor College of Medicine, Houston, TX, USA*
STEVEN M. RICHARDS • *Department of Pharmaceutical Sciences, MCPHS University, Worcester, MA, USA*
LUISA M. RUSSELL • *Department of Materials Science and Engineering, Johns Hopkins University, Baltimore, MD, USA; Institute for NanoBioTechnology, Johns Hopkins University, Baltimore, MD, USA*
GIUSEPPINA SALZANO • *Institute of Molecular Sciences, CNRS, Université Paris-Sud, Université Paris Saclay, Orsay, France*
PETER C. SEARSON • *Department of Materials Science and Engineering, Johns Hopkins University, Baltimore, MD, USA; Institute for NanoBioTechnology, Johns Hopkins University, Baltimore, MD, USA; Department of Oncology, Johns Hopkins University, Baltimore, MD, USA*
ILANCHEZHIAN SHANMUGAM • *Department of Physics, Northeastern University, Boston, MA, USA; Nanomedicine Science and Technology Center, Northeastern University, Boston, MA, USA*
MEE RIE SHEEN • *Department of Microbiology and Immunology, Geisel School of Medicine at Dartmouth, Hanover, NH, USA*
ALYSSA L. SIEFERT • *Department of Biomedical Engineering, Yale University, New Haven, CT, USA*
IGOR SOKOLOV • *Department of Mechanical Engineering, Tufts University, Medford, MA, USA; Department of Biomedical Engineering, Tufts University, Medford, MA, USA; Department of Physics, Tufts University, Medford, MA, USA*
VARUN K.A. SREENIVASAN • *Department of Physics and Astronomy, Macquarie University, Sydney, NSW, Australia*
SRINIVAS SRIDHAR • *Department of Physics, Northeastern University, Boston, MA, USA; Nanomedicine Science and Technology Center, Northeastern University, Boston, MA, USA*
JOAN SYOUFJY • *CVS Health, West Bloomfield, MI, USA*
SHIFALIKA TANGUTOORI • *Nanomedicine Science and Technology Center, Northeastern University, Boston, MA, USA*
VLADIMIR P. TORCHILIN • *Center for Pharmaceutical Biotechnology and Nanomedicine, Northeastern University, Boston, MA, USA; Department of Biochemistry, King Abdulaziz University, Jeddah, Saudi Arabia*
ANNE L. VAN DE VEN • *Department of Physics, Northeastern University, Boston, MA, USA; Nanomedicine Science and Technology Center, Northeastern University, Boston, MA, USA*
RUHUNG WANG • *Department of Biological Sciences, The University of Texas at Dallas, Richardson, TX, USA; Department of Chemistry and Biochemistry, The University of Texas at Dallas, Richardson, TX, USA*
ANDRE WATSON • *Ligandal Inc., Berkeley, CA, USA*

PEISHENG XU • *Department of Drug Discovery and Biomedical Sciences, University of South Carolina, Columbia, SC, USA*
QI YANG • *Division of Molecular Pharmaceutics, University of North Carolina at Chapel Hill, Chapel Hill, NC, USA*
REEMA ZEINELDIN • *School of Applied Sciences, Mount Ida College, Newton, MA, USA*
YUN ZHU • *Department of Radiology and Radiological Science, Medical University of South Carolina, Charleston, SC, USA*

Part I

Overviews

Chapter 1

Cancer Nanotechnology: Opportunities for Prevention, Diagnosis, and Therapy

Reema Zeineldin and Joan Syoufjy

Abstract

Nanotechnological innovations over the last 16 years have brought about the potential to revolutionize specific therapeutic drug delivery to cancer tissue without affecting normal tissues. In addition, there are new nanotechnology-based platforms for diagnosis of cancers and for theranostics, i.e., integrating diagnosis with therapy and follow-up of effectiveness of therapy. This chapter presents an overview of these nanotechnology-based advancements in the areas of prevention, diagnosis, therapy, and theranostics for cancer. In addition, we stress the need to educate bio- and medical students in the field of nanotechnology.

Key words Nanocarriers, Cancer, Targeting, Drug delivery, Theranostics, Education

1 Introduction

Nanotechnology has various applications in cancer including prevention, diagnosis, therapy, and the integration of diagnosis and therapy or theranostics. Various advancements in nanomaterials and design of nanocarriers or nano-based platforms have been tested for these applications. We present here an overview of these applications and we stress the need for partnership with biomedical scientists to focus on specific diseases in order to improve prevention, therapy, and theranostics of cancer.

2 Types of Nanocarriers and Nanomaterials

The first generation of nanocarriers included liposomes [1, 2] and simple polymers [3]. Liposomes are made of phospholipids, which have a polar head and a hydrophobic tail that self-assemble to form spheres ranging in size from tens of nanometers to hundreds of nanometers. Liposomes can be used to deliver hydrophilic or hydrophobic drugs [4–6] and they maybe functionalized with polyethylene glycol (PEG) to increase their half-life in circulation,

Reema Zeineldin (ed.), *Cancer Nanotechnology: Methods and Protocols*, Methods in Molecular Biology, vol. 1530,
DOI 10.1007/978-1-4939-6646-2_1, © Springer Science+Business Media New York 2017

and such liposomes are referred to as stealth liposomes [4, 7]. In general, nanocarriers that are used for drug delivery are usually functionalized by PEG with a molecular weight (MW) between 1 and 40 kDa [6]. This is a desirable coating for nanocarriers because it reduces their nonspecific interaction with serum proteins that tag them for internalization by cells within the reticuloendothelial system (RES). This reduces their immunogenicity and their non-specific uptake by cells within the RES, thus diminishing their phagocytosis and leading to prolonging the circulation time of nanocarriers [6]. In addition, functionalizing with PEG reduces toxicity and agglomeration of nanocarriers [8].

Simple polymers were also among the first generation of drug nanocarriers, and initially they comprised natural polymers such as polysaccharides [9] and polypeptides [10] made of natural building blocks, sugars and amino acids respectively. Examples of such polymers include chitosan and albumin, in addition to polylactic acid and polyglycolic acid or a combination of both. These natural polymers are also used to deliver non-soluble drugs after chemically conjugating them to the polymer. This way they mimic albumin in the circulation which transfers non-soluble molecules in the aqueous environment of the blood. Both liposomes and natural polymers have the advantages of being biocompatible and biodegradable.

More complex polymers that have been used as drug nanocarriers include micelles [11] which are made of self-assembling molecules that have hydrophobic and hydrophilic segments. In general nanocarriers with hydrophilic and hydrophobic domains are capable of transporting hydrophilic and hydrophobic drugs. The newer generations of nanocarriers include complex hydrogels made of a mixture of natural and nonnatural components [12], and other complex polymers like dendrimers [13, 14] which are branched polymers. Furthermore, stimuli-responsive polymers, such as those that change structure in response to a change in temperature or pH or even a physical stimulus have been incorporated into drug delivery systems [15, 16]. Newer nanocarriers include viruses [17, 18], metal- or oxide-based nanocarriers (gold, magnetic, quantum dots, titanium dioxide, zinc oxide, and silica) [19–27], carbon based nanocarriers (nanotubes and fullerenes) [28–30], and hybrids of materials such as lipid-coated or polymer-coated nanocarriers [31–33]. As new nanomaterials are generated and new nanocarriers are designed for various biomedical applications, it is important to characterize them for their physiochemical properties, toxicity, and biodistribution as described elsewhere [34].

3 Nanotechnology for Prevention and Diagnosis of Cancer

Prevention of cancer utilizes nanocarriers that deliver tumor-specific antigens to immune cells to elicit an immune response against cancer [35]. Diagnosis of cancer may be in the form of biosensing or diagnostic imaging [36]. Biosensing detects biomolecules that serve as biomarkers of cancers or detects cancer-specific cells such as cancer stem cells or circulating cancer cells. It may utilize the concept of lab-on-a-chip with employing nanocomponents or maybe based on utilizing nanomaterials to detect targets as reviewed elsewhere [37].

Imaging detects and monitors the cancer or may even assist in surgery to guide excision of cancerous tissue. Imaging that utilizes iron oxide, gold nanoparticles or carbon nanotubes may have a theranostic value because these nanomaterials may be employed for therapy in addition to imaging through their thermal ablation capabilities [38, 39]. The advantages of using nanomaterials in imaging include (1) their ability to generate and/or amplify imaging signals, (2) the development of new imaging technologies that are dependent on nanomaterial such as Raman imaging and photoacoustic imaging, (3) their targeting ability because their surface can be functionalized with cancer-targeting moieties, (4) their multimodality because some nanomaterials can produce signals for more than one imaging technology, (5) their utility in detecting micro-metastases usually missed by non-molecular imaging methods, and (6) some have a theranostic value.

4 Nanotechnology for Cancer Therapy

The traditional antineoplastic agents used with cancer patients are cytotoxic agents that are referred to as conventional chemotherapeutic agents. The common molecular drug targets of the conventional chemotherapeutic agents include DNA, RNA, enzymes, tubulin, or microtubules [40]. More recent therapies include molecularly targeted therapeutics that target specific cellular molecules within cancers (like inhibitors of receptors, transporters, signaling molecules, or transcription factors, antiangiogenic agents, and inhibitors of histone deacetylase) or immunotherapies that enhance the immune response to fight cancer [35, 41–44]. In general the use of conventional chemotherapeutic agents presents several problems and the use of nanocarriers for drug delivery overcomes these problems.

4.1 Challenges with Conventional Cancer Chemotherapeutic Agents

Treating the patient with the conventional chemotherapeutic agents may cause the patient to suffer from several side effects of the drug including loss of hair, reduced formation of blood cells, and sterility [40]. The reason for this is that the chemotherapeutic agents are toxic chemicals that kill cells nonspecifically so they are cytotoxic to both cancer and non-cancer cells. For example, if the chemotherapeutic agent used targets dividing cells, then normal actively dividing cells within the body such as hair cells, gastrointestinal cells, blood cells, and germ cells will be affected by the drug [40]. Alternatively, if the chemotherapeutic agent targets molecules in cells whether dividing or not dividing, this also means that non-disease cells in general will be affected by the drug [40].

Additional challenges of conventional chemotherapeutic agents include: (1) many of them have low aqueous solubility; (2) they get rapidly cleared by the liver and kidneys [40]; and (3) there may be a reduced effect of these drugs due to overexpression of a drug-efflux pump resulting in drug resistance [45]. These problems may limit the dose, frequency or duration of treatments with the conventional chemotherapeutic agents. Nano-based therapies have the potential to overcome all of these limitations.

4.2 Advantages of Nanocarriers in Drug Delivery to Cancers

Several of the above challenges can be counteracted through the use of different types of nanocarriers for drug delivery to cancers. The advantages of employing nanocarriers for drug delivery to cancers are summarized below.

4.2.1 Nanocarriers Can Deliver Hydrophobic Compounds

Using nanocarriers permits delivery of poorly soluble drugs as they may be enclosed within hydrophobic interfaces of the nanocarriers or they could be bound to molecules that can serve as their carriers in the blood.

4.2.2 Nanocarriers Are Multifunctional

Nanocarriers may be functionalized with various molecules through adsorption or chemical conjugations. Such molecules may include one or more drugs, an imaging agent, a targeting moiety such as a ligand or an antibody, and PEG. The loading of more than one drug is of importance in the case of drug resistance, so if the patient is not responsive to one drug, then presence of another or more drugs to which the patient appears to respond overcomes this problem. Carrying imaging agents in addition to drugs allows evaluating the responsiveness of cancer cells to the delivered drugs by visual evaluation of cancer tissue shrinkage, thus enabling theranostics. Adding a targeting ligand or antibody leads to specific active targeting of cancer cells by the drug-carrying nanocarriers with minimal effect on non-cancer cells.

4.2.3 Nanocarriers Passively and Actively Target Disease Cells

Nanocarriers within the size range 20–400 nm may accumulate at i.e., target the cancer site through passive targeting or enhanced permeability and retention (EPR) effect [46]. This results from the fact that the vascular endothelium lining the blood vessels at the cancer site exhibit large gaps in between cells and at the same time the cancer tissue lacks effective lymphatic drainage [47]. This causes leakage of nanocarriers through the gaps between endothelial cells into the cancer tissue where they get retained there because of defective lymphatic drainage, which results in targeting cancer tissue [46].

Not only can the nanocarriers carry more than one drug, but they can be loaded with high amounts of drugs especially if they are designed to target specific cancer cells through functionalization with targeting moieties so the nanocarriers serve as "magic bullets" [48]. A targeting moiety promotes active targeting of the cancer cells through molecules that are specifically expressed by the cancer cells, i.e., tumor markers, or by molecules that are overexpressed by the cancer cells. For example, folate receptor alpha (FRα) is a tumor marker expressed by certain epithelial cancers while in normal tissue it is not accessible through the blood [49]. Receptors overexpressed by cancer cells include epidermal growth factor receptor (EGFR), erbB2, αvβ3, CD20, and CD25 [41, 50–52]. In cancer, receptors on endothelial cells have been targeted to deprive cells from their blood supply. Examples for such receptors include integrins α2bβ3, αvβ3, and α5β1, and aminopeptidase-N [53, 54]. Actively targeting cancer cells or endothelial cells by nanocarriers results in more effective therapy while avoiding nonspecific toxicity to non-cancer cells.

The fact that nanocarriers can passively and/or actively target disease tissue while sparing normal tissue the side effects of drugs opens new areas for improving drug loading of nanocarriers with the aim of reducing the drugs' dose size. With traditional therapy it has been necessary to use high doses of drugs because drugs get metabolized by the liver or cleared through the liver and kidneys in addition to not being localized to the disease organ. In contrast, targeting of disease cells enhances the rate of bioavailability (through passive and active targeting) and intracellular delivery (through active targeting involving endocytosis) of the drug, which means smaller drug dose can be loaded onto nanocarriers.

4.2.4 Nanocarriers Prolong the Drug's Circulation Time

As discussed above modifying the nanocarriers with PEG is one way to prolong their blood circulation time. Other factors contributing to reducing the clearance of nanocarriers, thus prolonging their circulation time, include drug encapsulation and the nanocarriers' size. Drug encapsulation within a nanocarrier protects the drug from being metabolized by liver enzymes. The increased size of the nanocarriers decreases their clearance through the kidneys, although other factors such as charge may affect such clearance [55].

4.2.5 Nanocarriers Overcome Drug Resistance

Another advantage of using nanocarriers for drug delivery is that they promote overcoming drug resistance through more than one mechanism. One way is presented above and it is based on loading more than one drug onto nanocarriers, and the second results from the nanocarriers' avoidance of the drug efflux pump due to active targeting or the size of nanocarriers relative to pumped drug molecules [45].

4.2.6 Nanocarriers Promote Safety and Tolerability of Drugs

The use of nanocarriers increases the safety and tolerability of drugs as a result of the encapsulation of drugs in addition to the targeting to cancer site. Not all nanocarriers can be designed to encapsulate drugs, but the ones that do, prevent exposure of the blood and non-cancer cells to the drug and thus reduce the systemic side effects of drugs. The passive and the active targeting of the nanocarriers to the cancer site also prevent the unnecessary exposure of other cells to drugs and thus reduce the side effect of drugs. On the other hand, some nanocarriers may have their own toxicity and thus biocompatibility and studies on fate of nanocarriers are essential.

4.2.7 Nanocarriers Improve Other Technologies

Other existing technologies such as delivery of gene silencing inhibitory RNA (RNAi) benefit from the use of nanocarriers to specifically target disease cells while facilitating their entry into cells along with providing protection from cellular degradative nucleases. Different formulations of lipid nanocarriers and polymers have improved the delivery of RNAi [56–59]. More research is underway to improve their targeting to disease cells.

5 Opportunities for Research

There is not sufficient work on identifying mechanisms of uptake of nanocarriers and determining their fate within cells in addition to the fate of released drugs within cells. Active targeting of cell surface receptors usually leads to receptor-mediated endocytosis through endosomal pathway, in which a great percentage of the drug maybe trapped in the endosome or degraded. Releasing drugs from nanocarriers and endosomes may employ linkages that are cleavable within the environment of the endosome to which they are directed, and then the drug diffuses out of the endosome to reach its target within the cell. Release mechanisms for the drug from the nanocarriers include cleavage of thiolytic linkages or cleavage of acid labile linkages [60]. Alternatively when liposomes are used as nanocarriers, release of drugs can be triggered by employing mechanisms that destabilize phospholipids of liposomal nanocarriers such as applying heat [61], ultrasonication [62], or employing cancer-associated enzymes such as phospholipase A2 [63] and metalloproteases [64]. Release of drugs from endosomes can involve membrane penetrating peptides [65, 66] or proton sponges [67]. Membrane penetrating peptides such as HIV Tat-derived peptide usually have basic amino acids that allow the peptides to penetrate through lipid bilayers [65, 66]. When fused to drugs, they carry the drugs with them through the endosome's bilayer. Proton sponges are endosmolytically active polymers containing amine groups that get protonated in acidic endosomes. Replenishing the protons through their influx into endosomes along with chloride anions increases the osmotic pressure and ruptures the endosomes to release their content [67]. There are several other mechanisms for controlled release using stimuli-responsive "smart" polymers [68]. After the release of the drug from endosomes, it still needs to reach its target either in the cytoplasm or in another organelle. To achieve this goal nuclear targeting moieties such as nuclear signaling peptide [69] can be fused to drugs or nanocarriers that are designed not to release their cargo before reaching their destiny.

Future research is needed to address physical stability issues of nanocarriers including settling, changing particle size, aggregation, and stability of their biofunctional groups; in addition to evaluating the effect of conversion into dry form and sterilization. Finally, there are concerns about the toxicity of nanocarriers as several of them are made of nonbiodegradable materials. There is a need for animal studies not only to evaluate toxicity, but also to examine nanocarriers' fate, improving tumor penetration, and pharmacokinetic and pharmacodynamic studies, several of which are underway.

6 Partnership with Bio and Medical Personnel to Target Specific Diseases

Interdisciplinary collaborations are essential for advancing disease-oriented nano-based diagnosis and therapy rather than material-oriented research [70, 71]. However, there are not many educational graduate degree programs that provide a focused specialization in nanotechnology training for biomedical or health scientists. Most of the existing graduate degree programs target training engineers, physicists and chemists and such programs in the USA are listed on the website of the National Nanotechnology Initiative [72]. There are a few notable graduate degree programs that train bio and health professionals in the field and in the USA these include the University of Utah's graduate program that requires interactions of multiple disciplines [73], Louisiana Tech University [74], Radiological Technological University VT [75], and Northeastern University programs [76]. Examples of international graduate degree programs for bio-students include those offered by four European educational institutions in the form of an Erasmus Mundus Master of Nanoscience and Nanotechnology [77], Amrita Centre for Nanoscience in India [78], Universidad de Alicante in Spain [79], and Université de Bourgogne in France [80]. All the above are examples of graduate-level degree programs that attract bio-students into specialization in the area of nanotechnology. On the other hand, few programs offer nanotechnology courses that present case studies for tackling specific cancer issues through nanotechnology. The field still remains focused on new materials and designs and their potential for diagnosis and therapy rather than the other way around of focusing on studying a disease and its challenges with studying how nanotechnology can address these challenges. Thus partnerships with physicians and biomedical and health scientists remain lagging behind mainly due to the lack of educating such personnel in the field leading to their focus on fears of toxicity of materials rather than the potential of applying nanotechnology to address challenges of diseases.

References

1. Gregoriadis G (1976) The carrier potential of liposomes in biology and medicine (second of two parts). N Engl J Med 295(14):765–770
2. Gregoriadis G (1976) The carrier potential of liposomes in biology and medicine (first of two parts). N Engl J Med 295(13):704–710
3. Ringsdorf H (1975) Structure and properties of pharmacologically active polymers. J Polymer Sci Polymer Symp 51:135–153
4. Immordino ML, Dosio F, Cattel L (2006) Stealth liposomes: review of the basic science, rationale, and clinical applications, existing and potential. Int J Nanomedicine 1(3):297–315
5. Fenske DB, Chonn A, Cullis PR (2008) Liposomal nanomedicines: an emerging field. Toxicol Pathol 36(1):21–29
6. Ryan SM, Mantovani G, Wang X, Haddleton DM, Brayden DJ (2008) Advances in PEGylation of important biotech molecules: delivery aspects. Expert Opin Drug Deliv 5 (4):371–383
7. Torchilin VP (2005) Recent advances with liposomes as pharmaceutical carriers. Nat Rev Drug Discov 4(2):145–160
8. Allen C, Dos Santos N, Gallagher R, Chiu GN, Shu Y, Li WM, Johnstone SA, Janoff AS, Mayer LD, Webb MS, Bally MB (2002) Controlling the physical behavior and biological performance of liposome formulations through use of surface grafted poly(ethylene glycol). Biosci Rep 22(2):225–250
9. Liu Z, Jiao Y, Wang Y, Zhou C, Zhang Z (2008) Polysaccharides-based nanoparticles as drug delivery systems. Adv Drug Deliv Rev 60 (15):1650–1662
10. Hawkins MJ, Soon-Shiong P, Desai N (2008) Protein nanoparticles as drug carriers in clinical medicine. Adv Drug Deliv Rev 60 (8):876–885
11. Matsumura Y (2008) Polymeric micellar delivery systems in oncology. Jpn J Clin Oncol 38 (12):793–802
12. Hamidi M, Azadi A, Rafiei P (2008) Hydrogel nanoparticles in drug delivery. Adv Drug Deliv Rev 60(15):1638–1649
13. Kesharwani P, Iyer AK (2015) Recent advances in dendrimer-based nanovectors for tumor-targeted drug and gene delivery. Drug Discov Today 20(5):536–547. doi:10.1016/j.drudis.2014.12.012
14. Villalonga-Barber C, Micha-Screttas M, Steele BR, Georgopoulos A, Demetzos C (2008) Dendrimers as biopharmaceuticals: synthesis and properties. Curr Top Med Chem 8 (14):1294–1309
15. Taghizadeh B, Taranejoo S, Monemian SA, Salehi Moghaddam Z, Daliri K, Derakhshankhah H, Derakhshani Z (2015) Classification of stimuli-responsive polymers as anticancer drug delivery systems. Drug Deliv 22 (2):145–155. doi:10.3109/10717544.2014.887157
16. He C, Kim SW, Lee DS (2008) In situ gelling stimuli-sensitive block copolymer hydrogels for drug delivery. J Control Release 127 (3):189–207
17. Cattaneo R, Miest T, Shashkova EV, Barry MA (2008) Reprogrammed viruses as cancer therapeutics: targeted, armed and shielded. Nat Rev Microbiol 6(7):529–540
18. van Rijn P, Schirhagl R (2016) Viruses, artificial viruses and virus-based structures for biomedical applications. Adv Healthc Mater 5:1386–1400. doi:10.1002/adhm.201501000
19. Vallet-Regi M, Balas F, Arcos D (2007) Mesoporous materials for drug delivery. Angew Chem Int Ed Engl 46(40):7548–7558
20. Murakami T, Tsuchida K (2008) Recent advances in inorganic nanoparticle-based drug delivery systems. Mini Rev Med Chem 8 (2):175–183
21. Misra RD (2008) Quantum dots for tumor-targeted drug delivery and cell imaging. Nanomedicine (Lond) 3(3):271–274

22. Ghosh P, Han G, De M, Kim CK, Rotello VM (2008) Gold nanoparticles in delivery applications. Adv Drug Deliv Rev 60(11):1307–1315
23. Gobbo OL, Sjaastad K, Radomski MW, Volkov Y, Prina-Mello A (2015) Magnetic nanoparticles in cancer theranostics. Theranostics 5 (11):1249–1263. doi:10.7150/thno.11544
24. Liang R, Wei M, Evans DG, Duan X (2014) Inorganic nanomaterials for bioimaging, targeted drug delivery and therapeutics. Chem Commun (Camb) 50(91):14071–14081. doi:10.1039/c4cc03118k
25. Probst CE, Zrazhevskiy P, Bagalkot V, Gao X (2013) Quantum dots as a platform for nanoparticle drug delivery vehicle design. Adv Drug Deliv Rev 65(5):703–718. doi:10.1016/j.addr.2012.09.036
26. Sao R, Vaish R, Sinha N (2015) Multifunctional drug delivery systems using inorganic nanomaterials: a review. J Nanosci Nanotechnol 15(3):1960–1972
27. Rossi M, Pina CD, Falletta E (2016) Gold nanomaterials: from preparation to pharmaceutical design and application. Curr Pharm Des 22(11):1485–1493
28. Bakry R, Vallant RM, Najam-ul-Haq M, Rainer M, Szabo Z, Huck CW, Bonn GK (2007) Medicinal applications of fullerenes. Int J Nanomedicine 2(4):639–649
29. Pastorin G (2009) Crucial functionalizations of carbon nanotubes for improved drug delivery: a valuable option? Pharm Res 26:746–769
30. Chakrabarti M, Kiseleva R, Vertegel A, Ray SK (2015) Carbon nanomaterials for drug delivery and cancer therapy. J Nanosci Nanotechnol 15 (8):5501–5511
31. Vicent MJ, Dieudonne L, Carbajo RJ, Pineda-Lucena A (2008) Polymer conjugates as therapeutics: future trends, challenges and opportunities. Expert Opin Drug Deliv 5(5):593–614
32. Martins S, Sarmento B, Ferreira DC, Souto EB (2007) Lipid-based colloidal carriers for peptide and protein delivery–liposomes versus lipid nanoparticles. Int J Nanomedicine 2 (4):595–607
33. Nagahama K, Ouchi T, Ohya Y (2008) Biodegradable nanogels prepared by self-assembly of poly(L-lactide)-grafted dextran: entrapment and release of proteins. Macromol Biosci 8 (11):1044–1052
34. Hall JB, Dobrovolskaia MA, Patri AK, McNeil SE (2007) Characterization of nanoparticles for therapeutics. Nanomedicine (Lond) 2 (6):789–803. doi:10.2217/17435889.2.6.789
35. Moon JJ, Huang B, Irvine DJ (2012) Engineering nano- and microparticles to tune immunity. Adv Mater 24(28):3724–3746. doi:10.1002/adma.201200446
36. Zeineldin R (2013) Nanotechnology for cancer screening and diagnosis. In: Park K (ed) Biomaterials for cancer therapeutics: diagnosis, prevention and therapy. Woodhead Publishing Limited Philadelphia, PA, pp 137–164
37. Kim PS, Djazayeri S, Zeineldin R (2011) Novel nanotechnology approaches to diagnosis and therapy of ovarian cancer. Gynecol Oncol 120 (3):393–403. doi:10.1016/j.ygyno.2010.11.029
38. Chemburu S, Fenton K, Lopez GP, Zeineldin R (2010) Biomimetic silica microspheres in biosensing. Molecules 15(3):1932–1957
39. Doane TL, Burda C (2012) The unique role of nanoparticles in nanomedicine: imaging, drug delivery and therapy. Chem Soc Rev 41 (7):2885–2911
40. Chu E, Sartorelli A (2012) Cancer chemotherapy. In: Katzung B (ed) Basic and clinical pharmacology, 13th edn. Lange Medical Publications, Los Altos, CA, pp 918–945
41. Le Tourneau C, Faivre S, Raymond E (2008) New developments in multitargeted therapy for patients with solid tumours. Cancer Treat Rev 34(1):37–48
42. Rosato RR, Grant S (2003) Histone deacetylase inhibitors in cancer therapy. Cancer Biol Ther 2(1):30–37
43. Sivashankari PR, Prabaharan M (2015) Peptides to target tumor vasculature and lymphatics for improved anti-angiogenesis therapy. Curr Cancer Drug Targets 16:522–535
44. Manfredi GI, Dicitore A, Gaudenzi G, Caraglia M, Persani L, Vitale G (2015) PI3K/Akt/mTOR signaling in medullary thyroid cancer: a promising molecular target for cancer therapy. Endocrine 48(2):363–370. doi:10.1007/s12020-014-0380-1
45. Takara K, Sakaeda T, Okumura K (2006) An update on overcoming MDR1-mediated multidrug resistance in cancer chemotherapy. Curr Pharm Des 12(3):273–286
46. Maeda H (2001) The enhanced permeability and retention (EPR) effect in tumor vasculature: the key role of tumor-selective macromolecular drug targeting. Adv Enzyme Regul 41:189–207
47. Carmeliet P, Jain RK (2000) Angiogenesis in cancer and other diseases. Nature 407 (6801):249–257
48. Witkop B (1999) Paul Ehrlich and his magic bullets–revisited. Proc Am Philos Soc 143 (4):540–557

49. Sudimack J, Lee RJ (2000) Targeted drug delivery via the folate receptor. Adv Drug Deliv Rev 41(2):147–162
50. Robak T (2006) Current treatment options in hairy cell leukemia and hairy cell leukemia variant. Cancer Treat Rev 32(5):365–376
51. Uberall I, Kolar Z, Trojanec R, Berkovcova J, Hajduch M (2008) The status and role of ErbB receptors in human cancer. Exp Mol Pathol 84 (2):79–89
52. Mizejewski GJ (1999) Role of integrins in cancer: survey of expression patterns. Proc Soc Exp Biol Med 222(2):124–138
53. Silva R, D'Amico G, Hodivala-Dilke KM, Reynolds LE (2008) Integrins: the keys to unlocking angiogenesis. Arterioscler Thromb Vasc Biol 28(10):1703–1713
54. Sato M, Arap W, Pasqualini R (2007) Molecular targets on blood vessels for cancer therapies in clinical trials. Oncology (Williston Park) 21 (11):1346–1352, discussion 1354–1345, 1367, 1370 passim
55. Longmire M, Choyke PL, Kobayashi H (2008) Clearance properties of nano-sized particles and molecules as imaging agents: considerations and caveats. Nanomedicine (Lond) 3 (5):703–717
56. Whitehead KA, Langer R, Anderson DG (2009) Knocking down barriers: advances in siRNA delivery. Nat Rev Drug Discov 8 (2):129–138
57. Tiram G, Scomparin A, Ofek P, Satchi-Fainaro R (2014) Interfering cancer with polymeric siRNA nanomedicines. J Biomed Nanotechnol 10(1):50–66
58. Jhaveri AM, Torchilin VP (2014) Multifunctional polymeric micelles for delivery of drugs and siRNA. Front Pharmacol 5:77. doi:10.3389/fphar.2014.00077
59. Young SW, Stenzel M, Jia-Lin Y (2016) Nanoparticle-siRNA: a potential cancer therapy? Crit Rev Oncol Hematol 98:159–169. doi:10.1016/j.critrevonc.2015.10.015
60. West KR, Otto S (2005) Reversible covalent chemistry in drug delivery. Curr Drug Discov Technol 2(3):123–160
61. Bikram M, West JL (2008) Thermo-responsive systems for controlled drug delivery. Expert Opin Drug Deliv 5(10):1077–1091
62. Huang SL (2008) Liposomes in ultrasonic drug and gene delivery. Adv Drug Deliv Rev 60(10):1167–1176
63. Jensen SS, Andresen TL, Davidsen J, Hoyrup P, Shnyder SD, Bibby MC, Gill JH, Jorgensen K (2004) Secretory phospholipase A2 as a tumor-specific trigger for targeted delivery of a novel class of liposomal prodrug anticancer etherlipids. Mol Cancer Ther 3 (11):1451–1458
64. Tauro JR, Gemeinhart RA (2005) Matrix metalloprotease triggered delivery of cancer chemotherapeutics from hydrogel matrixes. Bioconjug Chem 16(5):1133–1139
65. Brooks H, Lebleu B, Vives E (2005) Tat peptide-mediated cellular delivery: back to basics. Adv Drug Deliv Rev 57(4):559–577
66. Torchilin VP (2008) Cell penetrating peptide-modified pharmaceutical nanocarriers for intracellular drug and gene delivery. Biopolymers 90(5):604–610
67. Yang S, May S (2008) Release of cationic polymer-DNA complexes from the endosome: a theoretical investigation of the proton sponge hypothesis. J Chem Phys 129(18):185105
68. Fogueri LR, Singh S (2009) Smart polymers for controlled delivery of proteins and peptides: a review of patents. Recent Pat Drug Deliv Formul 3(1):40–48
69. Pouton CW, Wagstaff KM, Roth DM, Moseley GW, Jans DA (2007) Targeted delivery to the nucleus. Adv Drug Deliv Rev 59 (8):698–717
70. Duncan R, Gaspar R (2011) Nanomedicine(s) under the microscope. Mol Pharm 8 (6):2101–2141. doi:10.1021/mp200394t
71. Youkhanna J, Syoufjy J, Rhorer M, Oladeinde O, Zeineldin R (2013) Toward nanotechnology-based solutions for a particular disease: ovarian cancer as an example. Nanotechnol Rev 2(4):473–484
72. http://www.nano.gov/education-training/university-college. Accessed April 2016
73. http://nanoinstitute.utah.edu/education-outreach/grads/index.php. Accessed April 2016
74. http://coes.latech.edu/grad-programs/msnt.php. Accessed April 2016
75. http://www.rtuvt.edu//nanomedicine-requirements.php. Accessed April 2016
76. http://www.igert.neu.edu/. Accessed April 2016
77. http://www.emm-nano.org/. Accessed April 2016
78. https://www.amrita.edu/program/m-tech-nanomedical-sciences. Accessed April 2016
79. http://www.uam.es/ss/Satellite/es/1242684629435/1242662105880/masteroficial/masterOficia/Master_Universitario_en_Nanociencia_y_Nanotecnologia_Molecular.htm. April 2016
80. http://www.u-bourgogne-formation.fr/-Nanotechnologies-et-h. Accessed April 2016

Chapter 2

Improved Targeting of Cancers with Nanotherapeutics

Christian Foster, Andre Watson, Joseph Kaplinsky, and Nazila Kamaly

Abstract

Targeted cancer nanotherapeutics offers numerous opportunities for the selective uptake of toxic chemotherapies within tumors and cancer cells. The unique properties of nanoparticles, such as their small size, large surface-to-volume ratios, and the ability to achieve multivalency of targeting ligands on their surface, provide superior advantages for nanoparticle-based drug delivery to a variety of cancers. This review highlights various key concepts in the design of targeted nanotherapeutics for cancer therapy, and discusses physicochemical parameters affecting nanoparticle targeting, along with recent developments for cancer-targeted nanomedicines.

Key words Targeting, Antibodies, Ligands, EPR, Cancer, Oncology, Nanoparticles, Nanotherapeutics, Nanomedicine, Multivalency, Drug delivery, Translation

1 Introduction

Cancer chemotherapy is fundamentally limited by dose-limiting toxicity. This has long been true of nonspecific cytotoxic agents that are still the most widely used anticancer therapies, which in addition suffer from a low therapeutic index. The last 20 years has seen the development of molecularly targeted agents, which have an improved toxicity profile, especially for acute events. However, these newer agents are often given continuously over longer time periods and chronic toxicity remains a key limiting factor [1, 2].

With our improved understanding of cancer biology and pathways, targeted agents and cancer immunotherapy approaches have gained considerable interest and investment, resulting in positive outcomes, and a rise in the use of these treatments. Targeted agents primarily include antibody drugs that are capable of specifically blocking proliferative cancer pathways, and immunotherapy approaches being aimed at priming the patient's own immune system to attack and destroy cancers [3, 4]. Surgery and radiotherapy are also still routinely used in the arsenal of anticancer treatments—along (or in combination) with chemotherapies,

Reema Zeineldin (ed.), *Cancer Nanotechnology: Methods and Protocols*, Methods in Molecular Biology, vol. 1530,
DOI 10.1007/978-1-4939-6646-2_2,

targeted therapies, immunotherapy or newer treatments such as adoptive cellular therapy [5]. Cancer nanomedicines are intended to add to this arsenal of therapeutics, by packaging and specifically delivering existing chemotherapies to where they are needed the most: within cancer cells.

Nanoparticles (NPs) enable the encapsulation of poorly soluble drugs, protection of a variety of therapeutic payloads from blood components, increase systemic circulation times and improve biodistribution, leading to minimized systemic toxicities [6]. These properties are ideal for oncology applications where systemic toxicity is a major issue. Doxil, which is the first anticancer nanomedicine to enter the clinic, is liposome-encapsulated doxorubicin, which was shown to drastically increase the systemic circulation half-life of doxorubicin (Dox) from 0.8 h to 2 days, in addition to reducing cardiotoxicity [7]. Albumin associated paclitaxel (nab-PTX) has also led to higher tolerated doses [8].

Once injected into systemic circulation, the localization of NPs within the body can be influenced via "passive" or "active" targeting strategies. The term passive targeting describes the accumulation of NPs bearing no affinity ligands at disease sites, where the degree of accumulation depends on their inherent physicochemical properties (size, shape, charge, flexibility, etc.). If suboptimal, these properties may also impede the effective concentration of NPs at active sites due to increased sequestration by the mononuclear phagocytic system (MPS), limiting their systemic concentration and potential to extravasate into target tissues [9]. Active targeting is a term used to describe the mode of action of NPs with surface-bound affinity ligands having specificity to diseased tissue and/or cells. Actively targeted particles rely on the principle of passive targeting discussed above, but targeting ligands have an additional effect, aiding accumulation in the tumor or uptake of NPs into cancer cells via endocytosis, or both.

The development of actively targeted NPs was facilitated by the maturation of antibody technologies, together with techniques for bioconjugation of targeting moieties including antibodies, antibody fragments, peptides, aptamers (Apts), sugars, and small molecule ligands to the surface of NPs [10–13]. Although more than 30 years has passed since the first targeted NPs were developed, only a handful have reached clinical translation, and none have yet been approved [14–17]. The lack of effective translation of targeted NPs could be attributed to the following limitations; (1) our insufficient understanding of events at the nano–bio interface both in vitro and in vivo; (2) our inadequate knowledge of the fate of NPs at the body, organ, and cellular levels; (3) difficulty in achieving reproducible and controlled synthesis of targeted NPs at larger scales; (4) lack of technologies enabling screening of a large number of targeted NP candidates under biologically relevant conditions that could be reliably correlated to clinical performance; (5) potential lack of or low occurrence of the so-called enhanced permeation and retention effect (EPR) in patient tumors, and; (6) inter- and intra-patient heterogeneity in receptor expression levels. In this review we discuss effective targeting of tumors via passive and active mechanisms, and highlight the various tumor biology and NP physicochemical properties that affect targeted nanodrug delivery for oncology applications.

2 Passive Targeting

The growth of a solid tumor requires development of a blood supply and lymphatic drainage. However, the development of these systems is pathological and this has profound implications for delivery of nanomedicines. Characteristics of the tumor vasculature such as excessive branching, chaotic structures, enlarged gaps between endothelial cell lining of vessel walls and associated breakdown of tight junctions, and a disrupted basement membrane, facilitate the extravasation of particulate materials from vessels into tumor tissues [18, 19]. An impaired lymphatic drainage system further entraps macromolecular particles and delays their clearance. Starting in the 1980s, the observation of increased accumulation of macromolecules and colloids such as the polymer-drug conjugate poly(styrene-co-maleic acid)-neocarzinostatin (SMANCS) in tumor tissues led to the term "enhanced permeability and retention" (EPR) effect [20]. Together with grafting of polyethylene glycol (PEGylation) to the surface of NPs (to enhance systemic circulation), this has become the most widely exploited concept in nano-oncology applications [20–24]. The EPR effect has been observed with a wide range of macromolecular agents such as: proteins, including immunoglobulin G (IgG); drug-polymer conjugates; micelles; liposomes; polymeric NPs and many other types of NPs [25–28].

The distribution of NPs within tumors begins with margination toward the vascular wall, followed by extravasation from the blood vessels, diffusion throughout the extravascular tissue and interaction with extracellular and intracellular targets [6]. The degree of vascular permeability in patients is far more heterogeneous than in pre-clinical models. Variable tumor microenvironments can affect the cutoff size for NP accumulation in tumors, restricting their effective penetration range, and accounting for the lack of observable EPR effects in certain tumor types [29, 30]. The negative pressure gradient present within the tumor interstitium can substantially limit the convection of NPs from the intravascular to the extravascular space within tumors, regardless of the presence of leaky vasculature [29, 31, 32].

The EPR effect is more highly multifaceted than first thought. Only recently are we beginning to understand the contribution of other tumor microenvironment (TME) related parameters such as blood circulation in tumors, extravasation to the perivascular tumor microenvironment, tumor-associated macrophages (TAMs), fibroblasts, collagen, penetration distance within tumor tissue, tumor cell internalization and intracellular trafficking (and other tumor matrix components). Although the EPR effect has been the main principle governing the use of nanomedicines for tumor therapy, a number of important limitations need to be considered. The main observations of EPR have been studied in small animal subcutaneous or orthotopic xenografts, and genetically engineered mouse models [33]. These settings are drastically different from tumors in humans where the EPR effect may not be present or manifested in a similar manner. Other than the observation of marginal progression-free survival in the case of ovarian cancer patients (receiving Doxil as a second line therapy or platinum-sensitive cohorts), passively targeted NPs up to now have not led to substantial improvement in patient survival rates, which may suggest patient populations with lowered tumor susceptibility to NPs and/or lack of EPR effect [6, 34–36]. More importantly, it appears that the EPR effect can also vary substantially between patients, with variability arising even within the same patient or tumor type [6]. To circumvent these problems, in the same manner that molecularly targeted treatments are currently offered to patients following genetic profiling of their tumors, more personalized approaches could be envisioned for the future where "nanomedicine-responsive" patient populations can also be identified. Research on companion diagnostics is helping to address this complex problem. In preclinical models, iodine loaded liposomes have been used to predict animal cohorts that were responsive to nanotherapeutics [37]. In another recent preclinical study magnetic resonance imaging (MRI) was used to predict treatment response and drug accumulation using co-administered 30 nm magnetic iron oxide NPs and paclitaxel encapsulated polymeric NPs in tumor-bearing mice [38]. In the clinic, a study was initiated to ascertain the safety of co-administering ferumoxytol as a tumor imaging agent, in addition to irinotecan-loaded liposomes (clinicaltrials.gov, NCT01770353). These approaches have yielded valuable insights into the in vivo kinetics of NP biodistribution and demonstrated how clinically relevant imaging modalities and agents can be utilized to select patients with high EPR and to predict therapeutic nanomedicine efficacy using companion diagnostics.

3 Active Targeting

Active targeting describes the use of affinity ligands to direct NP binding to antigens that are overexpressed in diseased tissue. Actively targeted particles rely on the principle of passive targeting

Table 1
Examples of targeting ligands and targeted NPs

Ligand Type	Nanoplatform	Target	Indication (Ref)
Antibodies and fragments			
• F(ab′)$_2$	Liposome	Non-muscle myosin heavy chain type A	Gastric cancer [63]
• F(ab′)	Liposome	HER2	Breast cancer [144]
• scFv	Liposome	HER2	Breast cancer [58]
Proteins			
• Transferrin	Polymeric NPs	Tf receptor	Cancer [59]
• Ankyrin repeat protein	siRNA complexes	EpCAM	Cancer [145]
• Affibodies	Polymeric NPs	HER2	Breast cancer [146]
Peptides			
• CGNKRTRGC (LyP-1)	Protein NPs	gC1qR (p32)	Cancer [147]
• F3 peptide	Iron oxide NPs	Nucleolin	Cancer (imaging) [148]
• iRGD	Iron oxide NPs	αvβ3/5	Cancer (imaging) [149]
• iRGD	Polymeric NPs	αvβ3/5	Cancer [150]
• KLWVLPKGGGC	Polymeric NPs	Collagen IV	Inflammation [151]
• KLWVLPK	Polymeric NPs	Collagen IV	Vascular wall [152]
• SSPIQGSWTWENGK-WTWRGIIRLEQ	Iron oxide	Fibronectin	Cancer (Imaging) [153]
• SSPIQGSWTWENGK-WTWRGIIRLEQ	Liposomes	Fibronectin	Cancer
Nucleic acid ligands			
• A10 aptamer	Polymeric NPs	PSMA	Prostate cancer [154]
• A9 CGA aptamer	Gold NPs	PSMA	Prostate cancer [155]
Small molecule ligands			
• Folic acid	Liposomes	FA receptor	Cancer [56]
• Folic acid	Polymeric NPs	FA receptor	Cancer [156]
• TPP	Polymeric NPs	Mitochondria	Various [157]
• ACUPA	Polymeric NPs	PSMA	Cancer [158]

HER2: human epidermal growth factor receptor 2. Tf: transferrin. EpCAM: epithelial cell adhesion molecule. PSMA: prostate specific membrane antigen. *FA* folic acid, *TPP* triphenyl phosphonium, *ACUPA* 2-[3-[5-amino-1-carboxypentyl]-ureido]-pentanedioic acid

discussed above, but the addition of ligands can aid accumulation in the tumor and uptake of NPs into cancer cells via endocytosis.

A wide variety of targeting ligands are used to create targeted NPs (Table 1). These ligands are often directed toward overexpressed receptors or antigens on proliferating cancer cells. Important parameters that should be taken into account when choosing a targeting ligand include binding affinity, ligand size, immunogenicity, and cost of manufacturing. The ideal ligand should also facilitate deeper tumor penetration.

The first antibody to be approved for clinical use was muromonab-CD3 (an immunosuppressive agent) in 1986 [39]. Since then numerous antibody platforms have been developed including murine, chimeric, humanized and human monoclonal antibodies (mAbs) [40]. For example, rituximab (Rituxan) is a chimeric mAb, which binds to CD20, and was approved for the treatment of non-Hodgkin's lymphoma in 1997 [41]. Trastuzumab (Herceptin) which was approved for the treatment of breast cancer in 1998 is a humanized mAb that binds to the HER2/neu antigen [42]. Natural or fully synthetic antigen-binding fragments (Fab and Fab′ ~ 50 kDa), variable fragments (Fv ~ 15 kDa), and single chain variable fragments (scFv ~ 30 kDa) of antibodies have been engineered and tested [43]. Antibody fragments are engineered to control properties such as affinity (K_D usually lower than 1 nM) or internalization capability. The advantage of antigen-binding fragments is that they lack the Fc-antibody region, which is the most immunogenic component of antibodies.

Several other classes of binding ligands, including antibody mimetics, peptides, nucleic acid ligands, and small molecules, have been developed against a number of target antigens [43]. These types of ligands can also be conjugated to radioisotopes or drug molecules to create more effective targeted imaging and therapeutic modalities [44–47]. Similar ligands can be conjugated to the surface of NPs in order to achieve antigen-specific active targeting [43, 48]. In contrast to antibody–drug conjugates, which typically carry 1–8 drug molecules, targeted NPs are capable of carrying up to 10^5 drug molecules, allowing for a higher amount of drug delivery per bio-recognition or binding event.

For effective cancer therapy, drug encapsulating NPs should ideally be delivered within cancer cells, and therefore therapies that act on intracellular active sites are most effectively delivered with targeted NPs since this facilitates uptake of NPs via either clathrin-dependent endocytosis, caveolin-assisted, cell adhesion molecule directed, or lipid raft associated mechanisms [49]. In the case of hydrophobic small molecule drugs that can easily permeate through the endosomal lipid bilayer, NP entrapment within endosomes following endocytosis can still lead to effective intracellular drug concentrations as the drug molecules are released from the carrier over time. In contrast, for the effective delivery of biological macromolecules such as nucleic acids (DNA, siRNA, miRNA), charged/and or hydrophilic small molecule drugs (that are impermeable to the endosomal membrane), endosomal escape is an important prerequisite [50]. This is crucial since intracellular payload release should occur prior to fusion of endosomes with lysosomes where biological payloads can be degraded as a result of low pH levels [51]. Studies to identify mechanisms that lead to endosomal escape based on pH buffering and osmotic swelling, which cause endosome bursting or endosomal membrane destabilization for the purposes of effective subcellular drug delivery are helping to further understand this effect [52–55].

Ligand mediated cell internalization can result in therapeutic benefits as compared to equivalent non-targeted NPs [56–59]. For example, accumulation of siRNA-loaded NPs at tumor sites is largely a function of effective EPR via passive targeting; however, cellular internalization and effective gene silencing are largely a function of targeting ligands, which facilitate intracellular uptake. Therefore, the colloidal properties of NPs determine their biodistribution, whereas the targeting ligand serves to facilitate and enhance cellular uptake at specific sites [60]. For effective tumor targeting and margination and extravasation of NPs for cancer therapy deeper tumor penetration and retention is important. Targeting strategies that focus on the TME can also be utilized to improve penetration. For example tumor-specific penetrating peptides such as iRGD with a R/KXXR/K C-terminal peptide motif have been used to stimulate neuropilin-1-mediated vascular permeability [61].

For targeting of nanomedicines in oncology applications parameters such as ligand binding affinity (K_D) and receptor expression levels throughout the treatment period also need to be considered.

3.1 Clinical Stage Actively Targeted Nanoparticles

Over the last four decades since the first actively targeted NPs were reported [62], only a handful have progressed to clinical trials (Table 2). MCC-465, the first targeted NP to enter trials, consists of liposome encapsulated Dox with surface bound PEG for immune shielding and dimers of F(ab′) fragments for targeting [15]. The $F(ab')_2$ used is a fragment of the tumor specific human mAb (GAH), which has shown affinity to >90 % of human stomach cancer cells [15]. MCC-465 exhibited significant antitumor response against GAH-positive xenografts leading to 80 % reduction in tumor mass [63]. Phase I trials with MCC-465 were carried out in order to determine the maximum tolerated dose and further dosing regimens. MCC-465 does not appear to have progressed through clinical development after phase I completion.

Anti-EGFR (epidermal growth factor receptor) immunoliposomes loaded with doxorubicin (anti-EGFR ILs-dox) have been tested in the clinic on patients with advanced solid tumors overexpressing EGFR no longer amenable to standard treatment and a maximal tolerated dose was defined (50 mg/m^2) from the phase I trial [64]. MM-302 is a HER-2-targeted PEGylated liposome that encapsulates doxorubicin for delivery to HER-2-overexpressing tumor cells, it is currently undergoing phase II and III trials for breast cancer and HER-2 positive breast cancer respectively [65]. MM-302 has been recently shown to improve the antitumor activity of oxaliplatin in HER-2 positive breast cancer, when administered after cyclophosphamide priming [66]. The overexpression of TfR, EGFR, and HER-2 occurs in a range of cancer types, making these cancer ligands attractive targeting strategies for drug delivery [67].

Table 2
Actively targeted nanoparticles in the clinic

Name	Nanoplatform	Targeting	API	Dose (Recommended)	Size (nm)	ζ potential (mV)	Ref
MCC-465	Liposomes	Metastatic gastric cancer, (Ab fragment)	Doxorubicin	6.5–45.5 mg/m^2 (32.5 mg/m^2)	143	-	[15]
anti-EGFR-ILs-dox	Liposomes (Doxil®/ Caelyx®)	Solid tumors, EGFR (Ab, cetuximab)	Doxorubicin	5–60 mg/m^2 (50 mg/m^2)	100–120	-	[64]
MM-302	Liposomes	HER2+ breast cancer, Her2 (Ab)	Doxorubicin	8–50 mg/m^2	80–100	-	[159] [65]
MBP-426	Liposomes	Gastric, esophageal, gastroesophageal Adenocarcinoma, Tf-Receptor (Tf)	Oxaliplatin	6–400 mg/m^2 (226 mg/m^2)	-	-	[66, 160]
SGT-53	Liposomes	Solid tumor, recurrent glioblastoma, metastatic pancreatic cancer, Tf-Receptor (Ab scFv)	p53 plasmid DNA	0.6–3.6 mg (2.4 mg)	114	28.2	[161]
SGT-94	Liposomes	Solid tumor Tf-Receptor (Ab scFv)	RB94 plasmid DNA	-	207	6.6	[162]
2B3-101	Liposomes	Brain metastases, glutathione transporter (glutathione)	Dox	-	95	-	[163]
BIND-014	Polymeric NPs	Non-small-cell lung, metastatic castration-resistant prostate cancer, others, PSMA (small molecule)	Docetaxel	15–75 mg/m^2 (60 mg/m^2)	100	−6	[158]
CALAA-01	Polymeric NPs	Tf-Receptor (Tf)	siRNA M2 subunit of ribonucleotide reductase	18–30 mg/m^2	70	15	[164]

Table adapted from refs. [6] and [75]. API: active pharmaceutical ingredient

SGT-53 is a transferrin receptor (TfR)-targeted liposome, which binds to TfRs on the surface of cancer cells using single-chain antibody fragments (TfRscFv). Its payload is a plasmid encoding wild type tumor suppressor P53 [68]. Preclinical studies showed that SGT-53 could sensitize tumors to the effects of radiation and chemotherapy [68]. It is currently undergoing phase I and II clinical trials in combination with Dox for treatment of solid tumors and metastatic breast cancer. SGT-94 is a similar formulation to SGT-53. In SGT-94 the P53 plasmid was replaced with an RB94 plasmid encoding a fragment of the wild-type retinoblastoma tumor suppressor protein. SGT-94 is undergoing Phase I trials in patients with RB negative tumor biopsies.

MBP-426 is another TfR-targeted liposome that encapsulates oxaliplatin [14]. In a phase I study, patients with advanced or metastatic solid tumors refractory to conventional therapy received MBP-426 as 2–4 h infusions every 3 weeks and it was well tolerated [14]. 2B3-101 is a targeted liposomal formulation of Dox using glutathione as a ligand. By targeting the glutathione receptor it is able to traverse the blood–brain and blood-CSF barriers. Phase II trials have taken place for glioma and for metastases of breast cancer to the brain or the leptomeninges.

BIND-014 is the first targeted, controlled-release polymeric NP for cancer chemotherapy to reach clinical development. It is composed of PLA-PEG diblock polymer, that targets prostate-specific membrane antigen (PSMA) and encapsulates a docetaxel (Dtxl) payload [69]. PSMA is a transmembrane protein that is overexpressed on the surface of prostate cancer cells and tumor-associated neovasculature of virtually all solid tumors [70, 71]. BIND-014 is currently in phase II trials for second-line therapy for patients with non-small-cell lung, metastatic castration-resistant prostate cancers, and squamous cell carcinoma of the head and neck [72].

CALAA-01 was the first targeted polymeric NP to reach clinical use for siRNA delivery in 2008 [73]. The CALAA-01 NP consists of siRNA that reduces the expression of the M2 subunit of ribonucleotide reductase (R2), cyclodextrin containing polymer (CDP) for siRNA condensation, adamantine-PEG (AD-PEG) for steric stabilization, and adamantine-PEG conjugated to human Tf (AD-PEG-Tf) to target the TfR which is overexpressed on the surface of many cancer cells [74, 75]. CALAA-01 currently has no further active trials after the completion of the phase I trial.

4 Optimal Biophysicochemical Parameters for Targeted Nanoparticles

Properties such as size, shape, surface charge, surface chemistry, hydrophobicity, roughness, rigidity, and composition are termed the physicochemical properties of NPs and can influence the uptake and/or targeting of NPs to tumors and cancer cells (Fig. 1) [76].

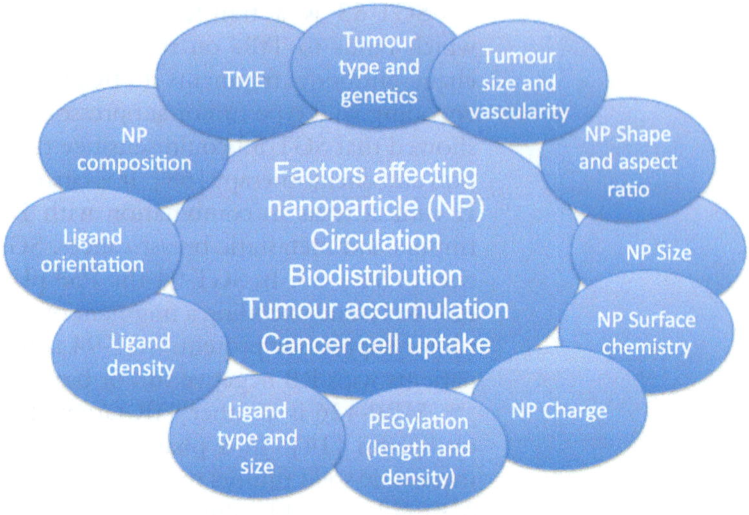

Fig. 1 Physicochemical properties of ligands and nanoparticles and the TME can affect their in vivo performance

Tumor targeted NPs must be able to effectively circulate, marginate, and successfully bind to vascular targets or extravasate into tumor interstitium and finally become internalized in cancer cells. The combination of these events requires that the NPs have optimal size, shape and surface properties, Each of these aspects merits investigation when developing optimal tumor targeted NPs. In this section, we discuss these properties, which generally affect both passively and actively targeted NPs.

NP biophysicochemical properties can significantly affect their cell uptake, cell cytotoxicity, pharmacokinetics (PK) and biodistribution (BD) in vivo. There is a strong interplay between each of these properties. Computational techniques ranging across scales from molecular dynamics through to simulation of fluid flow and tumor growth can help gain insight in to the optimal combination [77, 78]. However, the complexity of the bio–nano interface still demands a comprehensive experimental approach.

4.1 Influence of Nanoparticle Size

Nanoparticle size crucially effects three phases of biodistribution: circulation and clearance; diffusion into and through tumor tissue; and cellular internalization by tumor cells. NP sizes are most often given as hydrodynamic sizes, measured by dynamic light scattering. Other techniques, such as atomic force microscopy or electron microscopy are also sometimes used, and will generally measure smaller sizes for the same particles.

Based on many studies, 10–150 nm is a generally accepted size range for the development of NPs for in vivo applications with most favorable in vivo circulation and biodistribution, and tumor uptake patterns [79]. These upper and lower sizes are mostly determined because of interactions with the immune system and kidney filtration cutoffs, respectively. In general the larger the NP, the lower the curvature will be, which can lead to increased interactions of opsonins and more rapid in vivo clearance [80]. Larger NPs are more likely to be filtered by the sinusoids in the spleen and cleared by the MPS cells, which include the Kupffer cells of the liver [81]. Furthermore, NPs smaller than approximately 5.5 nm have been shown to be rapidly cleared by glomerular filtration in the kidneys [82].

For tumor accumulation, the upper limit for extravasation into solid tumors appears to be ~400 nm and it is generally observed that NPs <200 nm in size can accumulate effectively within tumor tissue, with the 70–200 nm range considered optimal for tumor passive targeting [83]. In relation to diffusion within the tumor, intercapillary distances must be considered, since it is important for NPs to reach tumor cells that are located further away from these microvessels. Tumor matrix components such as collagen fibers, extracellular proteins, increased interstitial fluid pressure, heterogeneous blood flow, and impaired lymphatics towards the tumor core present challenges for the effective passive diffusion of NPs within tumors [84, 85]. Work has shown that NPs of about ~10–20 nm are ideal for maximum tumor penetration [86].

Cellular internalization of NPs is highly dependent on the size of the NPs, and in general, particles in the 40–50 nm range exhibit maximal uptake in vitro [87]. For example, Herceptin (HER) gold NPs (2–100 nm) were synthesized and their size-dependent binding and uptake was investigated in ErbB2 receptor expressing cells [88]. Interestingly, studies have shown that NP uptake as a function of size can also be tumor cell type-dependent, and just a 10 nm deviation from an investigated optimal size, results in a significant decrease in NP uptake [88]. Firstly it was shown that the number of HER antibody binding sites on the NPs was dependent on the NP surface area and increased with particle radius. Surface antibody density also increased linearly with NP radius—demonstrating that these multivalent antibody-conjugated NPs can allow for a high degree of ErbB2 cross-linking and can be tuned by varying NP size. Therefore, NP shape and size can change ligand presentation, affecting NP binding avidity.

As noted above, animal models understate the extent of variability of the EPR found in patient tumors. Yet even examples from the preclinical literature clearly show that optimal size is dependent on the model chosen.

The size dependent accumulation of fluorescently labeled PLA-PEG polymeric NPs using two different tumor xenograft models, HT20 colon and A2780 ovarian carcinoma, which result in different tumor structures, growth rates, and microenvironments was investigated [89]. The biodistribution and accumulation of near-infrared dye-loaded PLA-PEG NPs was tracked using in vivo fluorescence imaging technique. NPs with sizes 111 and 141 nm accumulated efficiently in tumors and a larger 166 nm NP was shown to undergo rapid clearance in the liver. The pattern of accumulation was variable in both tumors, although fluorescence was mostly observed from the tumor core region in the case of HT29 tumors, which was not observed in the A2780 tumors. NP accumulation in the necrotic HT29 tumor core was shown to be size-independent, but size dependent in A2780 tumors, which were more vascularized. In general the larger NPs led to lower tumor accumulation.

Tumor permeability and degree of vascularization are key concepts for the assessment of NP biodistribution in tumors. In hyperpermeable murine colon adenocarcinoma polymeric micelles of sizes between 30 and 100 nm were found to be similar in their accumulation, tumor extravasation, and treatment efficacy [90]. However, in hypopermeable pancreatic tumors, only 30 nm micelles were shown to be effective [90]. Considering the diversity of nanomaterials and cell types used to investigate targeted NPs for cancer therapy, it is important that an optimal NP size be determined experimentally for a given NP type and cell type.

4.2 Influence of Nanoparticle Shape

The interaction between NP shape and hemodynamic forces (fluid dynamics of blood flow) affects circulation through the blood. The interaction between shape and cellular internalization affects both the rate of clearance by the MPS and the rate of uptake by target cells.

In relation to circulation of NPs in vivo, spherical NPs tend to be less susceptible to transport across streamlines by hemodynamic forces in the bloodstream. Certain studies, on the other hand, have shown that non-spherical particles with longitudinal lengths reaching cellular diameters and discoidal shapes can exhibit longer circulation times than spherical particles [91, 92]. Discoidal particles have highly oscillatory trajectories that can increase their contact with vessel walls. Oblate-shaped NPs are susceptible to torques resulting in tumbling and rotation, leading to an increase in the lateral drift of NPs towards blood vessel walls in microvessels [93]. Furthermore, oblate-shaped particles are less susceptible to uptake by macrophages leading to increased blood circulation [91, 94, 95]. Vascular endothelium or cancer cell targeting seems to also favor oblong and more elongated NPs since these shapes offer greater avidity towards targets due to an increased multivalency, maximizing NP surface contact with targets [96]. In particular for vascular targeting, geometrically enhanced targeting can avoid hemodynamic forces that can lead to NP detachment from the endothelium [97].

After systemic injection of a NP, before it reaches the cancer cells within tumors, it must first evade phagocytosis by macrophages, and marginate across the vascular wall against blood hemodynamic forces. This activity can be influenced by the tumbling rate of the NP which is affected by its buoyancy, drag, van der Waals interactions, electrostatic double layer interactions, and steric repulsive behavior [98]. The movement of spherical NPs and their margination is size dependent [99]. This is because transport of larger spherical NPs is dominated by advection while smaller NPs are more prone to diffusion, which facilitates their extravasation across blood vessels. For examples, 65 nm liposomes were more than three times likely to marginate than 130 nm liposomes [100].

Nanoparticle shape is also an important factor in the rate of cellular internalization [87], with shapes that can accommodate cellular membrane wrapping processes most effective at cellular uptake. Amongst NPs of either rod or sphere design, the spherical shaped NPs were taken up by cells more readily [101].

A wide variety of non-spherical NPs with different sizes and geometries have been manufactured using different methods [98]. A top-down fabrication method termed Particle Replication in Non-wetting Templates (PRINT) utilizes lithography techniques to create polymeric NPs of a wide variety of geometries, shapes and aspect ratios, and a study using cylindrical PLGA NPs created using this technique showed an increase in tumor levels of docetaxel with decreased liver and spleen uptake [102, 103]. However, typical processes used to fabricate therapeutic NPs (bottom-up fabrication, self-assembly) renders most nanomedicines spherical. In addition to further studies of the in vivo effects of shape, new methods of synthesis for non-spherical NPs suitable for industrial scale-up is therefore an important area for future research.

4.3 Influence of Nanoparticle Surface Charge

The degree of nonspecific binding of proteins to NPs in the blood is related to NP surface charge, because highly positively charged NPs are more rapidly cleared from circulation by cells of the MPS since they are more prone to opsonization [79]. Although cationic NPs promote cellular binding (due to interactions with the negatively charged phospholipids, proteins, and glycans on cell surfaces) and can be ideal for in vitro applications of drug delivery to cancer cells [104], in vivo this charge should be masked until the NPs are within the tumor. Negatively charged NPs can also exhibit selective cellular uptake compared to NPs with neutral surfaces [101]. Either the uptake of positively charged NPs could be an energy-dependent process involving the proteins dynamin and F-actin, or positively charged NPs can by-pass endocytic pathways and enter cells by creating holes in the cellular bilayer [104, 105].

In vitro studies have shown that amino terminated surfaces induce the highest levels of complement activation [106], and NPs with neutral methoxy surface groups were most immunocompatible. Post systemic administration, NPs with zeta (ζ) potential <15 mV exhibited minimal macrophage uptake and led to longer circulation times and overall tumor retention [107]. When near neutral polymeric micelles (ζ potential 1.3 mV) and anionic (ζ potential −10.6 mV) were compared, the more negatively charged NPs resulted in lower liver and spleen accumulation [108]. Cationically charged NPs have a high nonspecific uptake in a variety of cells, and can also facilitate endosomal release through the so-called "proton sponge effect" [109].

In summary, the charge of NPs, which is related to their surface chemistry influences the degree of opsonization, and circulation time of the NP, and interaction with macrophages within organs of the MPS. Positively charged NPs are more prone to uptake by macrophages in the lungs, liver, and spleen. Neutral and slightly negatively charged NPs exhibit prolonged circulation lifetimes and lowered uptake by the MPS.

4.4 Influence of NP Rigidity

Particle rigidity can highly influence both circulation and cellular uptake in vivo. This has long been studied in the case of larger structures, such as red blood cells. Synthetically engineered microparticles with both rigid and deformable properties were developed and their biodistribution evaluated in vivo [110]. The more deformable synthetic blood cells were eliminated 30 times more slowly than their rigid counterparts from blood, with the more rigid microparticles accumulating in the lungs 2 h post-injection.

More recently, attention has been paid to the rigidity of NPs although this is still a preliminary area of investigation [111, 112]. Rigidity affects circulation in capillaries. Healthy red blood cells tend to accumulate in the center of the capillary, leaving a cell-free sheath zone of several microns. In normal physiology this zone is also occupied by white blood cells and platelets that interact with the capillary wall. As referenced above, NPs tend to marginate toward the cell wall on the basis of size. Whether the correlation between stiffness and margination found for red blood cells extends down to the NP size regime is an open question.

In relation to cellular uptake there is in vitro evidence that macrophages take up harder particles more efficiently, by phagocytosis, and softer particles less efficiently by macropinocytosis [112]. Although evidence is more scant, the same in vitro preference for harder particles is found in endothelial cells. Cancer cell lines show much greater variation, which is not surprising in view of their heterogeneity [112]. It may be that tuning particle rigidity is another parameter for personalizing tumor treatment.

A key study which controlled for rigidity while holding other properties constant and investigated the NP size range was Zhang et al. who synthesized 120 nm poly(carboxybetaine) particles [113]. They used variable cross-linking of their zwitterionic monomers to achieve bulk moduli ranging from 180 to 1350 kPa. They showed that softest, more deformable NPs had a circulation half life of 20 h, more than twice that of the most rigid particles at 9 h. The softest particles also showed less than half as much spleen accumulation, probably aided by a capacity to squeeze through spleenic filtration. Another study found similar behavior with PEG based hydrogel particles, although at the upper end (greater than 200 nm) of the size range relevant to NP drug delivery [114].

Considering the highly flexible and deformable biconcave discoid shape of red blood cells, it is not surprising that the elastic modulus of NPs can also play an important role in their pharmacokinetics and biodistribution, with more flexible NPs navigating and traversing vessels and gaps more easily in vivo. Investigating targeted NPs with variable degrees of structural rigidity and flexibility could be of high interest for effective tumor targeting strategies.

4.5 Influence of Nanoparticle PEGylation

The large surface area-to-volume ratios of NPs can attract a "corona" type binding of blood proteins to their extremely curved surfaces [109], with up to hundreds of proteins adsorbing onto their surfaces [115]. Hydrophobic surfaces tend to lead to higher levels of protein adsorption, and IgG proteins (opsonins) have high affinities for hydrophobic surfaces [116].

In the case of small drug molecules plasma protein binding by abundant proteins such as albumin and alpha-1-acid glycoprotein can lead to increased bioavailability through the reduction of first pass hepatic extraction. However for NPs, this can lead to their enhanced blood clearance by the MPS [9]. Binding of plasma proteins onto the surface of NPs (opsonization) is extremely rapid once the NPs are injected into the blood stream. The ability to graft hydrophilic neutral polymers of polyethylene glycol (PEG) onto the surface of liposomes and polymeric NPs goes hand-in-hand with EPR discoveries and led to increased blood circulation times and improvements in tumor accumulation [12, 23, 75, 117]. The grafting of PEG molecules onto the surface of NPs is termed PEGylation and is currently the most utilized technique for improving the pharmacokinetics, plasma half-life, biodistribution, and elimination of NPs in vivo [118]. Indeed, uncoated NPs have been observed to be rapidly cleared by the MPS [116], and the density and thickness of the PEG layer can also influence opsonization and biodistribution of injected NPs. Surface-grafted PEG NPs exhibit reduced uptake by liver cells [119].

PEG configurations on the surfaces of NPs can present as extended brush-like structures, coiled mushroom or mushroom/brush intermediates. Brush-like PEG surfaces were shown to be more optimal to sterically suppress the approach and binding of opsonins such as the C3b protein [116]. PEGylation as a strategy for improving NP-based drug delivery has been recently discussed in an excellent review elsewhere [120].

5 Emerging Considerations for Improving Targeted Cancer Nanomedicines

The effective homing of targeted NPs to the required site of action faces numerous biological barriers, including the immune system and the TME. Opsonization driven sequestration, compromised vasculature, erratic blood flow and high interstitial fluid pressures all need to be overcome. In previous sections we discuss the variety of parameters that can be tailored and optimized in order to improve nanomedicine targeting to tumors and cancer cells. Further considerations that are more recently gaining momentum and interest are the realization of the importance of TME components and stimuli-responsive design elements for more controlled targeting and drug delivery to cancer cells—and are discussed in the following sections.

5.1 The Tumor Microenvironment

The tumor microenvironment (TME) includes subpopulations of genetically diverse cancer cells, genetically normal cells, vascular/endothelial cells, blood cells (e.g., erythrocytes, leukocytes, and thrombocytes) together with the tumor interstial medium—with all these components having a role in cancer progression [121]. TAMs, cancer-associated fibroblasts and endothelial cells have been shown to play a role in tumor progression. It is anticipated that reprogramming of the TME via non-cancerous cells can lead to tumor regression. For example targeting stromal cells has gained interest recently [122, 123]. Stromal cells play a major role in tumor growth and maintenance—and their reprogramming can be a potential next-generation cancer treatment approach [124]. Another striking example is the use of immune checkpoint blockade inhibitors to reprogram immunosuppressive TMEs. Nanotechnology can offer solutions for the effective targeting of each of these components, and pathways. In particular the combination delivery of multiple chemotherapeutics can be achieved using targeted NPs. Nano-enabled synergistic combination drug delivery to cancer cells can more effectively kills these cells and minimize resistance [125].

5.2 Stimuli-Responsive Nanomedicines

Cancer produces an inevitable shift in homeostatic chemical equilibrium, such as amplified or triggered enzymatic activity, a change towards acidic pH, reductive or oxidative states, or an increase in reactive oxygen species [126]. These differential biochemical signatures can be exploited for the development of more precise therapies through NPs which sense these differences ("endogenous stimuli") to trigger drug release. In addition to internally triggered drug release, externally controlled physical parameters ("exogenous stimuli") such as local induction of thermal, electrical, ultrasound, or magnetic energy can also be used to trigger release [127]. Interest is growing in adding biologically responsive elements to

NP design, to achieve more controlled output behaviors and therapeutic outcomes. Release can be triggered by causing structural changes such as NP building block degradation, shedding of surface layers (e.g., PEG) and charge switching (neutral to positive), which can ultimately allow for better uptake into cancer cells. As with targeting generally, the goal of stimuli-responsive drug delivery systems is to further minimize systemic toxicities and unfavorable drug-plasma interactions to allow more efficient dosing and treatment of disease.

A range of endogenous stimuli such as changes in pH, redox state and ionic content within tissues and cells can be utilized for the development of chemically triggered drug release from polymeric NPs. Solid tumors have acidic pH environments (pH 6.2–6.9) [128], that can be used to trigger chemical changes in the NP structure leading to increased drug release. Subcellular compartments also offer various low pH environments post uptake of NPs (endosome, lysosome, cytosol, etc.), which can cause either surface layer shedding or conformational changes in NPs, leading to site-specific and increased drug release.

5.3 Subcellular Targeting

Following cancer cell internalization through different endocytosis pathways, NPs need to release their therapeutic payload, which can further diffuse through the cellular compartments to reach the biological target. Cell cytosolic internalization is not always sufficient for drugs to reach their targets via diffusion alone [129–135]. The cytoplasm contains a cytoskeletal network and numerous dispersed organelles, with many dissolved macromolecules ranging in concentration between 50 and 400 g/L [136, 137]. In the case of drugs that are recognized by efflux pumps (e.g., P-glycoprotein) NPs that can be internalized by endocytosis and thus release their active drugs within specific subcellular organelles can be a way to reduce multidrug resistance in cancer cells [138, 139].

Folic acid, low-density lipoprotein, cholera toxin B, mannose-6-phosphate, Tf, riboflavin, the tripeptide RGD, ICAM-1 antibody, and nicotinic acid are suitable endocytic targeting ligands that can be useful for subcellular localization of NPs [49]. Cellular internalization with these ligands can occur via clathrin-dependent receptor mediated endocytosis, caveolin-assisted endocytosis, lipid raft-associated endocytosis, or cell adhesion molecule (CAM)-directed cellular uptake [49, 140, 141].

Encapsulation of Dox into liposomes bearing Tfs on the distal end of PEG chains was shown to increase Dox uptake into glioma cells (that overexpress TfRs) [142]. The dynamic subcellular fate of polymeric micelles formed from (1,2-diaminocyclohexane) platinum(II) (DACHPt/m), the parent complex of oxaliplatin, was investigated in tumor tissues [143]. Potent antitumor activity was shown and the micelles were able to overcome Pt resistance both in vitro and in vivo. The extravasation of DACHP/m NP was observed from blood vessels into tumors in addition to polymer dissociation within the cells. The polymeric NPs selectively dissociated in the late endosomes and facilitated Pt drug delivery to the nucleus relative to free oxaliplatin, by circumventing the cytoplasmic detoxification systems of metallothionein and methionine synthase, suggesting that NP intracellular targeting via compartmentalization is an effective strategy for drug delivery. It would be of interest to understand the exact mechanisms of subcellular transport of NPs in order to improve their design and targeting functions.

6 Conclusions and Outlook

Improving and fine-tuning our understanding of tumor heterogeneity and discovering EPR biomarkers can help identify "nanomedicine-responsive" patients and further improve their clinical outcomes. Our understanding of NP transport to tumors and factors involved in their biodistribution and uptake within the TME is constantly expanding and will result in safer and more efficacious nanotherapeutics. Investigating the challenges of controllable, reproducible and scalable NP synthesis, as well as large-scale NP screening and evaluation, will facilitate their more rapid clinical translation.

Oncology is one area where nanomedicine products are set to make the most impact, where cell and tissue targeting approaches can be used to efficiently deliver cytotoxic and molecularly targeted drugs to cancer cells. Ultimately physicochemical parameters need to be investigated for successful design of targeted NPs, which include optimization of NP biophysicochemical properties and the demonstration of the efficacy of targeted NPs in a clinical setting on their impact on patient treatment. Indeed, the value of tailoring these parameters with the purpose of minimizing toxicity, unfavorable interactions with the immune system, rapid renal clearance, and minimal accumulation in organs such as the liver and spleen is beginning to be more systematically recognized and more routinely investigated. Other than identification of optimal ligands and ligand targets suitable for highly selective NP targeting, other important practical challenges in the development of targeted therapeutic NPs should also be considered including: (1) the use of biocompatible, biodegradable/bioeliminable materials; (2) the use of simple, robust, and reproducible bioconjugation chemistries for the attachment of precursors and targeting ligands; (3) facile NP assemblies that avoid multistep NP preparation and purification steps; (4) optimization of NP biophysicochemical properties to achieve, optimal drug load/release, long circulation half-life, suitable biodistribution, differential target tissue accumulation, efficacious target tissue drug concentration and drug exposure kinetics;

(5) validation of NP stability and predictable shelf life; and (6) development or adaptation of scalable processes and units of operations amenable to the manufacturing of large quantities of targeted NPs for clinical development and commercialization. The field is steadily progressing and we will see targeted nanomedicines en route to becoming valuable therapeutics in oncology with greater impact in the near future.

Acknowledgments

Nazila Kamaly acknowledges support from the Technical University of Denmark (DTU), DTU Nanotech.

References

1. Ratain MJ (2015) Redefining the primary objective of phase I oncology trials. Nat Rev Clin Oncol 12(3):126
2. Thanarajasingam G, Hubbard JM, Sloan JA, Grothey A (2015) The imperative for a new approach to toxicity analysis in oncology clinical trials. J Natl Cancer Inst 107(10):djv216
3. Weiner GJ (2015) Building better monoclonal antibody-based therapeutics. Nat Rev Cancer 15(6):361–370
4. Scott AM, Wolchok JD, Old LJ (2012) Antibody therapy of cancer. Nat Rev Cancer 12 (4):278–287
5. Khalil DN, Smith EL, Brentjens RJ, Wolchok JD (2016) The future of cancer treatment: immunomodulation, CARs and combination immunotherapy. Nat Rev Clin Oncol 13:273–290
6. Bertrand N, Wu J, Xu X, Kamaly N, Farokhzad OC (2014) Cancer nanotechnology: the impact of passive and active targeting in the era of modern cancer biology. Adv Drug Deliv Rev 66:2–25
7. O'Brien ME et al (2004) Reduced cardiotoxicity and comparable efficacy in a phase III trial of pegylated liposomal doxorubicin HCl (CAELYX/Doxil) versus conventional doxorubicin for first-line treatment of metastatic breast cancer. Ann Oncol 15(3):440–449
8. Hoy SM (2014) Albumin-bound paclitaxel: a review of its use for the first-line combination treatment of metastatic pancreatic cancer. Drugs 74(15):1757–1768
9. McNeil SE (2005) Nanotechnology for the biologist. J Leukoc Biol 78(3):585–594
10. Leserman LD, Barbet J, Kourilsky F, Weinstein JN (1980) Targeting to cells of fluorescent liposomes covalently coupled with monoclonal antibody or protein A. Nature 288(5791):602–604
11. Heath TD, Fraley RT, Papahdjopoulos D (1980) Antibody targeting of liposomes: cell specificity obtained by conjugation of F(ab′)2 to vesicle surface. Science 210 (4469):539–541
12. Allen TM, Chonn A (1987) Large unilamellar liposomes with low uptake into the reticuloendothelial system. FEBS Lett 223 (1):42–46
13. Torchilin VP (1994) Immunoliposomes and PEGylated immunoliposomes: possible use for targeted delivery of imaging agents. Immunomethods 4(3):244–258
14. Sankhala KK et al (2009) A phase I pharmacokinetic (PK) study of MBP-426, a novel liposome encapsulated oxaliplatin. J Clin Oncol 27(2535):15S
15. Matsumura Y et al (2004) Phase I and pharmacokinetic study of MCC-465, a doxorubicin (DXR) encapsulated in PEG immunoliposome, in patients with metastatic stomach cancer. Ann Oncol 15(3):517–525
16. Nemunaitis J et al (2009) A phase I study of escalating doses of SGT-53 for intravenous infusion of patients with advanced solid tumors. Mol Ther 17:S226
17. Dawidczyk CM, Russell LM, Searson PC (2014) Nanomedicines for cancer therapy: state-of-the-art and limitations to pre-clinical studies that hinder future developments. Front Chem 2:69
18. Carmeliet P, Jain RK (2000) Angiogenesis in cancer and other diseases. Nature 407 (6801):249–257

19. Danquah MK, Zhang XA, Mahato RI (2011) Extravasation of polymeric nanomedicines across tumor vasculature. Adv Drug Deliv Rev 63(8):623–639
20. Matsumura Y, Maeda H (1986) A new concept for macromolecular therapeutics in cancer chemotherapy: mechanism of tumoritropic accumulation of proteins and the antitumor agent smancs. Cancer Res 46(12 Pt 1):6387–6392
21. Farokhzad OC, Langer R (2009) Impact of nanotechnology on drug delivery. ACS Nano 3(1):16–20
22. Maeda H (2010) Tumor-selective delivery of macromolecular drugs via the EPR effect: background and future prospects. Bioconjug Chem 21(5):797–802
23. Gref R et al (1994) Biodegradable long-circulating polymeric nanospheres. Science 263(5153):1600–1603
24. Rabanel JM, Aoun V, Elkin I, Mokhtar M, Hildgen P (2012) Drug-loaded nanocarriers: passive targeting and crossing of biological barriers. Curr Med Chem 19(19):3070–3102
25. Maeda H, Bharate GY, Daruwalla J (2009) Polymeric drugs for efficient tumor-targeted drug delivery based on EPR-effect. Eur J Pharm Biopharm 71(3):409–419
26. Acharya S, Sahoo SK (2011) PLGA nanoparticles containing various anticancer agents and tumour delivery by EPR effect. Adv Drug Deliv Rev 63(3):170–183
27. Saha RN, Vasanthakumar S, Bende G, Snehalatha M (2010) Nanoparticulate drug delivery systems for cancer chemotherapy. Mol Membr Biol 27(7):215–231
28. Torchilin VP (2010) Passive and active drug targeting: drug delivery to tumors as an example. Handb Exp Pharmacol 197:3–53
29. Chrastina A, Massey KA, Schnitzer JE (2011) Overcoming in vivo barriers to targeted nanodelivery. Wiley Interdiscip Rev Nanomed Nanobiotechnol 3(4):421–437
30. Hobbs SK et al (1998) Regulation of transport pathways in tumor vessels: role of tumor type and microenvironment. Proc Natl Acad Sci U S A 95(8):4607–4612
31. Jain RK (2001) Delivery of molecular and cellular medicine to solid tumors. Adv Drug Deliv Rev 46(1–3):149–168
32. Martini M, Vecchione L, Siena S, Tejpar S, Bardelli A (2012) Targeted therapies: how personal should we go? Nat Rev Clin Oncol 9(2):87–97
33. Taurin S, Nehoff H, Greish K (2012) Anticancer nanomedicine and tumor vascular permeability; where is the missing link? J Control Release 164(3):265–275
34. Prabhakar U et al (2013) Challenges and key considerations of the enhanced permeability and retention effect for nanomedicine drug delivery in oncology. Cancer Res 73 (8):2412–2417
35. Lammers T, Kiessling F, Hennink WE, Storm G (2012) Drug targeting to tumors: principles, pitfalls and (pre-) clinical progress. J Control Release 161(2):175–187
36. Staropoli N et al (2014) Pegylated liposomal doxorubicin in the management of ovarian cancer: a systematic review and metaanalysis of randomized trials. Cancer Biol Ther 15 (6):707–720
37. Karathanasis E et al (2009) Imaging nanoprobe for prediction of outcome of nanoparticle chemotherapy by using mammography. Radiology 250(2):398–406
38. Miller MA et al (2015) Predicting therapeutic nanomedicine efficacy using a companion magnetic resonance imaging nanoparticle. Sci Transl Med 7(314):314ra183
39. Hooks MA, Wade CS, Millikan WJ Jr (1991) Muromonab CD-3: a review of its pharmacology, pharmacokinetics, and clinical use in transplantation. Pharmacotherapy 11 (1):26–37
40. Peer D et al (2007) Nanocarriers as an emerging platform for cancer therapy. Nat Nanotechnol 2(12):751–760
41. James JS, Dubs G (1997) FDA approves new kind of lymphoma treatment. Food and drug administration. AIDS Treat News 284:2–3
42. Albanell J, Baselga J (1999) Trastuzumab, a humanized anti-HER2 monoclonal antibody, for the treatment of breast cancer. Drugs Today (Barc) 35(12):931–946
43. Toporkiewicz M, Meissner J, Matusewicz L, Czogalla A, Sikorski AF (2015) Toward a magic or imaginary bullet? Ligands for drug targeting to cancer cells: principles, hopes, and challenges. Int J Nanomedicine 10:1399–1414
44. Graham MM, Menda Y (2011) Radiopeptide imaging and therapy in the United States. J Nucl Med 52(Suppl 2):56S–63S
45. Sudimack J, Lee RJ (2000) Targeted drug delivery via the folate receptor. Adv Drug Deliv Rev 41(2):147–162
46. Qian ZM, Li H, Sun H, Ho K (2002) Targeted drug delivery via the transferrin receptor-mediated endocytosis pathway. Pharmacol Rev 54(4):561–587

47. Kue CS et al (2016) Small molecules for active targeting in cancer. Med Res Rev 36:494–575
48. Allen TM (2002) Ligand-targeted therapeutics in anticancer therapy. Nat Rev Cancer 2 (10):750–763
49. Bareford LM, Swaan PW (2007) Endocytic mechanisms for targeted drug delivery. Adv Drug Deliv Rev 59(8):748–758
50. Shete HK, Prabhu RH, Patravale VB (2014) Endosomal escape: a bottleneck in intracellular delivery. J Nanosci Nanotechnol 14 (1):460–474
51. Whitehead KA, Langer R, Anderson DG (2009) Knocking down barriers: advances in siRNA delivery. Nat Rev Drug Discov 8 (2):129–138
52. Schroeder A, Levins CG, Cortez C, Langer R, Anderson DG (2010) Lipid-based nanotherapeutics for siRNA delivery. J Intern Med 267 (1):9–21
53. Varkouhi AK, Scholte M, Storm G, Haisma HJ (2011) Endosomal escape pathways for delivery of biologicals. J Control Release 151 (3):220–228
54. Cheng X, Lee RJ (2016) The role of helper lipids in lipid nanoparticles (LNPs) designed for oligonucleotide delivery. Adv Drug Deliv Rev 99((Pt A)):129–137
55. Kauffman KJ, Webber MJ, Anderson DG (2015) Materials for non-viral intracellular delivery of messenger RNA therapeutics. J Control Release S0168-3659:30283
56. Kamaly N, Kalber T, Thanou M, Bell JD, Miller AD (2009) Folate receptor targeted bimodal liposomes for tumor magnetic resonance imaging. Bioconjug Chem 20 (4):648–655
57. Gallo J et al (2014) CXCR4-targeted and MMP-responsive iron oxide nanoparticles for enhanced magnetic resonance imaging. Angew Chem Int Ed Engl 53 (36):9550–9554
58. Kirpotin DB et al (2006) Antibody targeting of long-circulating lipidic nanoparticles does not increase tumor localization but does increase internalization in animal models. Cancer Res 66(13):6732–6740
59. Bartlett DW, Su H, Hildebrandt IJ, Weber WA, Davis ME (2007) Impact of tumor-specific targeting on the biodistribution and efficacy of siRNA nanoparticles measured by multimodality in vivo imaging. Proc Natl Acad Sci U S A 104(39):15549–15554
60. Pirollo KF, Chang EH (2008) Does a targeting ligand influence nanoparticle tumor localization or uptake? Trends Biotechnol 26 (10):552–558
61. Teesalu T, Sugahara KN, Ruoslahti E (2013) Tumor-penetrating peptides. Front Oncol 3:216
62. Gregoriadis G, Neerunjun ED (1975) Homing of liposomes to target cells. Biochem Biophys Res Commun 65(2):537–544
63. Hamaguchi T et al (2004) Antitumor effect of MCC-465, pegylated liposomal doxorubicin tagged with newly developed monoclonal antibody GAH, in colorectal cancer xenografts. Cancer Sci 95(7):608–613
64. Mamot C et al (2012) Tolerability, safety, pharmacokinetics, and efficacy of doxorubicin-loaded anti-EGFR immunoliposomes in advanced solid tumours: a phase 1 dose-escalation study. Lancet Oncol 13 (12):1234–1241
65. Espelin CW, Leonard SC, Geretti E, Wickham TJ, Hendriks BS (2016) Dual HER2 targeting with trastuzumab and liposomal-encapsulated doxorubicin (MM-302) demonstrates synergistic antitumor activity in breast and gastric cancer. Cancer Res 76(6): 1517–1527
66. Geretti E et al (2015) Cyclophosphamide-mediated tumor priming for enhanced delivery and antitumor activity of HER2-targeted liposomal doxorubicin (MM-302). Mol Cancer Ther 14(9):2060–2071
67. Cheng Z, Al Zaki A, Hui JZ, Muzykantov VR, Tsourkas A (2012) Multifunctional nanoparticles: cost versus benefit of adding targeting and imaging capabilities. Science 338 (6109):903–910
68. http://clinicaltrials.gov/ct2/show/NCT00470613
69. www.bindbio.com
70. Elsasser-Beile U, Buhler P, Wolf P (2009) Targeted therapies for prostate cancer against the prostate specific membrane antigen. Curr Drug Targets 10(2):118–125
71. Slovin SF (2005) Targeting novel antigens for prostate cancer treatment: focus on prostate-specific membrane antigen. Expert Opin Ther Targets 9(3):561–570
72. Sanna V, Pala N, Sechi M (2014) Targeted therapy using nanotechnology: focus on cancer. Int J Nanomedicine 9:467–483
73. Davis ME (2009) The first targeted delivery of siRNA in humans via a self-assembling, cyclodextrin polymer-based nanoparticle: from concept to clinic. Mol Pharm 6 (3):659–668
74. Heidel JD et al (2007) Potent siRNA inhibitors of ribonucleotide reductase subunit RRM2 reduce cell proliferation in vitro and in vivo. Clin Cancer Res 13(7):2207–2215

75. Kamaly N, Xiao Z, Valencia PM, Radovic-Moreno AF, Farokhzad OC (2012) Targeted polymeric therapeutic nanoparticles: design, development and clinical translation. Chem Soc Rev 41(7):2971–3010
76. Adiseshaiah PP, Hall JB, McNeil SE (2010) Nanomaterial standards for efficacy and toxicity assessment. Wiley Interdiscip Rev Nanomed Nanobiotechnol 2(1):99–112
77. Bao G et al (2014) USNCTAM perspectives on mechanics in medicine. J R Soc Interface 11(97):20140301
78. Li Y et al (2016) Cell and nanoparticle transport in tumour microvasculature: the role of size, shape and surface functionality of nanoparticles. Interface Focus 6(1):20150086
79. Wang J, Byrne JD, Napier ME, Desimone JM (2011) More effective nanomedicines through particle design. Small 7 (14):1919–1931
80. Vonarbourg A et al (2006) Evaluation of pegylated lipid nanocapsules versus complement system activation and macrophage uptake. J Biomed Mater Res A 78 (3):620–628
81. Moghimi SM, Hunter AC, Murray JC (2001) Long-circulating and target-specific nanoparticles: theory to practice. Pharmacol Rev 53 (2):283–318
82. Choi HS et al (2007) Renal clearance of quantum dots. Nat Biotechnol 25(10):1165–1170
83. Torchilin VP (2007) Targeted pharmaceutical nanocarriers for cancer therapy and imaging. AAPS J 9(2):E128–E147
84. Padera TP et al (2004) Pathology: cancer cells compress intratumour vessels. Nature 427 (6976):695
85. Boucher Y, Baxter LT, Jain RK (1990) Interstitial pressure gradients in tissue-isolated and subcutaneous tumors: implications for therapy. Cancer Res 50(15):4478–4484
86. Wong C et al (2011) Multistage nanoparticle delivery system for deep penetration into tumor tissue. Proc Natl Acad Sci U S A 108 (6):2426–2431
87. Gratton SE et al (2008) The effect of particle design on cellular internalization pathways. Proc Natl Acad Sci U S A 105 (33):11613–11618
88. Jiang W, Kim BY, Rutka JT, Chan WC (2008) Nanoparticle-mediated cellular response is size-dependent. Nat Nanotechnol 3 (3):145–150
89. Schadlich A et al (2011) Tumor accumulation of NIR fluorescent PEG-PLA nanoparticles: impact of particle size and human xenograft tumor model. ACS Nano 5(11):8710–8720
90. Cabral H et al (2011) Accumulation of sub-100 nm polymeric micelles in poorly permeable tumours depends on size. Nat Nanotechnol 6(12):815–823
91. Geng Y et al (2007) Shape effects of filaments versus spherical particles in flow and drug delivery. Nat Nanotechnol 2(4):249–255
92. Decuzzi P et al (2010) Size and shape effects in the biodistribution of intravascularly injected particles. J Control Release 141 (3):320–327
93. Lee SY, Ferrari M, Decuzzi P (2009) Shaping nano-/micro-particles for enhanced vascular interaction in laminar flows. Nanotechnology 20(49):495101
94. Chithrani BD, Ghazani AA, Chan WC (2006) Determining the size and shape dependence of gold nanoparticle uptake into mammalian cells. Nano Lett 6(4):662–668
95. Champion JA, Mitragotri S (2006) Role of target geometry in phagocytosis. Proc Natl Acad Sci U S A 103(13):4930–4934
96. Decuzzi P, Ferrari M (2006) The adhesive strength of non-spherical particles mediated by specific interactions. Biomaterials 27 (30):5307–5314
97. Peiris PM et al (2012) Imaging metastasis using an integrin-targeting chain-shaped nanoparticle. ACS Nano 6(10):8783–8795
98. Toy R, Peiris PM, Ghaghada KB, Karathanasis E (2014) Shaping cancer nanomedicine: the effect of particle shape on the in vivo journey of nanoparticles. Nanomedicine (Lond) 9 (1):121–134
99. Gentile F, Curcio A, Indolfi C, Ferrari M, Decuzzi P (2008) The margination propensity of spherical particles for vascular targeting in the microcirculation. J Nanobiotechnology 6:9
100. Toy R, Hayden E, Shoup C, Baskaran H, Karathanasis E (2011) The effects of particle size, density and shape on margination of nanoparticles in microcirculation. Nanotechnology 22(11):115101
101. Verma A, Stellacci F (2010) Effect of surface properties on nanoparticle-cell interactions. Small 6(1):12–21
102. Canelas DA, Herlihy KP, DeSimone JM (2009) Top-down particle fabrication: control of size and shape for diagnostic imaging and drug delivery. Wiley Interdiscip Rev Nanomed Nanobiotechnol 1(4):391–404
103. Chu KS et al (2013) Plasma, tumor and tissue pharmacokinetics of Docetaxel delivered via nanoparticles of different sizes and shapes in mice bearing SKOV-3 human ovarian carcinoma xenograft. Nanomedicine 9(5):686–693

104. Zhao F, Zhao Y, Liu Y, Chang X, Chen C (2011) Cellular uptake, intracellular trafficking, and cytotoxicity of nanomaterials. Small 7(10):1322–1337
105. Dausend J et al (2008) Uptake mechanism of oppositely charged fluorescent nanoparticles in HeLa cells. Macromol Biosci 8 (12):1135–1143
106. Salvador-Morales C, Zhang L, Langer R, Farokhzad OC (2009) Immunocompatibility properties of lipid-polymer hybrid nanoparticles with heterogeneous surface functional groups. Biomaterials 30(12):2231–2240
107. He C, Hu Y, Yin L, Tang C, Yin C (2010) Effects of particle size and surface charge on cellular uptake and biodistribution of polymeric nanoparticles. Biomaterials 31 (13):3657–3666
108. Yamamoto Y, Nagasaki Y, Kato Y, Sugiyama Y, Kataoka K (2001) Long-circulating poly (ethylene glycol)-poly(D, L-lactide) block copolymer micelles with modulated surface charge. J Control Release 77(1–2):27–38
109. Nel AE et al (2009) Understanding biophysicochemical interactions at the nano-bio interface. Nat Mater 8(7):543–557
110. Merkel TJ et al (2011) Using mechanobiological mimicry of red blood cells to extend circulation times of hydrogel microparticles. Proc Natl Acad Sci U S A 108(2):586–591
111. Best JP, Yan Y, Caruso F (2012) The role of particle geometry and mechanics in the biological domain. Adv Healthc Mater 1 (1):35–47
112. Anselmo AC, Mitragotri S (2016) Impact of particle elasticity on particle-based drug delivery systems. Adv Drug Deliv Rev http://dx.doi.org/10.1016/j.addr.2016.01.007
113. Zhang L et al (2012) Softer zwitterionic nanogels for longer circulation and lower splenic accumulation. ACS Nano 6 (8):6681–6686
114. Anselmo AC et al (2015) Elasticity of nanoparticles influences their blood circulation, phagocytosis, endocytosis, and targeting. ACS Nano 9(3):3169–3177
115. Anderson NL et al (2004) The human plasma proteome: a nonredundant list developed by combination of four separate sources. Mol Cell Proteomics 3(4):311–326
116. Vonarbourg A, Passirani C, Saulnier P, Benoit JP (2006) Parameters influencing the stealthiness of colloidal drug delivery systems. Biomaterials 27(24):4356–4373
117. Barenholz Y (2012) Doxil(R)–the first FDA-approved nano-drug: lessons learned. J Control Release 160(2):117–134
118. Hamidi M, Azadi A, Rafiei P (2006) Pharmacokinetic consequences of pegylation. Drug Deliv 13(6):399–409
119. Scherphof GL, Velinova M, Kamps J, Donga J, van der Want H, Kuipers F, Havekes L, Daemen T (1997) Modulation of pharmacokinetic behavior of liposomes. Adv Drug Deliv Rev 24(2-3):179-191
120. Suk JS, Xu Q, Kim N, Hanes J, Ensign LM (2016) PEGylation as a strategy for improving nanoparticle-based drug and gene delivery. Adv Drug Deliv Rev 99(Pt A):28–51
121. Spill F, Reynolds DS, Kamm RD, Zaman MH (2016) Impact of the physical microenvironment on tumor progression and metastasis. Curr Opin Biotechnol 40:41–48
122. Reisfeld RA (2013) The tumor microenvironment: a target for combination therapy of breast cancer. Crit Rev Oncog 18 (1–2):115–133
123. Wang LC et al (2014) Targeting fibroblast activation protein in tumor stroma with chimeric antigen receptor T cells can inhibit tumor growth and augment host immunity without severe toxicity. Cancer Immunol Res 2(2):154–166
124. Linton SS, Sherwood SG, Drews KC, Kester M (2016) Targeting cancer cells in the tumor microenvironment: opportunities and challenges in combinatorial nanomedicine. Wiley Interdiscip Rev Nanomed Nanobiotechnol 8 (2):208–222
125. Milane L, Duan Z, Amiji M (2011) Development of EGFR-targeted polymer blend nanocarriers for combination paclitaxel/ lonidamine delivery to treat multi-drug resistance in human breast and ovarian tumor cells. Mol Pharm 8(1):185–203
126. Mura S, Nicolas J, Couvreur P (2013) Stimuli-responsive nanocarriers for drug delivery. Nat Mater 12(11):991–1003
127. Kamaly N, Yameen B, Wu J, Farokhzad OC (2016) Degradable controlled-release polymers and polymeric nanoparticles: mechanisms of controlling drug release. Chem Rev 116(4):2602–2663
128. Kanamala M, Wilson WR, Yang M, Palmer BD, Wu Z (2016) Mechanisms and biomaterials in pH-responsive tumour targeted drug delivery: a review. Biomaterials 85:152–167
129. Torchilin VP (2006) Recent approaches to intracellular delivery of drugs and DNA and organelle targeting. Annu Rev Biomed Eng 8:343–375
130. Li S-D, Huang L (2008) Pharmacokinetics and biodistribution of nanoparticles. Mol Pharm 5(4):496–504

131. Kaufmann AM, Krise JP (2007) Lysosomal sequestration of amine-containing drugs: analysis and therapeutic implications. J Pharm Sci 96(4):729–746
132. Panyam J, Labhasetwar V (2003) Biodegradable nanoparticles for drug and gene delivery to cells and tissue. Adv Drug Deliv Rev 55 (3):329–347
133. Weissig V (2003) Mitochondrial-targeted drug and DNA delivery. Crit Rev Ther Drug Carrier Syst 20(1):1–62
134. Weissig V (2005) Targeted drug delivery to mammalian mitochondria in living cells. Expert Opin Drug Deliv 2(1):89–102
135. Weissig V, Boddapati SV, Jabr L, D'Souza GG (2007) Mitochondria-specific nanotechnology. Nanomedicine (Lond) 2(3):275–285
136. Minton AP (2006) How can biochemical reactions within cells differ from those in test tubes? J Cell Sci 119(14):2863–2869
137. Ellis RJ, Minton AP (2003) Cell biology: join the crowd. Nature 425(6953):27–28
138. Kim D, Lee ES, Oh KT, Gao ZG, Bae YH (2008) Doxorubicin-loaded polymeric micelle overcomes multidrug resistance of cancer by double-targeting folate receptor and early endosomal pH. Small 4 (11):2043–2050
139. Cho K, Wang X, Nie S, Chen ZG, Shin DM (2008) Therapeutic nanoparticles for drug delivery in cancer. Clin Cancer Res 14 (5):1310–1316
140. Seibel P et al (1995) Transfection of mitochondria: strategy towards a gene therapy of mitochondrial DNA diseases. Nucleic Acids Res 23(1):10–17
141. Weissig V, Torchilin VP (2001) Cationic bolasomes with delocalized charge centers as mitochondria-specific DNA delivery systems. Adv Drug Deliv Rev 49(1–2):127–149
142. Eavarone DA, Yu X, Bellamkonda RV (2000) Targeted drug delivery to C6 glioma by transferrin-coupled liposomes. J Biomed Mater Res 51(1):10–14
143. Murakami M et al (2011) Improving drug potency and efficacy by nanocarrier-mediated subcellular targeting. Sci Transl Med 3 (64):64ra2
144. Park JW et al (2002) Anti-HER2 immunoliposomes: enhanced efficacy attributable to targeted delivery. Clin Cancer Res 8 (4):1172–1181
145. Winkler J, Martin-Killias P, Pluckthun A, Zangemeister-Wittke U (2009) EpCAM-targeted delivery of nanocomplexed siRNA to tumor cells with designed ankyrin repeat proteins. Mol Cancer Ther 8(9):2674–2683
146. Alexis F et al (2008) HER-2-targeted nanoparticle-affibody bioconjugates for cancer therapy. ChemMedChem 3(12):1839–1843
147. Karmali PP et al (2009) Targeting of albumin-embedded paclitaxel nanoparticles to tumors. Nanomedicine 5(1):73–82
148. Park JH et al (2008) Magnetic iron oxide nanoworms for tumor targeting and imaging. Adv Mater 20(9):1630–1635
149. Sugahara KN et al (2009) Tissue-penetrating delivery of compounds and nanoparticles into tumors. Cancer Cell 16(6):510–520
150. Graf N et al (2012) Alpha(V)beta(3) integrin-targeted PLGA-PEG nanoparticles for enhanced anti-tumor efficacy of a Pt(IV) prodrug. ACS Nano 6(5):4530–4539
151. Kamaly N et al (2013) Development and in vivo efficacy of targeted polymeric inflammation-resolving nanoparticles. Proc Natl Acad Sci U S A 110(16):6506–6511
152. Chan JM et al (2010) Spatiotemporal controlled delivery of nanoparticles to injured vasculature. Proc Natl Acad Sci U S A 107 (5):2213–2218
153. Park J et al (2012) Fibronectin extra domain B-specific aptide conjugated nanoparticles for targeted cancer imaging. J Control Release 163(2):111–118
154. Cheng J et al (2007) Formulation of functionalized PLGA-PEG nanoparticles for in vivo targeted drug delivery. Biomaterials 28 (5):869–876
155. Kim D, Jeong YY, Jon S (2010) A drug-loaded aptamer-gold nanoparticle bioconjugate for combined CT imaging and therapy of prostate cancer. ACS Nano 4(7):3689–3696
156. Werner ME et al (2011) Folate-targeted nanoparticle delivery of chemo- and radiotherapeutics for the treatment of ovarian cancer peritoneal metastasis. Biomaterials 32 (33):8548–8554
157. Marrache S, Dhar S (2012) Engineering of blended nanoparticle platform for delivery of mitochondria-acting therapeutics. Proc Natl Acad Sci U S A 109(40):16288–16293
158. Hrkach J et al (2012) Preclinical development and clinical translation of a PSMA-targeted docetaxel nanoparticle with a differentiated pharmacological profile. Sci Transl Med 4 (128):128ra139
159. Wickham T, Futch K (2012) A phase I study of MM-302, a HER2-targeted liposomal doxorubicin, in patients with advanced, HER2- positive breast cancer. In: Thirty-Fifth Annual CTRC-AACR San Antonio Breast Cancer Symposium, Cancer Research, San Antonio, TX, pp Suppl 3 P5-18-09

http://cancerres.aacrjournals.org/content/72/24_Supplement/P5-18-09

160. Fernandes E et al (2015) New trends in guided nanotherapies for digestive cancers: a systematic review. J Control Release 209:288–307
161. Senzer N et al (2013) Phase I study of a systemically delivered p53 nanoparticle in advanced solid tumors. Mol Ther 21 (5):1096–1103
162. Pirollo KF et al (2008) Tumor-targeting nanocomplex delivery of novel tumor suppressor RB94 chemosensitizes bladder carcinoma cells in vitro and in vivo. Clin Cancer Res 14(7):2190–2198
163. Gaillard PJ et al (2014) Pharmacokinetics, brain delivery, and efficacy in brain tumor-bearing mice of glutathione pegylated liposomal doxorubicin (2B3-101). PLoS One 9(1): e82331
164. Davis ME et al (2010) Evidence of RNAi in humans from systemically administered siRNA via targeted nanoparticles. Nature 464:1067–1070

Part II

Nanotechnology-Based Platforms

Chapter 3

Multifunctional Liposomes

Bhawani Aryasomayajula, Giuseppina Salzano, and Vladimir P. Torchilin

Abstract

Liposomes have come a long way since their conception in the 1960s, when they were envisioned primarily for drug delivery. Besides serving the important function of the delivery of a variety of drugs, liposomes offer a platform for the co-delivery of a range of therapeutic and diagnostic agents with different physicochemical properties. They are also amenable to the addition of various targeting moieties such as proteins, sugars, and antibodies for selective targeting at a desired site, including tumors. Currently, the design of stimuli-sensitive liposomes for drug delivery is a lively area of research. Compared to conventional liposomes, stimuli-sensitive nanoplatforms respond to local conditions that are characteristics of the pathological area of interest, allowing the release of active agents at the targeted site. Acidic pH, abnormal levels of enzymes, temperature, altered redox potential, and external magnetic field are examples of internal and external stimuli exploited in the design of stimuli-sensitive liposomes. The penetration of the liposomes into the cells can be enhanced with the help of a variety of cell penetrating peptides, which can be incorporated into the liposomes with the help of various lipid–polymer conjugates. Liposomes are now being employed in diagnostics as well. Imaging of a tumor can be made easier by the inclusion of fluorescent probes. They can also be used for gamma or MR imaging using chelated reporter metals and incorporating them either into the core of the liposome or in the lipid bilayer facing outwards. In this chapter, we discuss methods that are commonly used for the preparation of liposomes with a vast range of functions to meet a variety of needs in diagnostics and drug delivery.

Key words Liposomes, Multifunctional, Long-circulating, Tumor-targeting, Temperature-sensitive, pH-sensitive, Redox-sensitive, MMP-sensitive, Magnetically sensitive, Cell-penetrating

1 Introduction

Liposomes are defined as microparticulate vesicles composed of a mixture of phospholipids, where the lipids form concentric bilayers and are capable of encapsulating an aqueous phase in their core [1, 2]. This property helps in the encapsulation of not only a wide range of therapeutic agents in the bilayer and hydrophilic agents in the aqueous core, but also enables the delivery of a high-payload of the intended drug. Liposomal technology has undergone tremendous change, since their development in the 1960s. First generation liposomes were lipid bilayers encapsulating many therapeutic

Reema Zeineldin (ed.), *Cancer Nanotechnology: Methods and Protocols*, Methods in Molecular Biology, vol. 1530,
DOI 10.1007/978-1-4939-6646-2_3,

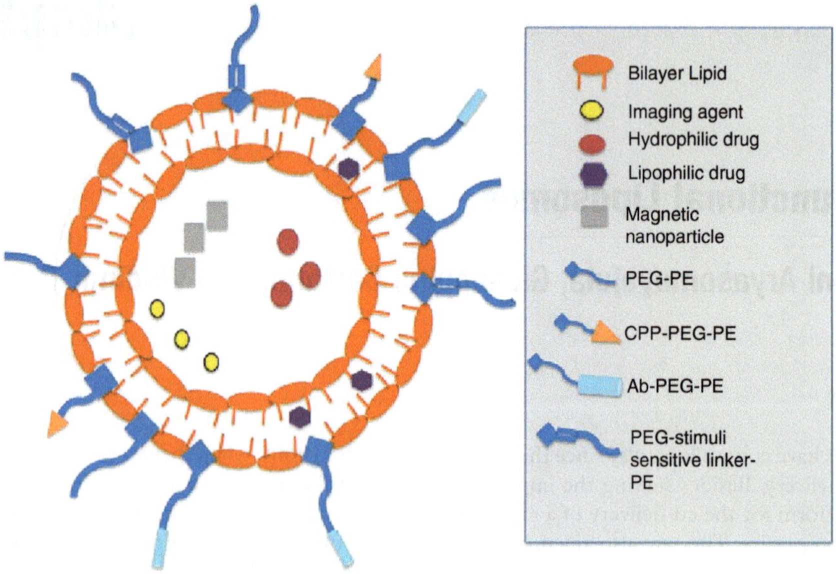

Fig. 1 Schematic representation of a multifunctional liposome

agents with a wide range of physicochemical properties. Second generation liposomes improved upon this concept and with the addition of polyethylene glycol (PEG) on their surface [3]. These liposomes acquired the property of "stealth," meaning that they could circulate in the body for a longer time by avoiding opsonization that causes recognition by the reticuloendothelial system (RES). This is a direct consequence of steric hindrance by the long PEG chains, resulting in increasing their circulation half-life. The third generation liposomes take it much further, allowing the engineering of complex liposomes which combined several functions at the same time, such as drug delivery, targeting at the site of action as well as cell organelles, penetration and accumulation at the site of action, stimuli-sensitive function, and imaging/diagnosis. Liposomes are now increasingly used in clinical settings and are very popular due to their salient properties. Numerous such formulations are now in the market and many more in clinical trials [4]. In this chapter we discuss the various types of novel, "smart" liposomes that are demonstrating promising potential for cancer therapy. *See* Fig. 1 for a schematic of a multifunctional liposome.

1.1 Preparation of Liposomes

The simplest method to prepare liposomes is by a technique known as thin-film hydration.

Briefly, an organic solution containing the desired lipid mixture is dried under vacuum by using a rotary evaporator, forming a film. This film is rehydrated using an aqueous buffer by simple agitation. Methods such as shaking, mixing using a vortex result in large multi-lamellar vesicles, which can be further broken down into small unilamellar vesicles using methods such a sonication or extrusion. These two methods yield liposomes with a narrow size distribution. Another method proposed by Szoka and Papahadjopoulos [2] known as reverse-phase evaporation relied on the creation of inverted micelles in an organic solvent and the slow removal of the organic solvent leading finally to the formation of unilamellar vesicles. The advantage of this technique is that it can encapsulate a large amount of drug but the use of an organic solvent might interfere with the encapsulation of proteins on account of denaturation.

1.2 Preparation of Long-Circulating "Stealth" Liposomes

Classical liposomes are susceptible to rapid clearance by the mononuclear phagocytic system also knows as the RES [5]. An effective way to prolong their circulation is to graft long chain poly ethylene glycol (PEG) on the surface of the liposomes. PEG chains confer many important traits such as decrease in hydrophobicity, decrease in immunogenicity, increase in stability and steric hindrance to protect against opsonization and clearance [3, 6]. Long chain PEG can range from 1 to10 KD and its hydroxyl terminal be coupled with a lipid anchor such as DSPE (1,2-distearoyl-sn-glycero-3-phosphoethanolamine) and DOPE (1,2-dioleoyl-sn-glycero-3-phosphoethanolamine). via various chemical reactions. These PEG chains can be incorporated into the liposomes either during the preparation of the liposomes [7], or after they have been manufactured via a technique known as post insertion [8]. The use of PEG not only helps in sterically stabilizing the liposomes but also provides an opportunity for the attachment of various targeting ligands, cell-penetrating peptides, stimuli-sensitive linkers, etc. by the use of functionalized PEG polymers [9–11]. This chapter describes a simple method to insert PEG into prepared liposomes using a technique known as post insertion.

1.3 Preparation of Liposomes Functionalized with Specific Ligands for Selective Targeting to Tumors

To selectively target liposomes to tumor tissues, a plethora of targeting ligands have been used. The strategy of active targeting is based on attaching a ligand to the liposomes surface, which can bind to specific components that are either selectively or overexpressed in tumor cells. These targeting moieties includes ligands such as folate for targeting folic acid receptors [12], transferrin for transferrin receptors [13], and antibodies such as anti-HER2 [14], nucleosome specific antibodies [9] to name a few. In this section we describe an efficient way of grafting an antibody known as 2C5, which targets the nucleosomes that are overexpressed on the surface of cancer cells [15, 16], onto a PEG chain of a chosen length, which can be subsequently incorporated into liposomes as described by Torchilin et al. [15].

1.4 Preparation of Liposomes Containing Stimuli-Sensitive Moieties

Tumor tissue differs from normal tissue in numerous ways such as an acidic and reducing environment, overexpression of a specific enzymes including matrix metallo-proteases (MMPMetallo-protease), receptors such as transferrin receptors, folate receptors to name a few [12, 13, 17–19]. Designing liposomes with lipids and polymers that respond to these stimuli is an effective way to target them to the site of action and achieve a selective release of the drug. Moreover, the use of external triggers such as temperature and magnetic stimulus can also guide the liposomes externally, thereby making the therapy more effective. In this chapter we describe a few methods to render the liposomes sensitive to various types of stimuli, internal and external.

1.4.1 pH-Sensitive Liposomes

Anaerobic glycolysis in tumor tissue causes lactate secretion and its accumulation, giving rise to a lower pH in the tumor tissue [20]. Furthermore, one of the predominant mechanisms of uptake of the liposomes into the cells is their incorporation into the endocytic pathway wherein, the pH steadily decreases from about 6.5 to 4.5 depending on the stage of the endocytic vesicles [21]. This phenomenon can be exploited to bring about site-specific delivery of the drug by the use of lipids that are shaped conically and inverted conically at neutral pH. At a more acidic pH, these lipids undergo protonation, change their shape from conical to cylindrical and hence destabilize the liposomes, thereby losing the liposome's lamellar structure [22]. DOPE is frequently used in such formulations, owing to its conical shape, in conjunction with lipids such as cholesterolhemisuccinate (CHEMS), long chain fatty acids such as oleic acid. Another method of creating a stimuli sensitive nanocarrier is by the use of pH sensitive lipid–polymer conjugates such as PEG-HZ-PE (a hydrazone based acid sensitive PEG-PE [23]) to provide an outer shell for imparting long circulation function by warding off opsonins via steric hindrance, and eventually losing the PEG shell upon encountering a low pH environment for imparting enhanced penetration. Shown here is an example of a simple pH sensitive liposome as detailed by Ishida et al., using DOPE, CHEMS, and PEG-PE for steric stabilization, although more complex lipid compositions have been optimized to fit various needs [24].

1.4.2 Redox-Sensitive Liposomes

There exists a huge difference between the redox potentials of extracellular and intracellular environments. The extracellular space is known to be oxidizing, and intracellular, reducing [25, 26]. This is attributed to the presence of a large amount of GSH (glutathione), cysteine and other such reducing agents. In tumor tissue as well, GSH levels have been found to be about 100 fold higher than extracellular GSH levels [27]. When nanocarriers are designed with special polymers that contain bonds that can undergo reduction, such as disulfide bonds, then the GSH destabilizes the liposomes and releases their payload. The most commonly used polymers for designing these kinds of liposomes consist of a disulfide linkage, which is a covalent linkage formed by the oxidation of two sulfhydryl (SH) groups. These linkages are reversible and make use of the disulfide to thiol reduction reaction. PEG chains with a disulfide linkage are redox sensitive PEG and their incorporation into liposomes results in designing nanocarriers with a sheddable PEG coating. Polymers such as 1,2-Dioleoyl-sn-glycero-3-phosphoethanolamine (DOPE)/CHEMS (3β-hydroxy-5-cholestene 3-hemisuccinate)/mPEG-DTP-DSPE (PEG coupled with 1,2-distearoyl-sn-glycero-3-phosphoethanolamine using 3,3′-dithiopropionate as the linker) [28], PEG-DTH-DSPA (PEG coupled with 1,2-distearoyl-*sn*-glycerol-3-phosphatidic acid using the linker dithio-3-hexanol) [29], PEG-DTB-DSPE (PEG coupled with 1,2-distearoyl-sn-glycero-3-phosphoethanolamine using dithiobenzyl carbamate linkers) [30], and PEG-S–S-DSPE (PEG coupled with 1,2-distearoyl-sn-glycero-3-phosphoethanolamine using a thiolytic cleavable spacer) [31] are frequently employed in designing such liposomes. In this chapter, we describe a simple chemical reaction for the synthesis of a dilsufide bond between DOPE and PEG-SH as described by Maeda et al. [31].

1.4.3 MMP-Sensitive Liposomes

The presence of altered levels of certain local enzymes in cancer cells, such as matrix metallo proteinases (MMPs) have been used to develop enzyme-triggered nanoplatforms for drug delivery. Overexpression of MMPs, especially MMP2 and MMP9, have been found in the tumor microenvironment, where they promote invasion, progression, and metastasis of most human tumors due to the degradation of the surrounding connective extracellular matrix [32]. Recently, Torchilin et al. successfully synthesized multifunctional MMP2-sensitive liposomes for enhanced penetration of chemotherapeutic drugs into tumors [33]. Amino acid sequences that are sensitive to MMP2 can be introduced into PEG2000-lipid derivatives and used to prepare MMP2-sensitive PEGylated liposomes. The introduction of a stimulus-sensitive moiety between the PEG chain and the liposome allows to have long-circulation liposomes with local tissue environment controlled release mechanisms. The presence of PEG on the surface of nanocarriers results in reduced cellular uptake and hinders the endosomal release of a carrier, the well-known "PEG dilemma" [34]. Hence, the incorporation of MMP2-sensitive PEG derivatives on the surface of liposome has the aim to "de-shield" the protective PEG function once in the tumor microenvironment, where the overexpressed levels of the proteolytic enzymes cleave the enzyme-sensitive linkage, allowing for efficient liposomes cellular uptake. In this chapter, we describe a simple chemical reaction for the synthesis of a MMP2-sensitive PEG derivative and its incorporation in liposomes as described by Zhu Lin et al. [33].

1.4.4 Temperature-Sensitive Liposomes (TSL)

The ultimate goal of any chemotherapeutic agent is to penetrate across the vasculature and accumulate at the site of action to bring about cytotoxicity. Mild hyperthermia (heating up to 43 °C) is known to bring about tumor shrinkage via various mechanisms, making it a viable tool for combination therapy with radiation, chemotherapy, etc. Mild hyperthermia has been shown to increase the tumor perfusion and vascular permeability, making it a great tool for also increasing the accumulation of liposomes in the tumor tissue. It was found that the use of certain lipids in the liposomes makes the liposomes thermally sensitive causing the release of drug at the tumor site, further enhancing the effect. This involves the use of lipids that undergo gel-liquid crystalline phase transition at temperatures (T_C) slightly higher than the body temperature. Such liposomes were first described by Yatvin and Weinstein in 1970s. These liposomes employed the use of the lipid dipalmitoyl phosphatidylcholine (DPPC) with T_C of 41 °C [35] as the thermosensitive component, along with the use of distearoyl phosphatidylcholine (DSPC) with a higher T_C of 54 °C [35] in the ratio of DPPC: DSPC 3:1, to yield liposomes with T_C around 41 °C [36]. Since then great strides have been made with regard to temperature-sensitive liposomes. One such formulation, Thermodox® is currently in the Phase 3 trial for the treatment primary liver cancer (hepatocellular carcinoma). Thermodox was developed by optimizing various lipid ratios for maximum release of the contents. They discovered that the incorporation of a highly bilayer compatible lysolipid, 1-palmitoyl-2-hydroxy-*sn*-glycero-3-phosphocholine (MPPC) instead of the frequently used DSPC, in DPPC liposomes, confers the liposomes a better drug release profile [37]. TSLs now include a wide range of lipids (such as egg phosphatidyl choline and cholesterol) to suit specific requirements and frequently include PEG for long circulation. This chapter presents a simple protocol for manufacturing the traditional TSLs as reported by Gaber et al. This method makes is a departure from the first TSL as it includes cholesterol for increased stability and improved release kinetics [38].

1.4.5 Magnetic-Sensitive Liposomes

Magnetic metals and alloys such as iron [39], cobalt [40], iron oxides such as magnetite (Fe_3O_4) and maghemite (Fe_2O_3) are frequently used for designing nanoparticles which can be manipulated with an external magnetic field. Coating with biocompatible polymers such as dextran, PEG or encapsulation inside a lipid vesicle provides the construct with not just the ability to be guided to the target site of action by the use of an external magnetic field, but also enables imaging of the nanoparticles using MRI and also allows for treatment by magnetic hyperthermia. The commonly used super-paramagnetic nanoparticles are made of iron oxide, earning them the name super-paramagnetic iron-oxide nanoparticles (SPIONS). SPIONS can either be synthesized by breaking down larger particles using mechanical attrition, or by the more efficient and more frequently used method of building up from smaller particles using chemical methods. One of the more widely used chemical methods is known as co-precipitation, where iron oxide is synthesized from Fe^{2+} or Fe^{3+} salt solutions (chlorides, sulfates, nitrates) by the addition of a base at either room or elevated temperatures [41]. Synthesis of liposomes using magnetic nanoparticles is a two-step process that first includes the synthesis of the magnetic nanoparticles, and then their incorporation into the liposomes. Alternatively, magnetic nanoparticles such as magnetite can be purchased to fit various needs such as size, dispersion, and functionalized coating. The synthesis of magnetic nanoparticle by co-precipitation has been described in details in various papers [42, 43] and hence we focus on the preparation of liposomes using them.

1.5 Adding Cell Penetration Function

It is well known that the plasma membrane of the cell presents a formidable barrier to the penetration of a plethora of nonessential molecules and drugs. To improve the penetration of drugs and nanoparticles across the cell membrane, the use of cell penetrating peptides (CPPs) is increasingly gaining popularity. CPPs are usually short (less than 40) amino acid sequences that are amphipathic and mostly positively charged [44]. The first CPP to be identified was the Transactivator of Transcription of human immunodeficiency virus (TAT peptide) isolated from the HIV virus in the 1980s [45]. Since then, a large number of CPPs such as R8, transportan, and Pep-1 have been discovered and widely used for transporting drug molecules, peptides, proteins, oligonucleotides, nanoformulations, etc. across the cell membrane [46]. In this chapter, we describe the conjugation of the CPP known as TAT peptide, to a PEG chai, which can be introduced into the liposomes via post-insertion.

1.6 Adding an Imaging Function

Liposomes can be used for various imaging modalities such as magnetic resonance imaging (MRI), computed tomography [40], ultrasound, and gamma scintillography. A wide range of agents such as Technetium (Tc), Gadolinium (Gd), Indium (In), microbubbles made of Argon (Ar), and air can be encapsulated into the liposomes for this purpose. Imaging requires a sufficient amount of signal being emitted from the tissue to allow for a contrast between normal tissue and the tissue under investigation. This demands a high payload of the contrast agent, and liposomes are an efficient way to deliver them. Positron Emission Tomography (PET) is a widely used modality in medical imaging. This technique employs radioactive tracers attached to biologically active molecules such as 18-fluorine fluorodeoxyglucose (FDG), ^{64}Cu diacetyl-bis(N^4-methylthiosemicarbazone), and technetium-99 m. Upon uptake into the organ of interest, the radioactive tracers undergo decay and emit positrons, which undergo annihilation by electrons, thereby emitting photons which have energies and can be detected by imaging [47]. PET is heavily employed in imaging tumors and is increasingly making its way into liposomal technology [48, 49]. In this chapter we present incorporation of FDG into a liposomal formulation, which is frequently used for imaging tumor tissue.

1.7 Characterization of "Conventional" Liposomes and Stimuli-Sensitive Liposomes

The mean diameter and the size distribution of liposomes are usually determined by dynamic light scattering (DLS). The size distribution of multifunctional liposomes is generally unimodal, in the range of 150–200. Interestingly, the size of liposomes does not change significantly after the introduction of stimuli-sensitive conjugates. To confirm the results obtained from dynamic light scattering, it is recommended to evaluate the size distribution and the morphology by transmission electron microscopy (TEM). The presence of the ligands on the surface of the liposomes can be investigated by surface charge analysis performed using a Zeta Phase Analysis Light Scattering (PALS) UltraSensitive Zeta Potential Analyzer instrument.

2 Materials

1. Handheld extruder.
2. Rotary evaporator.
3. Probe sonicator.
4. Freeze dryer.
5. Bath sonicator.
6. PEG_{2000}-DSPE.
7. 1,2-dioleoyl-sn-glycero-3-phosphoethanolamine (DOPE).
8. p-nitrophenyl carbonate PEG_{3400} (PNP-PEG_{3400}-PNP).
9. Sepharose CL4B.
10. 2C5 antibody was synthesized and purified in-house.
11. Cholesterolhemisuccinate (CHEMS).
12. PEG-Hz-PE was prepared in house using the technique described by Torchilin et al. [23].
13. Succinimidyl 3-(2-pyridyldithio)propionate (SPDP).
14. mPEG-SH.
15. MMP2-cleavable peptides (NH2-Gly-Pro-Leu-Gly-Ile-Ala-Gly-Gln-COOH) are synthetized by Tufts University Core Facility (Boston, MA).

16. Maleimide-polyethylene glycol (3400)-N-hydroxysuccinimide ester (NHS-PEG3400-maleimide) and maleimide-polyethyleneglycol1000-N-hydroxysuccinimide ester (NHS-PEG1000-maleimide).
17. L-α-phosphatidylcholine (egg PC).
18. 1,2-dioleoyl-sn-glycero-3-phosphoethanolamine-N-(lissamine rhodamine B sulfonyl) (ammonium salt) (Rh-PE).
19. 4-dimethylaminopyridine (DMAP).
20. Dialysis tubing (MWCO 2000 Da).
21. 1,2-dipalmitoyl-sn-glycero-3-phosphocholine (DPPC).
22. L-α-phosphatidylcholine, hydrogenated (Soy) (HSPC).
23. Cholesterol.
24. 1,2-dipalmitoyl-sn-glycero-3-phosphoethanolamine-PEG (DPPE-PEG).
25. Iron oxide nanoparticles.
26. TAT cysteine peptide (TATp-Cys) (12-mer: CysTyrGlyArgLys-LysArgArgGlnArgArgArg) was obtained from Tufts University Core Facility (Boston, MA).
27. [18 F]-2-fluoro-2-deoxy-d-glucose is synthesized from 2-deoxyglucose (Sigma-Aldrich, St. Louis, MO) by a chemical reaction substituting the hydrogen with F^{18} in the 2-position using a technique described by Barrios et al. [50].
28. Coulter® N4-Plus Submicron Particle Sizer and Zeta Phase Analysis Light Scattering (PALS) UltraSensitive Zeta Potential Analyzer instrument.
29. Human MMP2.
30. Hoechst 33342.
31. Immunodeficient mice, e.g., NU/NU nude mice.
32. TissueTek O.C.T Compound.
33. TissueTek Cryomold.

3 Methods

3.1 Preparation of Liposomes by Thin Film Hydration Method

1. In a round-bottomed flask (RBF) add the desired lipids (*see* **Note 1**) dissolved in an organic phase such as a mixture of chloroform and methanol (*see* **Note 2**).
2. Evaporate the organic phase using nitrogen or a rotary evaporator, to form a thin film. To ensure complete evaporation of the organic phase, freeze-dry the flask for a few hours (*see* **Note 3**).
3. Hydrate the lipid film using an aqueous buffer such as phosphate buffered saline pH 7.4 (PBS) and HEPES buffered saline

pH 7.4 (HBS) and using mechanical agitation, detach the film from the flask to form a milky dispersion.

4. Using a mechanical extrusion assembly, extrude the multilamellar vesicles (MLVs) through filters of descending pore-size ranging from 400 to 50 nm. Optimize the range for optimal size distribution (a particle size distribution under 0.2 is considered optimal).
5. Alternatively, using a probe sonicator, the MLVs can be broken down into small unilamellar vesicles (SUVs). Immerse the flask in an ice bath. Immerse the tip of the sonicator into the RBF such that the tip is 1 cm above the bottom of the flask, while still immersed in the dispersion. Sonicate the dispersion for 10–60 min till the dispersion turns opalescent. Remove the titanium particles via centrifugation at 12,000 RCF for 10–15 min (*see* **Note 4**).

3.2 Preparation of Drug-Encapsulated Liposomes Using Reverse Phase Evaporation Method

1. In a round-bottomed flask (RBF), add the desired lipids in powder form or in an organic phase. The method described by Szoka and Papahadjopoulos uses 33 mmol of phospholipid and 33 mmol of cholesterol.
2. Remove the organic phase using a rotary evaporator.
3. Redissolve the lipid mixture in 3 ml diethyl ether. Up to 250 μL of chloroform or methanol can be added to the mixture to increase solubility.
4. Add 1 ml of the aqueous phase/hydrophilic drug that is to be encapsulated in the liposomes. Keep the mixture under nitrogen or any other inert gas at all times.
5. Sonicate the mixture for a few minutes to form a homogenous, stable mixture of inverted micelles. Keep the sonication temperature under 10 °C (*see* **Note 5**).
6. Remove the organic solvent using the rotary evaporator at around 200 rpm at low pressure. No bubbles should be seen during the process. In case of bubbles, restart the procedure. Once the solvent has evaporated, a viscous gel will form at the bottom of the RBF. This gel will eventually collapse into an aqueous suspension. Reduce the pressure and keep on the rotary evaporator for a few more minutes (*see* **Note 6**).
7. Remove the un-encapsulated material using dialysis, centrifugation or column chromatography.

3.3 Preparation of Long-Circulating "Stealth" Liposomes

1. Make a stock solution of PEG_{2000}-DSPE in chloroform (25–50 mg/ml) in a glass vial.
2. In a glass vial/RBF (depending on the quantity of the formulation), add PEG_{2000}-DSPE solution equivalent to 2 mol % of the lipid content. (*see* **Note** 7).

3. Remove the organic solvent under a stream of nitrogen gas or by using a rotary evaporator, to form a uniform thin film.
4. Ensure complete solvent removal by freeze-drying for about 4 h.
5. Remove from the freeze dryer and add the required amount of liposomes to the RBF.
6. Place in a suitable holder such a beaker, and in allow the sample to incubate overnight at 37 °C with constant shaking.

3.4 Synthesis of pNP-PEG$_{3400}$-PE to Attach a Targeting Moiety

1. Dissolve pNP-PEG$_{3400}$-pNP [800 mg, 213 μmole, 4.8× excess over PE] **in** 10 ml dry $CHCl_3$ (80 mg/ ml) in a 25 ml pear-shaped flask and start stirring at RT (*see* **Note 8**).
2. Add DOPE (33 mg, 44 μmole, 1310 μl of $CHCl_3$ solution (at 25 mg/ml) to solution with magnetic stirring.
3. Add fresh TEA (20 μl, 143 μmole, 3× excess over PE) to solution with magnetic stirring.
4. Incubate overnight at RT under argon, with constant stirring.
5. Monitor the reaction using TLC. (*see* **Note 9**).
6. Remove the organic solvent under the rotary evaporator and freeze-dry for 4 h. This flask approximately yields 180 mg of product, and contains about 630 mg excess PEG.
7. Hydrate the film using about 4 ml of 0.001 M HCl (pH 3) to form micelles, with bath sonication.
8. Separate the unconjugated PEG using column chromatography with 220 ml of Sepharose CL-4B column saturated in 0.001 M HCl (pH 3). Set up an automatic fraction collector using 13 small test tubes and collecting about 4 ml per fraction. Use no more than 300 ml of the eluent.
9. Apply the entire sample to the column. Product loading onto column is thus about 1.8 % v/v and 0.4 % w/v. After draining the void volume of the column (about 25 % column volume), start collecting 2 ml fractions. Analyze the fractions using TLC (using ½ of a 20 × 20 cm aluminium-backed sheet, and using a larger tank with 10 min development. As the product is a micelle, it is larger than the excess PEG, and will elute first.
10. Pool the fractions of interest and freeze under −80 °C.
11. Freeze-dry the frozen product to obtain a powder. Weigh and dissolve the powder in chloroform and store at −80 °C.

3.5 Attachment of Antibody 2C5 to pNP-PEG$_{3400}$-PE

1. Dissolve octyl-glucoside [34] in 5 mM Na-citrate, 150 mM NaCl pH 5, to obtain a 10 mg/ml solution.
2. In a glass vial, dissolve 40 M excess of pNP$_{3400}$-PEG-PE over the antibody (2C5 in our case) in the OG solution.

3. Dissolve the antibody in Tris-buffered saline pH 8.5 to get a 1 mg/ml solution.
4. Dissolve equal volumes of the PEG and antibody solution and raise the pH to 8.5.
5. Incubate at overnight at 4 °C.
6. Dialyze using a 300 kDa membrane, against PBS pH 7.4, for 4 h at RT. Use bicinchoninic acid assay (BCA) to determine conjugation efficiency (*see* **Note 10**).
7. Add the required amount of the 2C5-PEG_{3400}-PE micelles to the liposomes (optimize the mol% of PEG) and incubate overnight at 4 °C (*see* **Note 11**).

To prepare liposomes, use the methods described in the earlier sections and optimize for the quantity of 2C5-PEG2000-PE using in vitro association studies described in Subheading 3.16, for achieving a significant increase in active targeting without affecting the uptake of the liposomes by the cells.

3.6 Preparation of pH-Sensitive Liposomes Using CHEMS

1. In a round-bottom flask, prepare a mixture DOPE and CHEMS (with CHEMS more than 20 mol % of the total lipid).
2. Remove the organic solvent using a rotary evaporator or by drying under nitrogen in case of a smaller sample. Freeze-dry the sample to remove the organic solvent completely.
3. Rehydrate the film with an aqueous buffer such as HEPES buffer by sonication in a sonication bath for a few minutes.
4. Transfer to a sealed tube and freeze using liquid nitrogen. Thaw at room temperature and repeat the procedure three times (*see* **Note 12**).
5. Extrude the preparation using a 200 nm pore size filter 11–21 times. Optimize the number for a uniform size distribution.

3.7 Preparation of pH-Sensitive Liposomes Using PEG-HZ-PE

1. In a round-bottom flask, prepare a mixture of the desired lipids dissolved in an organic solvent such as chloroform or a mixture of chloroform and methanol 2:1 v/v.
2. Evaporate the organic solvent under a rotary evaporator or nitrogen and subsequently, freeze-dry the flask for at least 1 h.
3. Hydrate the film with HEPES buffered saline (pH. 7.4) or a similar buffer.
4. Sonicate the liposomes with a probe-type sonicator at 11 W power for 30 min or use the methods previously described in the chapter to produce a dispersion with a uniform size distribution.
5. Incubate the dispersion overnight with 15 mol % PEG2000-HZ-PE (*see* **Note 13**).
6. Dialyze against water (MWCO 3500–5000) to remove unreacted reagents.

3.8 Preparation of Redox-Sensitive Liposomes

1. In an RBF, dissolve DOPE (79 μmol) DOPE in a solution of chloroform (5 ml) containing triethylamine (11 μL), and add succinimidyl 3-(2-pyridyldithio)propionate (170.9 μM). Dissolve and let the reaction proceed at RT for 5 h.
2. Remove the methanol by evaporation under reduced pressure. Dissolve in 5 ml chloroform.
3. To separate the product i.e., PDP-DOPE, size exclusion chromatography can be employed using Sepharose CL-4B. Apply the sample and wash the silica gel column with 4 ml chloroform followed by 4 ml of each of the chloroform–methanol mixtures ranging from 4:0.25, 4:0.5, 4:1, to 4:1.25 (v/v). Collect 2 ml fractions and analyze by TLC. Pool the fractions containing the product and dry under reduced pressure.
4. Weigh the fractions and dissolve in chloroform.
5. For every 1.5 times of the product, add 1 mol mPEG-SH. Allow to react for 2 days at RT.
6. Confirm the reaction completion using TLC with silica gel plates and chloroform–methanol–water (65:25:4) as the eluent (*see* **Note 14**).
7. Recrystallize the polymer using diethyl ether and dry under reduced pressure. Recrystallization involves pouring hot solvent over the impure substance, enough to just about dissolve the solute and the impurities. The solution is then cooled under air first and ice water next, to start the process of recrystallization. The pure polymer thus obtained is purified by vacuum filtration.

For the preparation of liposomes, use the methods described in Subheading 3.1, optimizing for the amount of redox sensitive PEG. Optimization parameters includes optimal size distribution and stability of liposomes.

3.9 Synthesis of MMP2-Sensitive PEG-Lipid Conjugate

1. Mix the MMP2-cleavable peptide (NH2-Gly-Pro-Leu-Gly-Ile-Ala-Gly-Gln-COOH) and a heterobifunctional PEG derivative maleimide-PEG(3400)–NHS at a molar ratio of 1.2:1, in carbonate buffer (pH 8.5) and stir at 4 °C for overnight.
2. Remove the excess of peptides by dialysis (MWCO 2,000 Da) against distilled water.
3. Identify the MAL-PEG(3400)–peptide conjugate by RP-HPLC on a reverse phase C18 column at 214 nm using gradient solvent conditions. The chromatographic conditions for the analysis are: solvent A—0.1 % TFA in acetonitrile (ACN); solvent B—0.1 % TFA in water. 0–15 min: 5–75 % ACN, 15–15.1 min: 75–100 % ACN, 15.1–20 min: 100 % ACN, 20–20.1 min: 100–5 % ACN, 20.1–25 min: 5 % ACN,

with a flow rate of 1.0 ml/min at room temperature. After the reaction and purification process, peaks of the peptide (Retention Time = ~9.0 min) and MAL-PEG(3400)–NHS (Retention Time = ~11 min) will completely disappear while a new peak of MAL-PEG(3400)–peptide will be detected (Retention time = ~12.1 min). This change indicates the completion of the product purification.

4. Freeze-dry the product for the next step.

3.10 Synthesis of an MMP2-Sensitive PEG3400-Lipid Conjugate

1. Activate the MAL-PEG(3400)–peptide conjugate with a 20-fold molar excess of N-hydroxysuccinimide (NHS)–1-ethyl-3-(3-dimethylaminopropyl)carbodiimide (EDC) (1:1 molar ratio) in an anhydrous chloroform–methanol mixture (9:1, v/v) for 2 h.
2. Mix the MAL-PEG-peptide activated with an excess of DOPE in the presence of 1 % v/v of TEA under nitrogen protection at room temperature for overnight.
3. Monitor the reaction by using TLC followed by the Molybdenum Blue Spray Reagent staining. (*see* **Note 15**).
4. Purify MAL-PEG(3400)-peptide-DOPE by preparative TLC (use a mobile phase of chloroform–methanol 80:20 % v/v.

3.11 Incorporation of MMP2-Sensitive PEG-Lipid Conjugate into Liposomes

1. Dissolve a lipid mixture of egg PC (60 % mol), cholesterol (39 % mol), and MAL-PEG(3400)-peptide-DOPE (1 % mol) in chloroform.
2. Make a lipid film by rotary evaporation and freeze-dry overnight, followed by hydration of the film with phosphate buffer at room temperature for 20 min.
3. Pass the lipid dispersion 40 times through polycarbonate filters (pore size 200 nm) using a Micro Extruder.

3.12 Preparation of Temperature-Sensitive Liposomes (TSL)

1. In an RBF, add DPPC, HSPC, cholesterol, and DPPE-PEG (50:25:15:3 mol %). Add a mixture of chloroform–methanol (4:1) to dissolve the lipids. Add the lipophilic drug at this stage.
2. Remove the organic solvents using a rotary evaporator, followed by freeze drying for 4 h to overnight, to form a thin lipid film.
3. Hydrate the film using an aqueous buffer such as PBS. Add the hydrophilic drug at this stage. Keep the temperature of the buffer around 60 °C.
4. Detach the lipid film using pipetting, sonication or mixing by a vortex for 5–20 min.
5. Extrude through polycarbonate filters of decreasing pore size starting from 400 to 200 nm, 11–21 times. Optimize for a narrow size distribution.

3.13 Preparation of Magnetic-Sensitive Liposomes

1. In a round-bottom flask, prepare a mixture of the desired lipids dissolved in an organic such as chloroform or a mixture of chloroform and methanol 2:1 v/v. Add the hydrophobic drugs at this stage. Hydrophobic drugs will dissolve along with the lipids in the organic solvent. This makes it easier to incorporate them into the bilayer upon the evaporation of the organic solvent and addition of the aqueous dispersion medium.
2. Using an aqueous dispersion of the magnetic nanoparticles in a buffer or 0.9 % (w/v) saline, rehydrate the lipid film. Add the hydrophilic drug at this stage. Optimize for the quantity of iron oxide to be added. Too much iron oxide will interfere with the extrusion. Multiple studies report a wide range of values [51–53]. A wide range of toxicity studies have also been performed and can be used as reference while deciding on the concentration (*see* **Note 16**).
3. Agitate the dispersion mechanically to detach the film from the flask. Heat the dispersion to a temperature slightly above the transition temperature of the lipids.
4. Using a handheld extruder, pass the dispersion through polycarbonate filters of decreasing pore sizes (from 400 to 200 nm). This results in the formation of unilamellar magnetic liposomes.
5. Centrifuge for 15 min at 1000 × *g* to separate the iron-oxide encapsulated liposomes (supernatant) from the un-encapsulated iron oxide.
6. Store the liposomes at 4 °C till further use.

3.14 Preparation of a TAT-PEG-PE Conjugate

1. In an RBF or a glass vial, stir a mixture of DOPE and maleimide-PEG_{1000}-NHS (1.5 times molar excess) in chloroform with a three times molar excess of triethylamine.
2. After 2 h of continuous stirring at room temperature, add TAT-cys (2 times molar excess) and stir overnight at room temperature.
3. Remove the organic solvent using the rotary evaporator or drying under nitrogen, and freeze for a few hours.
4. Using dialysis (MWCO 2,000), remove the unreacted TAT-Cys. Analyze each fraction using thin layer chromatography on silica plates (mobile phase chloroform–methanol 80:20 % v/v). Visualize the conjugate with Dragendorff agent and phosphomolybdenic acid (*see* **Note 17**).
5. Use this TAT-PEG_{1000}-PE conjugate for post insertion into liposomes formed by the methods described in Subheading 3.3.

3.15 Preparation of FDG Liposomes

1. Prepare a lipid film using the methods mentioned in Subheading 3.1, and hydrate it with 0.45 M sodium gluconate or another isotonic solution such as 0.9 M glucose.
2. Vortex well to detach the film.
3. Heat in a water bath, to a temperature higher than the Tm (phase transition temperature) of the lipids for 3 min.
4. Add a solution of [18 F]-2-fluoro-2-deoxy-d-glucose in saline (up to 2 ml) and freeze thaw for three cycles using liquid nitrogen.
5. Extrude the solution through polycarbonate membrane filters with decreasing cut off sizes from 400 to 100 nm. Optimize for a uniform size distribution.
6. Centrifuge the resulting liposomes at 180,000 × *g* for 15 min (after dilution with saline) to remove the untrapped [18 F]-2-fluoro-2-deoxy-d-glucose.
7. Resuspend in an isotonic buffer of choice.

3.16 Interaction of Multifunctional Liposomes with Cancer Cells

1. Grow cancer cells on coverslips in 24-well culture plates at the density of 1×10^5 cells/well.
2. When the cells reach 60–70 % of confluence, wash the cells twice with pH 7.4 PBS and treat the cells with a fluorescent dye such as Rhodamine coupled with a phospholipid group (Rh-PE) labeled liposomes in serum containing media. For pH-sensitive liposomes, pre-incubate samples at pH 5.0 to cleave the pH-sensitive PEG conjugate. In the case of MMP2-sensitive liposomes, pre-incubate samples with 5 ng/μL of human MMP2 overnight, at 37 °C to "deshield" the liposomes from the PEG chains or use cells which overexpress MMP2 in the culture media, such as HT1080 cells, a fibrosarcoma cell line [54].
3. After fixed incubation times, add Hoechst 33342 nuclear stain (2.5 μg/ml) for 30 min at room temperature.
4. Remove the cell culture medium and wash the cells at least three times with phosphate buffer at pH 7.4.
5. Mount coverslips cell-side down on glass slides using fluorescence-free glycerol-based mounting medium (Fluoromount-G), visualize with a confocal microscope system and analyze using an image browser software.

3.17 Evaluation of the In Vivo Tumor Internalization of Stimuli-Sensitive-Based Nanopreparations

The therapeutic activity of different anticancer drugs incorporated in multifunctional liposomes can be evaluated in mouse xenograft models. A typical example is demonstrated here.

1. Grow the required tumor cell line in a flask. Detach and count the cells.

2. Inject a known number of cells into the left or right flank of immunodeficient mice.
3. When the tumors reach a size in the range of 100–200 mm^3, inject 100–200 μl of liposome suspensions in phosphate buffer i.v. via the tail vein at different time points. For FACS studies, inject Rh-labeled liposomes.
4. At the end of the study (approximately 2 h for FACS and confocal studies and a few weeks for tumor regression studies), anesthetize the mice, sacrifice them by cervical dislocation, excise the tumors to evaluate the tumor weight and cryofix them for further biological examination (*see* **Notes 18** and **19**).

4 Notes

1. A typical liposome comprises of a mixture of neutral phospholipids such as phosphatidyl cholines and phosphatidyl ethanolamines along with a certain amount of cholesterol, which imparts fluidity to the bilayer. The amount of cholesterol is optimized to impart stability to the liposome without destroying the stability of the bilayer. In some cases, positively or negatively charged lipids are also added to the mixture. For this example we use a mixture of EPC (egg L-α-phosphatidylcholine) and cholesterol in the molar ratios 70:30.
2. Storage of lipids: The lipids should be stored in an amber glass vial with a Teflon lined cap under an inert gas at −20 °C ± 4 °C. Saturated lipids can be stored as powders, but unsaturated lipids should be stored as solutions in an organic solvent.
3. Only high quality borosilicate glass tubes or flasks must be used. Care should be taken to wash the glassware multiple times with detergent, and subsequently with chloroform or methanol. The glassware should be dried thoroughly to get rid of contaminants that may cause oxidation of the lipids.
4. Keep the flask in an ice bath while using the probe sonicator.
5. Ice cold water can be used in a bath sonicator. Alternatively, while using a probe sonicator, the glass flask should be constantly in an ice bath.
6. Bubbles will interfere with the formation of a smooth film.
7. Optimize the quantity of PEG to prevent aggregation. Values can range from 0.5 to 5 % depending on the ligands attached to the PEG chain.
8. PNP-PEG_{3400}-PNP (polyoxyethylene(MW 3400)-bis(*p*-nitrophenyl carbonate) is a homobifunctional PEG moiety with a reactive nitrophenyl carbonate group at both ends. This makes the crosslinking agent especially valuable for the conjugation of

a variety of ligands at one end and the incorporation of a PE group at the other, for insertion into liposomes.

9. Monitor reaction with TLC (Silica Gel 60 F 254). Use 80: 20 $CHCl_3$–MeOH as the mobile phase. Use UV light for general visualization. For specific visualization, use Dragendorff reagent for PEG spots, molybdenum blue for PE spots (phosphorous derivative) and ninhydrin reagent for primary amine spots. Compare reaction spots with standards to detect total elimination of PE spot from reaction sample and appearance of combined PEG/PE spot.

10. Biocinchonic assay measures the total protein content in the formulation by using the peptide bonds present in the formulation to reduce cupric ions to cuprous ions, which are detectable using colorimetry. This can quantitatively detect the amount of 2C5 present in the conjugate.

11. Confirm the post insertion and immunological activity using an ELISA for 2C5.

12. Freeze-thawing is another example of a technique to synthesize liposomes with high encapsulation efficiency. This technique is often employed for synthesizing liposomes containing a mixture of phosphatidyl cholines with anionic or cationic lipids.

13. If there is another moiety such as a targeting agent, e.g., 2C5, or a Cell Penetrating Peptide, e.g., TAT (derived from the transactivator of transcription of the human immunodeficiency virus) involved, use a PEG chain of a greater length to provide a shielding effect. Here we have shown the use of PEG2000.

14. The DOPE will upon reaction with SPDP, convert to a faster running product, PDP-DOPE, which can be detected using molybdenum blue.

15. Monitor the reaction by using TLC followed by the Molybdenum Blue Spray Reagent staining to detect the phospholipid moiety. The conjugation of MAL-PEG(3400)-peptide with DOPE delays its migration compared to free DOPE in the TLC plate stained by Molybdenum Blue Spray Reagent.

16. Optimize for the quantity of iron oxide to be added. This is done by trial and error, to ensure easy extrusion.

17. Visualize the conjugate with Dragendorff agent and phosphomolybdenic acid for the detection of PEG chains and lipids, respectively.

18. To follow liposome-to-cell interactions, Rh-PE (0.5 % mol) can be added to the liposomal formulations.

19. For confocal analysis, frozen sections (6 μm) are cut on a Cryostats microtome, placed on glass slides and stained by Hoechst 33342 for nuclei visualization. The presence of

Rh-labeled liposomes in the tumor tissues is analyzed by confocal microscopy. The slides will be visualized by light microscopy at 40× magnification. For FACS analysis, Rh-labeled liposomes are injected iv in tumor-bearing mice. At 2 h after injection, and fresh tumor tissues will be minced into small pieces and incubated in 400 U/ml collagenase D solution for 30 min at 37 °C to dissociate cells. The single-cell suspension is analyzed immediately by FACS.

References

1. Torchilin VP (2005) Recent advances with liposomes as pharmaceutical carriers. Nat Rev Drug Discov 4(2):145–160
2. Szoka F, Papahadjopoulos D (1978) Procedure for preparation of liposomes with large internal aqueous space and high capture by reverse-phase evaporation. Proc Natl Acad Sci 75 (9):4194–4198
3. Harris JM, Chess RB (2003) Effect of pegylation on pharmaceuticals. Nat Rev Drug Discov 2(3):214–221
4. Fan Y, Zhang Q (2013) Development of liposomal formulations: from concept to clinical investigations. Asian J Pharm Sci 8(2):81–87
5. Senior J (1986) Fate and behavior of liposomes in vivo: a review of controlling factors. Crit Rev Ther Drug Carrier Syst 3(2):123–193
6. Nissander UK et al (1990) Liposomes. In: Langer R (ed) Biodegradable polymers as drug delivery systems. Marcel Deker Inc., New York
7. Yang T et al (2007) Enhanced solubility and stability of PEGylated liposomal paclitaxel: in vitro and in vivo evaluation. Int J Pharm 338:317–326
8. Suzuki S et al (1995) Preparation of long-circulating immunoliposomes containing adriamycin by a novel method to coat immunoliposomes with poly (ethylene glycol). Biochim Biophys Act (BBA)-General Subjects 1245:9–16
9. Lukyanov AN et al (2004) Tumor-targeted liposomes: doxorubicin-loaded long-circulating liposomes modified with anti-cancer antibody. J Control Release 100 (1):135–144
10. Glorioso J, DeLuca N, Fink D (1995) Development and application of herpes simplex virus vectors for human gene therapy. Annu Rev Microbiol 49(1):675–710
11. Zhu L et al (2013) Enhanced anticancer activity of nanopreparation containing an MMP2-sensitive PEG-drug conjugate and cell-penetrating moiety. Proc Natl Acad Sci 110(42):17047–17052
12. Sudimack J, Lee RJ (2000) Targeted drug delivery via the folate receptor. Adv Drug Deliv Rev 41(2):147–162
13. Ishida O et al (2001) Liposomes bearing polyethyleneglycol-coupled transferrin with intracellular targeting property to the solid tumors in vivo. Pharm Res 18(7):1042–1048
14. Park J et al (2001) Tumor targeting using anti-her2 immunoliposomes. J Control Release 74 (1):95–113
15. Iakoubov LZ, Torchilin VP (1996) A novel class of antitumor antibodies: nucleosome-restricted antinuclear autoantibodies (ANA) from healthy aged nonautoimmune mice. Oncol Res 9(8):439–446
16. Iakoubov LZ, Torchilin VP (1997) Nucleosome-releasing treatment makes surviving tumor cells better targets for nucleosome-specific anticancer antibodies. Cancer Detect Prev 22(5):470–475
17. Trudel D et al (2003) Significance of MMP-2 expression in prostate cancer an immunohistochemical study. Cancer Res 63 (23):8511–8515
18. Schafer FQ, Buettner GR (2001) Redox environment of the cell as viewed through the redox state of the glutathione disulfide/glutathione couple. Free Radic Biol Med 30 (11):1191–1212
19. Gerweck LE, Seetharaman K (1996) Cellular pH gradient in tumor versus normal tissue: potential exploitation for the treatment of cancer. Cancer Res 56(6):1194–1198
20. Kato Y et al (2013) Acidic extracellular microenvironment and cancer. Cancer Cell Int 13 (1):89
21. Sorkin A, Zastrow MV (2002) Signal transduction and endocytosis: close encounters of

many kinds. Nat Rev Mol Cell Biol 3 (8):600–614

22. Ellens H, Bentz J, Szoka FC (1984) pH-induced destabilization of phosphatidylethanol amine-containing liposomes: role of bilayer contact. Biochemistry 23(7):1532–1538
23. Kale AA, Torchilin VP (2007) Design, synthesis, and characterization of pH-sensitive PEG-PE conjugates for stimuli-sensitive pharmaceutical nanocarriers: the effect of substitutes at the hydrazone linkage on the ph stability of PEG-PE conjugates. Bioconjug Chem 18(2):363–370
24. Ishida T et al (2003) Development of pH-sensitive liposomes that efficiently retain encapsulated doxorubicin (DXR) in blood. Int J Pharm 309(1):94–100
25. Go YM, Jones DP (2008) Redox compartmentalization in eukaryotic cells. Biochim Biophys Acta 1780(11):1273–1290
26. Wu G et al (2004) Glutathione metabolism and its implications for health. J Nutr 134 (3):489–492
27. Torchilin VP (2009) Multifunctional and stimuli-sensitive pharmaceutical nanocarriers. Eur J Pharm Biopharm 71(3):431–444
28. Ishida T et al (2001) Targeted delivery and triggered release of liposomal doxorubicin enhances cytotoxicity against human B lymphoma cells. Biochim Biophys Acta 1515 (2):144–158
29. Zhang JX et al (2004) Pharmaco attributes of dioleoylphosphatidylethanolamine/cholesterylhemisuccinate liposomes containing different types of cleavable lipopolymers. Pharmacol Res 49(2):185–198
30. Romberg B, Hennink WE, Storm G (2008) Sheddable coatings for long-circulating nanoparticles. Pharm Res 25(1):55–71
31. Maeda T, Fujimoto K (2006) A reduction-triggered delivery by a liposomal carrier possessing membrane-permeable ligands and a detachable coating. Colloids Surf B Biointerfaces 49(1):15–21
32. Mansour AM et al (2003) A new approach for the treatment of malignant melanoma: enhanced antitumor efficacy of an albumin-binding doxorubicin prodrug that is cleaved by matrix metalloproteinase 2. Cancer Res 63 (1):4062–4066
33. Zhu L, Kate P, Torchilin VP (2012) Matrix metalloprotease 2-responsive multifunctional liposomal nanocarrier for enhanced tumor targeting. ACS Nano 6(1):3491–3498
34. Hama S et al (2015) Overcoming the polyethylene glycol dilemma via pathological environment-sensitive change of the surface property of nanoparticles for cellular entry. J Control Release 206:67–74
35. Mabrey S, Sturtevant JM (1976) Investigation of phase transitions of lipids and lipid mixtures by sensitivity differential scanning calorimetry. Proc Natl Acad Sci 73(11):3862–3866
36. Yatvin MB et al (1978) Design of liposomes for enhanced local release of drugs by hyperthermia. Science 202(4374):1290–1293
37. Anyarambhatla GR, Needham D (1999) Enhancement of the phase transition permeability of DPPC liposomes by incorporation of MPPC: a new temperature-sensitive liposome for use with mild hyperthermia. J Liposome Res 9(1):491–506
38. Gaber MH et al (1995) Thermosensitive sterically stabilized liposomes: formulation and in vitro studies on mechanism of doxorubicin release by bovine serum and human plasma. Pharm Res 12(10):1407–1416
39. Park SJ et al (2000) Synthesis and magnetic studies of uniform iron nanorods and nanospheres. J Am Chem Soc 122(35):8581–8582
40. Puntes VF, Krishnan KM, Alivisatos AP (2001) Colloidal nanocrystal shape and size control: the case of cobalt. Science 291 (5511):2115–2117
41. Lu AH, Salabas EL, Schüth F (2007) Magnetic nanoparticles: synthesis, protection, functionalization, and application. Angew Chem Int Ed 46(8):1222–1244
42. Pan C et al (2009) Novel and efficient method for immobilization and stabilization of β-d-galactosidase by covalent attachment onto magnetic Fe 3 O 4–chitosan nanoparticles. J Mol Catal B Enzym 61(3):208–215
43. Hamada S, Matijević E (1982) Formation of monodispersed colloidal cubic haematite particles in ethanol + water solutions. J Chem Soc Faraday Trans 1 78(7):2147–2156
44. Zorko M, Langel Ü (2005) Cell-penetrating peptides: mechanism and kinetics of cargo delivery. Adv Drug Deliv Rev 57(1):529–545
45. Frankel AD, Pabo CO (1988) Cellular uptake of the tat protein from human immunodeficiency virus. Cell 55(6):1189–1193
46. Bechara C, Sagan S (2013) Cell-penetrating peptides: 20years later, where do we stand? FEBS Lett 587(12):1693–1702
47. Kapoor V, McCook BM, Torok FS (2004) An Introduction to PET-CT Imaging 1. Radiographics 24(2):523–543

48. Oku N et al (1995) Real-time analysis of liposomal trafficking in tumor-bearing mice by use of positron emission tomography. Biochim Biophys Acta 1238(1):86–90
49. Seo JW et al (2008) A novel method to label preformed liposomes with 64Cu for positron emission tomography (PET) imaging. Bioconjug Chem 19(12):2577–2584
50. Iwata R et al (1984) Automated synthesis system for production of 2-deoxy-2-[18 F] fluoro-D-glucose with computer control. Int J Appl Radiat Isot 35(6):445–454
51. Skouras A et al (2011) Magnetoliposomes with high USPIO entrapping efficiency, stability and magnetic properties. Nanomedicine 7 (5):572–579
52. Sabaté R et al (2008) Preparation and characterization of extruded magnetoliposomes. Int J Pharm 347(1):156–162
53. Martina MS et al (2005) Generation of superparamagnetic liposomes revealed as highly efficient MRI contrast agents for in vivo imaging. J Am Chem Soc 127(30):10676–10685
54. Maeda-Yamamoto M et al (1999) Effects of tea polyphenols on the invasion and matrix metalloproteinases activities of human fibrosarcoma HT1080 cells. J Agric Food Chem 47 (6):2350–2354

Chapter 4

Multifunctional Concentric FRET-Quantum Dot Probes for Tracking and Imaging of Proteolytic Activity

Melissa Massey, Jia Jun Li, and W. Russ Algar

Abstract

Proteolysis has many important roles in physiological regulation. It is involved in numerous cell signaling processes and the pathogenesis of many diseases, including cancers. Methods of visualizing and assaying proteolytic activity are therefore in demand. Förster resonance energy transfer (FRET) probes offer several advantages in this respect. FRET supports end-point or real-time measurements, does not require washing or separation steps, and can be implemented in various assay or imaging formats. In this chapter, we describe methodology for preparing self-assembled concentric FRET (cFRET) probes for multiplexed tracking and imaging of proteolytic activity. The cFRET probe comprises a green-emitting semiconductor quantum dot (QD) conjugated with multiple copies of two different peptide substrates for two target proteases. The peptide substrates are labeled with different fluorescent dyes, Alexa Fluor 555 and Alexa Fluor 647, and FRET occurs between the QD and both dyes, as well as between the two dyes. This design enables a single QD probe to track the activity of two proteases simultaneously. Fundamental cFRET theory is presented, and procedures for using the cFRET probe for quantitative measurement of the activity of two model proteases are given, including calibration, fluorescence plate reader or microscope imaging assays, and data analysis. Sufficient detail is provided for other researchers to adapt this method to their specific requirements and proteolytic systems of interest.

Key words Assay, Fluorescence, FRET, Imaging, Microscopy, Peptide, Peptidase, Protease, Proteinase, Quantum dot

1 Introduction

1.1 Proteases

Proteases, which are also known as peptidases or proteinases, are enzymes that catalyze the hydrolysis of peptide bonds. Their activity is important in numerous physiological processes and the pathogenesis of diseases [1–4]. For example, numerous proteases and their cascaded activation are involved in cellular processes that are associated with the growth and progression of cancer [5]. One group of proteases associated with cancers is the caspases, which are members of the cysteine protease family. These proteases are the key effectors of apoptosis (i.e., programmed cell death) and their activation is often inhibited in tumorigenesis [6, 7]. Another relevant group of

Reema Zeineldin (ed.), *Cancer Nanotechnology: Methods and Protocols*, Methods in Molecular Biology, vol. 1530,
DOI 10.1007/978-1-4939-6646-2_4,

proteases is the matrix metalloproteinases (MMPs), which are members of the zinc-dependent metalloprotease family. The activity of MMPs in the extracellular matrix is important in cancer cell invasion and metastasis, and MMPs can affect signaling pathways, including the induction of apoptosis [8, 9]. Other proteases implicated in cancer include cathepsin B (a cysteine protease) and urokinase-type plasminogen activator (a serine protease), among many others [5, 10, 11]. Given the foregoing, it is not surprising that proteases are targets of both assay and imaging methods [12, 13], as well as therapeutics [14–16]. While many of the assay and imaging probes developed for protease activity utilize traditional materials such as fluorescent dyes and fluorescent proteins, often in combination with Förster resonance energy transfer (FRET) [17–19], there has been substantial and growing interest in utilizing nanomaterials and their unique properties for protease detection [20, 21].

1.2 Quantum Dots

Quantum dots (QDs) are among the most prolific nanomaterials for biological applications. These colloidal semiconductor nanocrystals are less than 10 nm in diameter and exhibit bright photoluminescence (PL; *see* **Note 1**) as a result of a nanoscale phenomenon called *quantum confinement* [22]. This PL is in many ways superior to the fluorescence exhibited by molecular dyes and fluorescent proteins [23], and QDs thus offer several advantages when substituted for fluorescent dyes and proteins in biological applications [22]. The combination of the optical and physical properties of QDs can also enable new methods that are not possible with molecular dyes and fluorescent proteins alone.

The most common QD materials are CdSe/ZnS core/shell nanocrystals. These QDs exhibit visible PL that can be tuned from blue (~450 nm) through red (~650 nm) as the core nanocrystal size is varied from ~2 to 7 nm in diameter [22]. Related $CdSe_{1-x}S_x$/ZnS alloyed core/shell QDs have PL that can be tuned over a similar wavelength range through control of the core semiconductor composition. QD PL is more spectrally narrow and symmetric (25–35 nm full-width-at-half-maximum) than the fluorescence from molecular dyes, and light absorption by QDs is more spectrally broad (extending over a 200–400 nm range) and stronger (molar absorption coefficients, ~10^4–10^7 M^{-1} cm^{-1}) than that of molecular dyes [22, 23]. QDs are frequently 10–100-fold brighter than fluorescent dyes and proteins, and are also more resistant to photobleaching [22, 23]. A physical property of QDs that is leveraged with their optical properties is their nontrivial surface area, which supports both chemical and biological functionalization, the latter including multivalent conjugates with peptides, nucleic acids, antibodies, and other biomolecules [24]. High-quality QD-bioconjugates have been found to be relatively nontoxic in cultured cells and animal models [25–27], and a multitude of biological assay and imaging applications for QDs have been reported in the literature [28–30]. Some of the most exciting of these applications utilize QDs in combination with FRET [31–33], including the multifunctional concentric FRET probes for proteolytic activity that are described in this chapter.

1.3 Förster Resonance Energy Transfer

FRET can modulate QD PL 'on' and 'off', and probes that operate on this principle have been developed for assaying many different proteases [20]. Basic QD-FRET probes for protease activity are the progenitors to the concentric FRET probes described in this chapter.

FRET is a nonradiative energy transfer process that occurs between an excited-state donor and a ground-state acceptor [34, 35]. The excitation energy of the donor (D) is transferred to the acceptor (A) through resonant interactions between the transition dipoles associated with donor relaxation and acceptor excitation. FRET decreases the PL intensity and lifetime of the donor, and increases the PL intensity of a fluorescent acceptor. The Förster formalism describes FRET quantitatively and can be summarized by Eqs. 1–3 [34]:

$$k_{\mathrm{FRET}} = \frac{1}{\tau_{\mathrm{D}}}\left(\frac{R_0}{r}\right)^6 = k_{\mathrm{D}}\left(\frac{R_0}{r}\right)^6 \tag{1}$$

$$R_0^6 = \left(8.79 \times 10^{-28}\ \mathrm{mol}\right) n^{-4} \Phi_{\mathrm{D}} \kappa^2 J \tag{2}$$

$$J = \frac{\int I_{\mathrm{D}}(\lambda)\varepsilon_{\mathrm{A}}(\lambda)\lambda^4 \mathrm{d}\lambda}{\int I_{\mathrm{D}}(\lambda)\mathrm{d}\lambda} \tag{3}$$

Equation 1 is the rate of energy transfer, k_{FRET}, where $\tau_{\mathrm{D}} = k_{\mathrm{D}}^{-1}$ is the excited state lifetime of the donor, r is the donor-acceptor separation distance, and R_0 is the Förster distance. Equation 2 is used to calculate R_0 (in units of cm), where n is the refractive index of the medium, Φ_{D} is the donor quantum yield, κ^2 is the orientation factor, and J is the spectral overlap integral. The overlap integral is calculated from Eq. 3, where $I_{\mathrm{D}}(\lambda)$ is the wavelength-dependent donor emission intensity, $\varepsilon_{\mathrm{A}}(\lambda)$ is the wavelength-dependent molar absorption coefficient of the acceptor, and λ is the wavelength. The terms in these equations can be calculated with data from experimental measurements, including the absorption spectrum of the acceptor, and the emission spectrum, quantum yield, and lifetime of the donor (*see* **Notes 2–4**).

The efficiency of FRET, E, is given by Eq. 4, and can be measured experimentally through changes in the emission intensity or lifetime of the donor as per Eq. 5, where I_{D} (or τ_{D}) and I_{DA} (or τ_{DA}) are the intensity (or lifetime) of the donor in the absence and presence of acceptor(s), respectively [34]. If the donor and acceptor quantum yields, Φ_D and Φ_A, are known, then the acceptor/donor PL intensity ratio, I_{AD}/I_{DA}, can be related to the FRET efficiency using Eq. 6.

$$E = \frac{k_{FRET}}{k_D + k_{FRET}} = \frac{R_0^6}{r^6 + R_0^6} \quad (4)$$

$$E = 1 - (I_{DA}/I_D) = 1 - (\tau_{DA}/\tau_D) \quad (5)$$

$$\frac{I_{AD}}{I_{DA}} = \frac{\Phi_A E}{\Phi_D(1 - E)} = \frac{\Phi_A}{\Phi_D}\left(\frac{R_0}{r}\right)^6 \quad (6)$$

The properties of QDs make them ideal for FRET, and energy transfer with these materials is consistent with the Förster formalism [32, 33]. Although there are some examples with QDs as FRET acceptors, the majority of applications utilize QDs as donors with fluorescent dye or fluorescent protein acceptors [32, 33]. The ability to use a QD donor as a scaffold to array multiple acceptors is one of the many advantages that QDs have over conventional fluorescent dye and protein donors. When there are multiple acceptors per QD donor, Eqs. 1, 4, and 6 are modified to Eqs. 7, 8, and 9, where a is the number of equivalent acceptors. Tuning of both QD PL properties and the number of acceptors per QD offers a level of control over FRET that is not possible with other materials.

$$k_{FRET} = \frac{a}{\tau_D}\left(\frac{R_0}{r}\right)^6 \quad (7)$$

$$E = \frac{a k_{FRET}}{k_D + a k_{FRET}} = \frac{a R_0^6}{r^6 + a R_0^6} \quad (8)$$

$$\frac{I_{AD}}{I_{DA}} = a\left(\frac{\Phi_A}{\Phi_D}\right)\left(\frac{R_0}{r}\right)^6 \quad (9)$$

QD-FRET probes for proteolytic activity attach multiple copies of an acceptor dye to a QD donor through peptide linkers that are substrates for a target protease. Changes in the number of acceptors per QD with hydrolysis of the peptide linkers results in changes in FRET that can be tracked through recovery of QD PL, loss of FRET-sensitized acceptor PL, or the ratio of these signals.

1.4 Concentric FRET

Concentric FRET (cFRET) is a multifunctional extension of conventional FRET that has been enabled by the surface area and optical properties of QDs. Rather than arraying multiple copies of one acceptor per QD donor, multiple copies of two or more types of acceptor are arrayed, as shown in Fig. 1a. The "concentric" terminology refers to the position of these acceptors on the surface of an imaginary sphere larger in diameter and concentric with the QD. A cFRET configuration with a QD donor and two types of

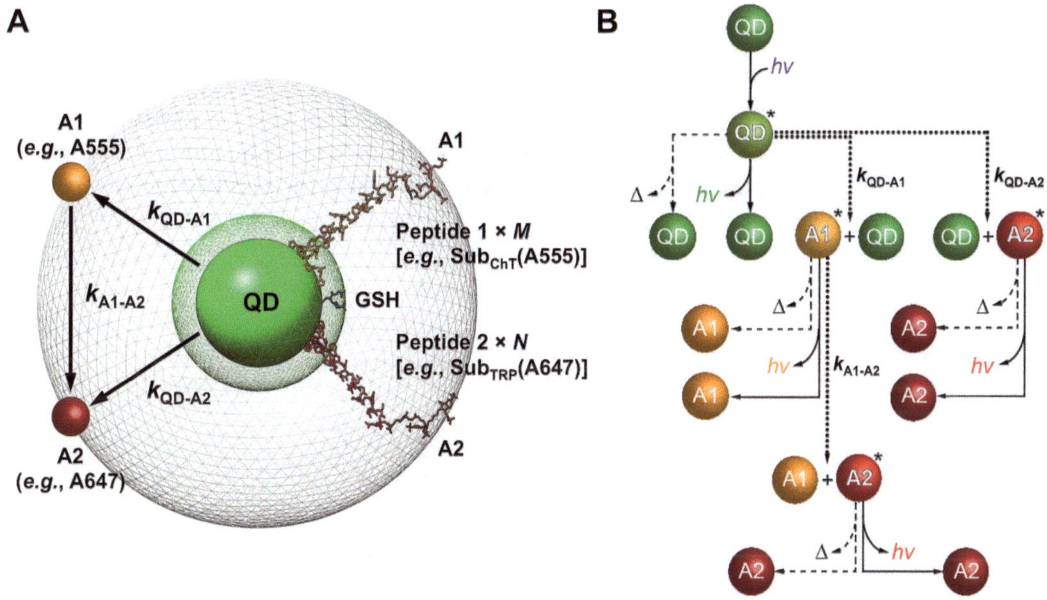

Fig. 1 (**a**) Simplified schematic of a QD-(A1)$_M$-(A2)$_N$ cFRET configuration showing a prototypical example with peptide substrates for chymotrypsin and trypsin, and A555 and A647 as fluorescent acceptor dyes. The *right-hand side* of the figure shows the assembly of the cFRET configuration, including the QD, hydrophilic glutathione (GSH) ligand coating, and A1- and A2-labeled peptides self-assembled to the QD through polyhistidine tags. The *left-hand side* of the figure depicts the three FRET rates, $k_{QD\text{-}A1}$, $k_{QD\text{-}A2}$, and $k_{A1\text{-}A2}$, in the cFRET configuration. (**b**) Flow chart showing the energy transfer and relaxation pathways in the cFRET configuration after initial photoexcitation of the QD. The *asterisk* denotes an excited state, *hv* is a photon, and Δ is heat. Adapted with permission from ref. 36. Copyright 2015 American Chemical Society

fluorescent dye acceptor has multiple energy transfer pathways to consider. These pathways include energy transfer from the QD to the first type of dye acceptor (A1), from the QD to the second type of dye acceptor (A2), and between the two types of dye acceptor, where A1 serves as a donor for A2 [36]. The flowchart in Fig. 1b shows how these pathways compete with and follow one another, as well as the intrinsic luminescent and nonluminescent relaxation pathways of each emitter.

In a cFRET configuration, the QD PL intensity, I_{QD}, is quenched as a result of FRET to both A1 and A2. The quenching efficiency, Q_{QD}, is given by Eq. 10 where M and N represent the number of A1 and A2 per QD, k_{QD} is equivalent to k_D in Eq. 4, and $k_{QD\text{-}A1}$ and $k_{QD\text{-}A2}$ are FRET rates analogous to k_{FRET} in Eq. 1 [36].

$$Q_{QD} = 1 - \left(\frac{I_{QD\text{-}A1\text{-}A2}}{I_{QD}}\right) = \frac{M k_{QD}^{-1} k_{QD\text{-}A1} + N k_{QD}^{-1} k_{QD\text{-}A2}}{1 + M k_{QD}^{-1} k_{QD\text{-}A1} + N k_{QD}^{-1} k_{QD\text{-}A2}} \tag{10}$$

The FRET efficiency between A1 and A2 can be empirically approximated by Eq. 11 (*see* **Note 5**) [36, 37]:

$$E_{\text{A1-A2}} = \frac{N k_{\text{A1}}^{-1} k_{\text{A1-A2}}}{1 + N k_{\text{A1}}^{-1} k_{\text{A1-A2}}} \tag{11}$$

Two PL ratios, $I_{\text{A1}}/I_{\text{QD}}$ and $I_{\text{A2}}/I_{\text{QD}}$, can be measured for the cFRET configuration. These ratios approximately follow Eqs. 12 and 13, which are derived from first principles [36].

$$\begin{aligned}\frac{I_{\text{A1}}}{I_{\text{QD}}} &= \left(\frac{\Phi_{\text{A1}}}{\Phi_{\text{QD}}}\right) \frac{E_{\text{QD-A1}}(1 - E_{\text{A1-A2}})}{1 - E_{\text{QD-A1}} - E_{\text{QD-A2}}} \\ &= \left(\frac{\Phi_{\text{A1}}}{\Phi_{\text{QD}}}\right) M k_{\text{QD}}^{-1} k_{\text{QD}-\text{A1}} \left(\frac{1}{1 + N k_{\text{A1}}^{-1} k_{\text{A1-A2}}}\right)\end{aligned} \tag{12}$$

$$\begin{aligned}\frac{I_{\text{A2}}}{I_{\text{QD}}} &= \left(\frac{\Phi_{\text{A2}}}{\Phi_{\text{QD}}}\right) \frac{E_{\text{QD-A2}} + E_{\text{QD-A1}} E_{\text{A1-A2}}}{1 - E_{\text{QD-A1}} - E_{\text{QD-A2}}} \\ &= \left(\frac{\Phi_{\text{A2}}}{\Phi_{\text{QD}}}\right) \left[N k_{\text{QD}}^{-1} k_{\text{QD-A2}} + M k_{\text{QD}}^{-1} k_{\text{QD-A1}} \left(\frac{N k_{\text{A1}}^{-1} k_{\text{A1-A2}}}{1 + N k_{\text{A1}}^{-1} k_{\text{A1-A2}}}\right)\right]\end{aligned} \tag{13}$$

The rate terms, ${k_{\text{QD}}}^{-1} k_{\text{QD-A}x}$, in Eqs. 10–13 can be determined from experiments with nonconcentric QD-A1 and QD-A2 FRET systems, and the ${k_{\text{A1}}}^{-1} k_{\text{A1-A2}}$ term can be determined from direct excitation of A1 in a cFRET configuration [36]. Prediction of the QD quenching (Eq. 10) is more robust than prediction of the emission ratios (Eqs. 12 and 13), although the latter remain useful first approximations. Overall, these equations are helpful in designing and optimizing cFRET probes, but they are not strictly required for the practical application of cFRET probes.

1.5 Tracking Proteolytic Activity with Concentric FRET

We have used cFRET configurations to quantitatively track the activation of pro-chymotrypsin to chymotrypsin by trypsin [38], to image spatially heterogeneous trypsin and chymotrypsin activities [39], and to simultaneously measure both the activity and concentration of thrombin [40]. These studies, and the methods outlined in this chapter, utilized a prototypical cFRET configuration with a green-emitting QD donor and multiple copies of both an Alexa Fluor 555 (A555)-labeled peptide and an Alexa Fluor 647 (A647)-labeled peptide conjugated to the QD. FRET occurs from the QD to the A555, to a lesser extent from the QD to the A647, and from the A555 to the A647 [36]. The A555 and A647 are thus equivalent to A1 and A2 in the equations in Subheading 1.4. Proteolysis is tracked through changes in the A555/QD and A647/QD PL ratios as the peptides are hydrolyzed by their respective proteases and the number of each dye acceptor per QD changes. This chapter describes how to use this prototypical cFRET configuration for assaying and imaging the activity of two proteases. Detailed procedures for empirical calibration of cFRET PL ratios, assays, and data analysis are presented using trypsin and chymotrypsin as widely accessible model proteases. Subheading 4 provides additional tips and information that enable the methodology to be extended to other proteases of interest and different experimental formats.

2 Materials

2.1 Reagents

1. Hydrophilic (i.e., water-soluble), ligand-coated QDs with green PL centered between 520 and 525 nm (*see* **Notes 6–9**). Here, we use CdSe/CdS/ZnS core/shell/shell QDs with peak PL at 520 nm, which are denoted simply as "QD" from this point forward. We have also successfully used CdSeS/ZnS and CdSe/ZnS core/shell QDs with peak PL between 520 and 525 nm [36, 38, 39].
2. Peptides with a hexahistidine sequence at one terminus and a suitable dye label (*see* **Notes 10** and **11**) at the opposite terminus. The amino acid sequence contains a series of residues recognized and hydrolyzed by the target proteases (*see* **Note 12**). Examples of dye-labeled peptide sequences that we use with chymotrypsin and trypsin are given in Table 1, and are denoted as Sub_{ChT}(A555) and Sub_{TRP}(A647), respectively.
3. Borate buffer (BB1): 100 mM borate, pH 8.5 (*see* **Note 13**).
4. Borate buffer (BB2): 50 mM borate, pH 8.5, 50 mM NaCl (*see* **Note 13**).
5. Agarose: molecular biology grade, low electroendoosmosis.
6. 10× Tris-borate-EDTA (TBE) buffer: 0.89 M Tris, 0.89 M boric acid, 20 mM EDTA.
7. 1× Tris-borate-EDTA (TBE) buffer diluted from 10× TBE stock: 89 mM Tris, 89 mM boric acid, 2 mM EDTA.
8. Aqueous glycerol solution (50 % v/v) prepared with ultrapure water.
9. α-Chymotrypsin from bovine pancreas (TLCK treated, Type VII, salt-free, lyophilized powder, ≥40 units/mg protein).
10. Trypsin from bovine pancreas (TPCK treated, ≥10,000 BAEE units/mg protein).

Table 1
Dye-labeled peptide sequences (written N-terminal to C-terminal)

Peptide sequence	Abbreviation
A555–CSA**Y**AATDEGNQGTSP$_6$SH$_6$	Sub_{ChT}(A555)
A647–CST**R**TDEGNQGGTSSP$_6$ SH$_6$	Sub_{TRP}(A647)

The target protease hydrolyzes the peptide C-terminal to the bold residue

2.2 Equipment

1. Agarose gel electrophoresis system: gel casting unit, tank, tray, combs, and power supply.
2. Black, flat-bottom 96-well microtiter plates with nonbinding surface (for microtiter plate assays; *see* **Note 14**).
3. Clear, UV-transparent, flat-bottom 96-well microtiter plates (for microscope imaging; *see* **Note 15**).
4. Fluorescence plate reader (for microtiter plate assays). We use an Infinite M1000 Pro plate reader (Tecan US, Inc., Morrisville, NC, USA). The main requirements are that the fluorescence plate reader is able to provide excitation at ~400 nm and measure three different emission wavelengths (~520 nm, ~570 nm, and ~650 nm) with bandwidths of ~5 nm or less. For real-time measurements, the plate reader should be able to make these measurements in an automated and repetitive fashion. Other plate reader instruments may also be suitable (*see* **Note 16**).
5. Fluorescence microscope (for imaging assays). We use an IX83 Inverted Microscope (Olympus, Richmond Hill, ON, Canada) equipped with a broad spectrum metal-halide light source (X-Cite 120XL, Excelitas Technologies, Mississauga, ON, Canada), a 405/20 (center line/bandwidth in nm) excitation filter (Chroma Technology Corp., Bellow Falls, VT, USA), either a 425 nm-cutoff or 470 nm-cutoff dichroic mirror (Chroma), a 4.0×/0.16NA objective lens, a motorized emission filter wheel (Olympus) with 520/40, 565/30, and 665 nm longpass (LP) filters (Chroma), and a sCMOS camera (Orca-Flash 4.0 V2, C11440; Hamamatsu Photonics, Hamamatsu, SZK, Japan). Our microscope is operated with MetaFluor software (Molecular Devices, Sunnyvale, CA, USA). Other microscope systems and specifications may also be suitable (*see* **Note 17**).
6. Other instruments capable of PL measurements may also be substituted for the plate reader and microscope systems noted above (*see* **Note 18**).
7. Image processing software. We use Image J software (National Institutes of Health, Bethesda, MD, USA).
8. Spreadsheet software. We use Excel (Microsoft, Redmond, WA, USA).
9. Data analysis software capable of fitting data to custom mathematical functions and mixed global and local fitting (*see* **Note 19**). We use pro Fit (QuantumSoft, Uetikon am See, Switzerland) and/or MatLab (MathWorks, Natick, MA, USA).

3 Methods

3.1 Calibration Samples

To calibrate the cFRET system, a series of QD-[Peptide1(A1)]$_M$-[Peptide2(A2)]$_N$ samples with different values of M and N are required. For the prototypical cFRET configuration with chymotrypsin and trypsin as model proteases, the configurations are QD-[Sub$_{ChT}$(A555)]$_M$-[Sub$_{TRP}$(A647)]$_N$. The procedure described below is a simple empirical calibration procedure that assumes negligible nonspecific adsorption of hydrolyzed peptide fragments on the QD (*see* **Note 20** for an alternative calibration strategy that does not make this assumption). The quantities are intended for preparation of samples with 100 μL volumes and 0.10 μM concentration for use in a 96-well microtiter plate. The quantities can be scaled to accommodate other measurement formats (*see* **Note 21**).

1. Obtain stock solutions of Sub$_{ChT}$(A555) and Sub$_{TRP}$(A647). The product of the volume (μL) and concentration (μM) of the solutions should be greater than 3800 pmol for Sub$_{ChT}$(A555) and 4350 pmol for Sub$_{TRP}$(A647), with minimum concentrations of 8.0 μM. These amounts will be sufficient for calibration samples and 12 samples for enzyme assays (*see* **Note 22**).
2. Prepare 400 and 900 μL substock solutions of 1.0 and 2.0 μM Sub$_{ChT}$(A555) in BB2 in 1.7 mL microcentrifuge tubes (*see* **Note 22**).
3. Prepare 150, 350, and 425 μL substock solutions of 1.0, 2.0, and 4.0 μM Sub$_{TRP}$(A647) in BB2 in 1.7 mL microcentrifuge tubes (*see* **Note 22**).
4. Obtain a stock solution of QDs. The product of the volume (μL) and concentration (μM) of the solution should be greater than 560 pmol with a minimum concentration of 1.0 μM. This amount will be sufficient for the calibration samples and 12 samples for enzyme assays.
5. Prepare a 800 μL substock solution of 0.50 μM QD in BB2 in a 1.7 mL microcentrifuge tube (*see* **Note 22**).
6. Set up an array of microcentrifuge tubes with six rows and six columns in a microcentrifuge tube rack. These tubes will hold the 36 samples specified in Fig. 2. An additional 12 samples may be warranted if utilizing a cFRET configuration different from the prototypical QD-(A555)$_M$-(A647)$_N$ configuration or utilizing an instrument or settings different from those specified (*see* **Note 23**).
7. Add M equivalents of Sub$_{ChT}$(A555) to each sample tube as specified in Fig. 2 (*see* **Note 24**).
8. Add N equivalents of Sub$_{TRP}$(A647) to each sample tube as specified in Fig. 2 (*see* **Note 24**).

[Sub_{TRP}(A647)] Sub-Stock Solution	N \ M	[Sub_{ChT}(A555)] Sub-Stock Solution: 1.0 µM						2.0 µM					
		0 A555		2 A555		4 A555		6 A555		8 A555		10 A555	
	0 A647	0	20	20	20	40	20	30	20	40	20	50	20
		0	80	0	60	0	40	0	50	0	40	0	30
1.0 µM	2 A647	0	20	20	20	40	20	30	20	40	20	50	20
		20	60	20	40	20	20	20	30	20	20	20	10
2.0 µM	4 A647	0	20	20	20	40	20	30	20	40	20	50	20
		20	60	20	40	20	20	20	30	20	20	20	10
	6 A647	0	20	20	20	40	20	30	20	40	20	50	20
		30	50	30	30	30	10	30	20	30	10	30	0
4.0 µM	9 A647	0	20	20	20	40	20	30	20	40	20	50	20
		23	57	23	37	23	17	23	27	23	17	23	7
	12 A647	0	20	20	20	40	20	30	20	40	20	50	20
		30	50	30	30	30	10	30	20	30	10	30	0

Volumes (µL): QD (green) A555 (pink) A647 (blue) Buffer (white)

Fig. 2 Example of a calibration sample preparation matrix with 36 different (*M*, *N*) combinations. Suggested concentrations of Sub_{ChT}(A555) and Sub_{TRP}(A647) substock solutions are indicated. The concentration of the QD substock solution is 0.5 µM. The value of *M* varies across the matrix rows and the value of *N* varies down the matrix columns. The volume (µL) of each solution to add per calibration sample is indicated in each *box*

9. Add BB2 to each sample tube as specified in Fig. 2. All solutions will have the same total volume at this step.
10. Add 20 µL of the 0.50 µM QD substock solution to each sample tube as specified in Fig. 2 (*see* **Note 24**). Mix each sample after adding the QD. The final volume of each sample is 100 µL. Each sample has 10 pmol of QD at a concentration of 0.10 µM with *M* and *N* equivalents of Sub_{ChT}(A555) and Sub_{TRP}(A647).
11. Incubate the samples at room temperature for 2 h and protect from light (*see* **Note 25**).

12. Proceed to Subheading 3.2 for plate reader measurement of the calibration samples. Alternatively, proceed to Subheading 3.3 for microscope imaging of the calibration samples.

3.2 Plate Reader Calibration

1. Set the plate reader to an excitation wavelength of ~400 nm. This wavelength minimizes direct excitation of the A555 and A647 (*see* **Note 26**).
2. Load a black, flat-bottom 96-well microtiter plate with the calibration samples prepared in Subheading 3.1 and at least one buffer blank.
3. Use the plate reader to measure either the complete emission spectrum of each sample or, alternatively, to measure the emission intensities at only 520, 570, and 670 nm (*see* **Notes 27** and **28**).
4. Proceed to Subheading 3.4 (optional) or Subheading 3.5.

3.3 Microscope Imaging Calibration

1. Set the microscope excitation filter to 405/20. This wavelength range minimizes direct excitation of the A555 and A647 (*see* **Note 26**).
2. Set the microscope dichroic mirror to a 425 nm- or 470 nm-cutoff.
3. Load a clear, UV-transparent, flat-bottom 96-well microtiter plate with the calibration samples prepared in Subheading 3.1 and at least one buffer blank.
4. Position the microtiter plate on the microscope stage so that a single sample well or group of sample wells is centered in the field of view.
5. Acquire PL images of the calibration samples with 520/40, 565/30, and 665LP filters (*see* **Notes 29** and **30**).
6. Repeat **steps 4** and **5** for any remaining sample wells.
7. Proceed to Subheading 3.4 (optional) or Subheading 3.5.

3.4 Confirmation of Peptide Binding to QDs

Agarose gel electrophoresis is used to confirm binding of dye-labeled peptides to the QDs. This step may be considered optional (proceed to Subheading 3.5 if skipping this step) but is good practice for quality control. Aliquots from the samples prepared and measured in Subheading 3.1 can be utilized (*see* **Note 31**). Gel electrophoresis can also be used to estimate the peptide loading capacity of the QDs (i.e., maximum average number of peptides per QD; *see* **Note 32**).

1. Prepare a 1.0 % w/v agarose gel with 1× TBE buffer.
2. Mix selected sample aliquots (20 μL) with 5 μL of 50 % v/v aqueous glycerol (*see* **Note 33**).

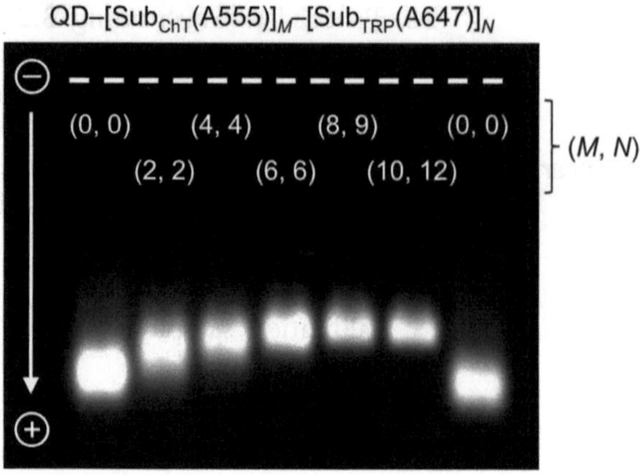

Fig. 3 Example of a 1.0 % w/v agarose gel to confirm the self-assembly of polyhistidine-terminated peptides to QDs. The glutathione-coated QDs migrate toward the anode and their electrophoretic mobility decreases as peptides are assembled. Adapted with permission from ref. 36. Copyright 2015 American Chemical Society

3. Load between 10 and 20 μL of the samples into the wells of the agarose gel. Use a consistent volume between wells.
4. Run the gel at a field strength of ~7–8 V/cm for ~25–35 min (*see* **Note 34**). Glutathione (GSH)-coated QDs are negatively charged and therefore migrate toward the anode (positive electrode). The self-assembly of peptides generally adds size to the QD without adding significant net charge. QDs with a greater number of peptides assembled will thus have a decreased electrophoretic mobility and will travel at a slower rate through the gel (*see* **Note 35**).
5. Image the gel using PL (*see* **Note 36**). A representative example of a gel is shown in Fig. 3.

3.5 Data Analysis of Calibration Samples

If analyzing plate reader data (from Subheading 3.2), proceed to Subheading 3.5.1 to correct this data for crosstalk and to calculate PL ratios. If analyzing imaging data (from Subheading 3.3), it is likely that regions of interest (ROIs) will need to be defined before proceeding to Subheading 3.5.1. Most image analysis programs support the definition and analysis of multiple ROIs within or between images and image stacks. For time-lapse imaging, we use Image J to import a stack of images for each channel (QD520, A555, and A647, where each image in a stack is taken at a specific time point), define common ROIs between each stack, and calculate average PL intensities for each ROI. Once the data has been extracted from ROIs, it can be corrected for crosstalk and the PL ratios can be calculated.

3.5.1 Crosstalk Corrections

1. Background correct all data by subtracting the appropriate value(s) from the buffer blank(s) or suitable ROIs of images (*see* **Note 37**).
2. For all (M, N) calibration samples, record the PL intensity at 520 nm (plate reader) or with the 520/40 bandpass filter (microscope) as I_{520}. The QD PL is not subject to significant crosstalk from the A555 or A647 PL (*see* **Note 38**) and therefore Eq. 14 applies, where I_{QD} is the QD emission intensity.

$$I_{QD}(M,N) = I_{520}(M,N) \tag{14}$$

3. For the (M, N) = (0, 0) calibration sample (i.e., QD only), record the PL intensity at 570 nm (plate reader) or with the 565/30 filter (microscope) as I_{570}. For the (0, 0) sample, this value represents the crosstalk from the QD when attempting to measure the A555 PL intensity. Calculate the crosstalk coefficient, ${}_{A555}\sigma_{QD}$, according to Eq. 15.

$${}_{A555}\sigma_{QD} = \frac{I_{570}(0,0)}{I_{QD}(0,0)} \tag{15}$$

4. For the (0, 0) calibration sample, record the PL intensity at 670 nm (plate reader) or with the 665LP filter (microscope) as I_{670}. This value represents the crosstalk from the QD when attempting to measure the A647 PL intensity. Calculate the crosstalk coefficient, ${}_{A647}\sigma_{QD}$, according to Eq. 16.

$${}_{A647}\sigma_{QD} = \frac{I_{670}(0,0)}{I_{QD}(0,0)} \tag{16}$$

5. For all (M, N) calibration samples, record the PL intensity at 570 nm (plate reader) or with the 565/30 filter (microscope) as I_{570}. Convert this value to the A555 PL intensity, I_{A555}, using the ${}_{A555}\sigma_{QD}$ crosstalk correction coefficient using Eq. 17.

$$I_{A555}(M,N) = I_{570}(M,N) - {}_{A555}\sigma_{QD} I_{QD}(M,N) \tag{17}$$

6. For the ($M >$ 0, 0) calibration samples, record the PL intensity at 670 nm (plate reader) or with the 665LP filter (microscope) as I_{670}. This value represents the crosstalk from both the QD and A555 when attempting to measure the A647 PL. Correct this value for the QD crosstalk using Eq. 18 and the ${}_{A647}\sigma_{QD}$ crosstalk coefficient. The new value is ${}_{A647}\sigma_{A555} I_{A555}$, which is the crosstalk from only the A555 when attempting to measure the A647 PL.

$${}_{A647}\sigma_{A555} I_{A555}(M,0) = I_{670}(M,0) - {}_{A647}\sigma_{QD} I_{QD}(M,0) \tag{18}$$

Calculate the crosstalk coefficient, ${}_{A647}\sigma_{A555}$, according to Eq. 19 (*see* **Note 39**). Average the values of all (M, 0) samples with sufficient signal-to-noise ratios.

$$ {}_{A647}\sigma_{A555} = \frac{I_{670}(M,0) - {}_{A647}\sigma_{QD} I_{QD}(M,0)}{I_{A555}(M,0)} \quad (19)$$

7. For all (M, N) calibration samples, record the PL intensity at 670 nm (plate reader) or with the 665LP filter (microscope) as I_{670}. Convert this value to the A647 PL intensity, I_{A647}, using the crosstalk correction coefficients and Eq. 20.

$$ I_{A647}(M,N) = I_{670}(M,N) - {}_{A647}\sigma_{QD} I_{QD}(M,N) - {}_{A647}\sigma_{A555} I_{A555}(M,N) \quad (20)$$

8. For all (M, N) calibration samples, calculate the I_{A555}/I_{QD} and I_{A647}/I_{QD} PL ratios.
9. We use one of two methods for analyzing the crosstalk-corrected PL ratio calibration data. If software capable of three-dimensional surface fitting is available, then optionally proceed to Subheading 3.5.3 (i.e., fitting data on a plot with x, y, and z axes). Otherwise, proceed to Subheading 3.5.2 for two-dimensional fitting (i.e., fitting data on a plot with x and y axes).

3.5.2 Two-Dimensional Fitting

1. We use Excel or pro Fit software for this analysis.
2. For a given value of N, plot the A555/QD PL ratio on the y-axis versus the values of M on the x-axis.
3. Repeat **step 2** for the remaining values of N and plot the data on the same graph. A representative example of data is shown in Fig. 4a(i).
4. Identify the general function, $f(M)$, that will fit each data subset (i.e., variable M for fixed N). In our experience, a linear function or a parabolic function is typically satisfactory (*see* **Note 40**). The data shown in Fig. 4a(i) can be fit with quadratic functions of the type shown in Fig. 4a(ii).
5. Fit each data subset (i.e., variable M for fixed N) with the function from **step 4**. Record the equations of fit. The fitting process may use only local variables (i.e., different values for each value of N) or a combination of local and global (i.e., same value regardless of N) variables. For the data in Fig. 4a(i), a scaled quadratic equation is used where the b and c coefficients are global variables and the a coefficient is a local variable. The fitted data is shown in Fig. 4a(iii).

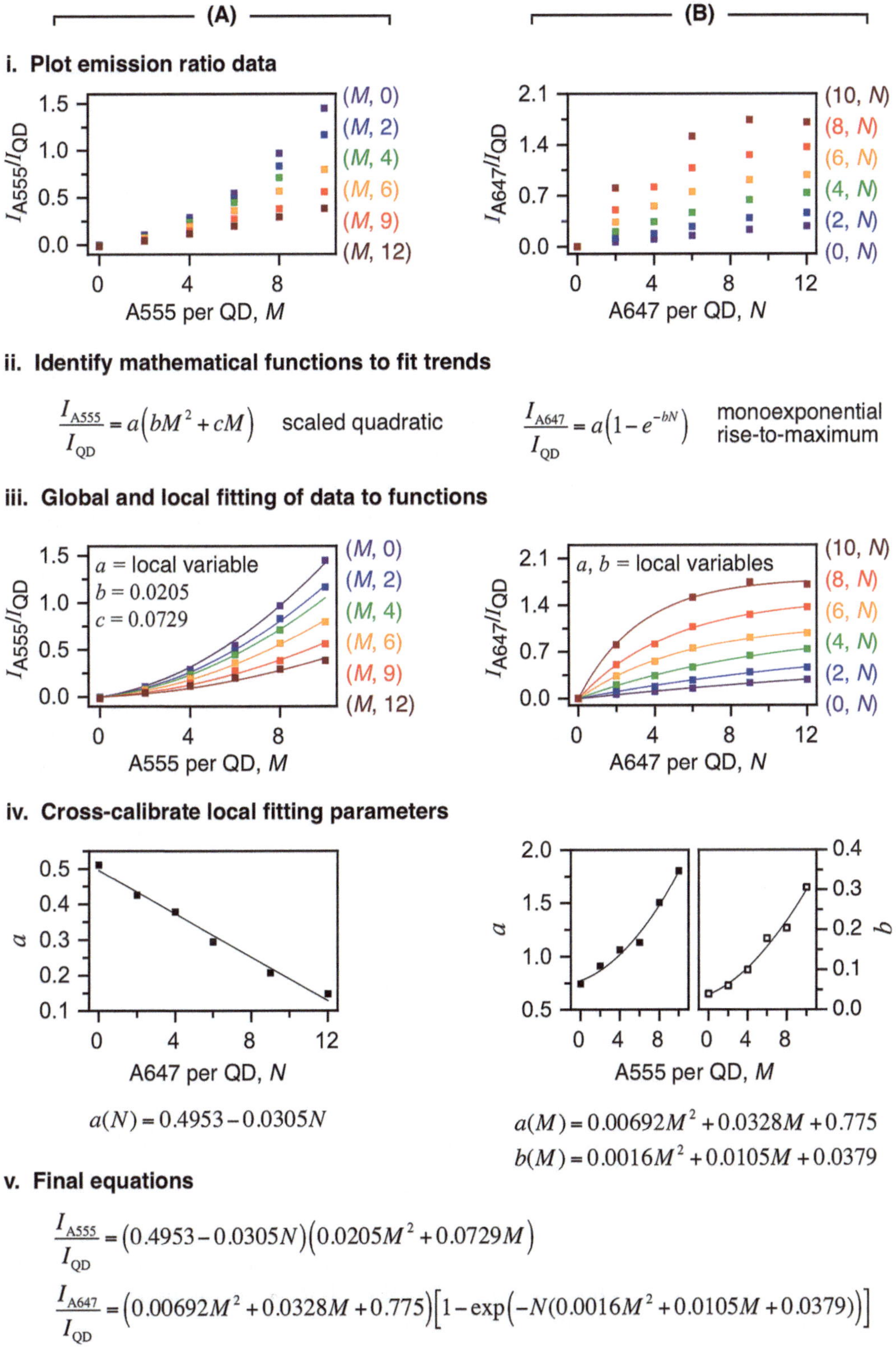

Fig. 4 An example of cFRET calibration data for QD520-[Sub_{ChT}(A555)]$_M$-[Sub_{TRP}(A647)]$_N$ samples and its five-step (*i*–*v*) analysis with coupled two-dimensional fitting. Analysis of (**A**) the A555/QD PL ratio and (**B**) A647/QD PL ratio is separated until the final step. Subheading 3.5.2 describes each step in detail. Data adapted from ref. 36

6. For each locally fit coefficient in the fitted functions from **step 5**, plot the values of the coefficient on the *y*-axis versus the values of *N* on the *x*-axis. For the fitted data in Fig. 4a(iii), the value of the *a* coefficient is plotted versus *N* in Fig. 4a(iv).
7. For each coefficient value plotted versus *N*, fit the data with a satisfactory function (*see* **Note 41**). Record the function. For the data in Fig. 4a(iv), the trend in the *a* coefficient as a function of *N* is approximately linear.
8. Substitute the function from **step 7** into the general function from **step 4**. The resulting calibration equation is the A555/QD PL ratio as a function of *M*, *N*, and numerical coefficients, as shown in Fig. 4a(v).
9. For a given value of *M*, plot the A647/QD PL ratio on the *y*-axis versus the values of *N* on the *x*-axis of a new graph.
10. Repeat **step 9** for the remaining values of *M* and plot the data on the same graph. A representative example of data is shown in Fig. 4b(i) (this data is from the same calibration experiment as the data in Fig. 4a).
11. Identify the general function, *f*(*N*), that will fit each data subset (i.e., variable *N* for fixed *M*). In our experience, a linear function or a monoexponential rise-to-maximum function is typically satisfactory (*see* **Note 40**). The data in Fig. 4b(i) can be fit with monoexponential rise-to-maximum functions of the type shown in Fig. 4b(ii).
12. Fit each data subset (i.e., variable *N* for fixed *M*) with the function from **step 11**. Record the equation of fit. For the data in Fig. 4b(i), an exponential rise-to-maximum equation is used where the *a* and *b* coefficients are both local variables. The fitted data is shown in Fig. 4b(iii).
13. For each locally fit coefficient in the fitted functions from **step 12**, plot the values of the coefficient on the *y*-axis versus the values of *M* on the *x*-axis. For the fitted data in Fig. 4b(iii), the *a* and *b* coefficients are plotted versus *M*.
14. For each coefficient value plotted versus *M*, fit the data with a satisfactory function (*see* **Note 41**). Record the function. For the data in Fig. 4b(iii), both the *a* and *b* coefficients are quadratic functions of *M* in Fig. 4b(iv).
15. Substitute the function from **step 14** into the general function from **step 11**. The resulting calibration equation is the A647/QD PL ratio as a function of *M*, *N*, and numerical coefficients, as shown in Fig. 4b(v).
16. The two calibration equations of fit obtained from **steps 8** and **15** will enable back-calculation of *M* and *N* from PL ratios measured during enzyme assays.

3.5.3 Three-Dimensional Fitting

1. We use MatLab for this analysis.
2. Plot the A555/QD PL ratio on the *z*-axis with *M* and *N* on the *x*-axis and *y*-axis, respectively.
3. Fit the data with a polynomial surface and record the equation of fit, which is the A555/QD PL ratio as a function of *M*, *N*, and numerical coefficients. Figure 5a(i) shows the data from Fig. 4a, plotted in three dimensions and fit with a polynomial surface that is third degree in *M* and third degree in *N*.
4. Repeat **steps 2** and **3** with the A647/QD emission ratio on the *z*-axis instead. The resulting equation is the A647/QD PL ratio as a function of *M*, *N*, and numerical coefficients. Figure 5a(ii) shows the data from Fig. 4b, plotted in three dimensions and fit with a polynomial surface that is third degree in *M* and third degree in *N*.
5. The two calibration equations of fit obtained from **steps 2** and **3** will enable back-calculation of *M* and *N* from emission ratios measured during enzyme assays. Examples of equations are shown in Fig. 5a. Figure 5b shows the correlation between experimental PL ratios and the PL ratios calculated from the calibration equations of fit derived in this section (three-dimensional fitting) and Subheading 3.5.2 (two-dimensional fitting).

3.6 Enzyme Assays and Data Analysis

Microtiter plate-based enzyme assays are carried out by first preparing a batch of cFRET probes and aliquoting the probes into a row of wells in a microtiter plate. To initiate the assays, protease solution is added to each of the wells. In the case of real-time assays, repetitive PL measurements are started immediately. For end-point assays, the samples are left to incubate for a defined period of time prior to PL measurements. The following steps are sufficient to assay 12 samples (i.e., one row of a 96-well microtiter plate; *see* **Note 42**). For imaging assays, the same general procedure applies, but the quantities and other details will need to be adapted to the imaging format (*see* **Note 43**).

1. Prepare or obtain a 200 μL substock solution of 8.0 μM Sub_{ChT}(A555) in BB2. Use the same stock solution used in Subheading 3.1 (*see* **Note 44**).
2. Prepare or obtain a 225 μL substock solution of 8.0 μM Sub_{TRP}(A647) in BB2. Use the same stock solution used in Subheading 3.1 (*see* **Note 44**).
3. Prepare or obtain a 150 μL substock solution of 1.0 μM QD in BB2. Use the same stock solution used in Subheading 3.1 (*see* **Note 44**).
4. Prepare a substock solution of cFRET probes with values of *M* and *N* within the range used for calibration experiments. If

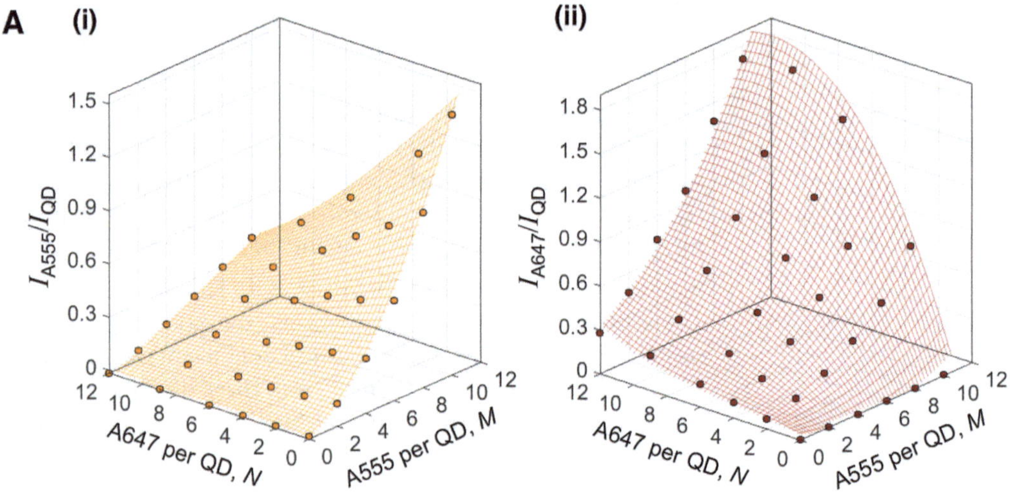

$$\frac{I_{A555}}{I_{QD}} = (-6.51\times10^{-5})M^3 + (7.59\times10^{-5})N^3 - (8.96\times10^{-4})M^2N + (2.93\times10^{-4})MN^2 + (1.18\times10^{-2})M^2 - (1.97\times10^{-3})N^2 + (3.19\times10^{-2})M + (1.15\times10^{-2})N - (3.18\times10^{-3})MN - (1.38\times10^{-2})$$

$$\frac{I_{A647}}{I_{QD}} = (1.21\times10^{-4})M^3 + (2.61\times10^{-4})N^3 + (3.57\times10^{-4})M^2N - (1.74\times10^{-3})MN^2 + (2.63\times10^{-3})M^2 - (2.72\times10^{-3})N^2 - (3.22\times10^{-2})M + (1.99\times10^{-2})N + (2.86\times10^{-2})MN + (3.70\times10^{-2})$$

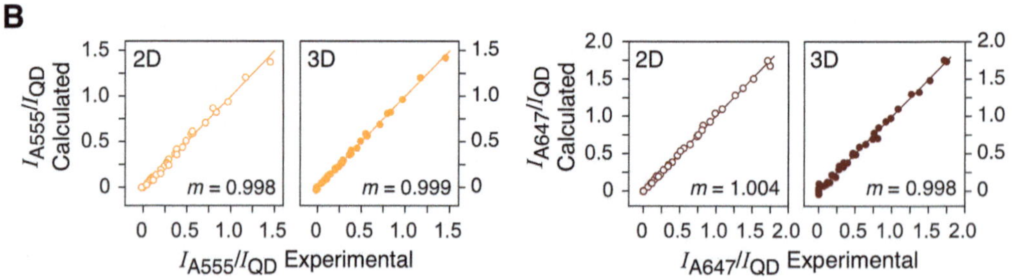

Fig. 5 (**a**) The same cFRET calibration data shown in Fig. 4i but plotted in three dimensions instead of two dimensions. The data is fit with the polynomial functions shown. (**b**) Plots showing the correlation between the calculated and experimental PL ratios. The calculated PL ratios were derived from the equations of best fit for the calibration data. Correlations are shown for both two-dimensional (2D) fitting (Fig. 4) and three-dimensional (3D) fitting (panel **a** of this figure). A good correlation is indicated by slopes (*m*) that are very close to unity. Data adapted from ref. 36

using QD-[Sub_{ChT}(A555)]$_{10}$-[Sub_{TRP}(A647)]$_{12}$ conjugates (the highest values of *M* and *N* in the calibration samples; *see* **Note 45**) and 96-well microtiter plates (*see* **Note 43**), add 175 μL of 8.0 μM Sub_{ChT}(A555), 210 μL of 8.0 μM Sub_{TRP}(A647), 175 μL of BB2, and, lastly, 140 μL of 1.0 μM QDs to a microcentrifuge tube. Mix immediately and let stand for

2 h. The cFRET probe solution will be diluted by a factor of 2 in a subsequent step.

5. Prepare solutions of proteases to be assayed. The protease solution will be diluted by a factor of 2 in a subsequent step.
6. Set up the plate reader or microscope with the same parameters and settings used for the calibration experiment (*see* Subheading 3.2 or 3.3).
7. Add 50 μL of the QD-[Sub_{ChT}(A555)]$_{10}$-[Sub_{TRP}(A647)]$_{12}$ cFRET probes from **step 4** to each well in a row of a microtiter plate.
8. Add 50 μL of BB2 to at least one of the wells in **step** 7 as a negative control.
9. Add 50 μL of the desired protease solution(s) to the remaining wells from **step** 7.
10. For a real-time assay, begin making PL measurements immediately after adding the last aliquot of enzyme. The time interval between measurements should be much longer than the time required for measurement of the PL intensities in the three wavelength channels. The time required for complete hydrolysis should be much longer than the time interval between measurements. For end-point assays, incubate the samples for the desired period of time before making PL measurements in all three channels.
11. Convert the raw emission data into crosstalk-corrected A555/QD and A647/QD PL ratios. If the data is from a real-time assay, perform this analysis at each time point.
12. Using the two calibration equations from Subheading 3.5.2 or 3.5.1, calculate the values of M and N from the measured A555/QD and A647/QD PL ratios. The two equations need to be solved simultaneously. In many cases, an analytic solution will be either inconvenient or impossible and a numerical method should be used (*see* **Note 46**).
13. If using Excel for data analysis, rearrange the two calibration equations so that the left-hand side is equal to zero (i.e., subtract the PL ratio from both sides of the equation). Input the initial values for M and N (from **step 4**) in two cells (e.g., columns A and B). Input the rearranged equations for the A555/QD and A647/QD PL ratios in two cells (e.g., columns C and D).
14. Open the Solver function in Excel. For end-point data or real-time data at a particular time-point, set the Solver objective so that the cell containing the equation for the A555/QD PL ratio will have a value of zero (e.g., in column C). Set the cells containing the values of M and N (e.g., columns A and B) to the variable cells that are changed by Solver. Apply the

constraint that the cell containing the A647/QD PL ratio (e.g., column D) must also have a value of zero. Use Solver to solve the system of equations and determine the values of *M* and *N*.

15. For real-time assays, plot the values of *M* and *N*, or, alternatively, the change in the values of *M* and *N* from their initial values (*see* **Note 47**) versus time. The resulting progress curves can be analyzed and correlated to protease activity. For end-point assays, a similar analysis can be done.

Figure 6 shows an example of data from a plate reader-based pro-chymotrypsin activation assay with trypsin [38]. Figure 7 shows an example of data from a microscope-based imaging assay with a mixture of chymotrypsin and trypsin [39].

4 Notes

1. Photoluminescence (PL) refers to the emission of a photon (i.e., luminescence) from the excited state of a material (e.g. dye molecule, QD) following the absorption of a photon to generate that excited state (i.e. photoexcitation). Fluorescence is an example of a type of PL that is generally associated with dye molecules.
2. Calculation of the spectral overlap integral, *J*, and the Förster distance, R_0, are not strictly required for cFRET assays or imaging since an empirical calibration procedure is used (*see* Subheading 3.1). Refer to **Notes 3** and **4** if interested in calculation of these parameters.
3. The spectral overlap integral, *J*, can be calculated from a full PL spectrum of the donor and the absorption spectrum of the acceptor. To measure the full donor PL spectrum, excite the donor on the short-wavelength side of the absorption maximum. Measure the absorption spectrum for the acceptor over the same wavelength range with the same wavelength step as the PL measurement. Background correct both spectra. Divide the acceptor absorption spectrum by its peak absorbance value (i.e., normalize the acceptor absorption spectrum). The shape of the spectrum will not change, but the peak value will be unity. Multiply the full absorption spectrum by the peak molar absorption coefficient for the dye (typically provided by the dye manufacturer or vendor). Convert the wavelength values to units of cm. For molar absorption coefficients with units of M^{-1} cm^{-1}, further multiplication by 1000 is required to have the correct units for Eq. 2 (mol^{-1} cm^2). The value of the numerator integrand of Eq. 3 can be calculated for each measured wavelength and the full integral evaluated

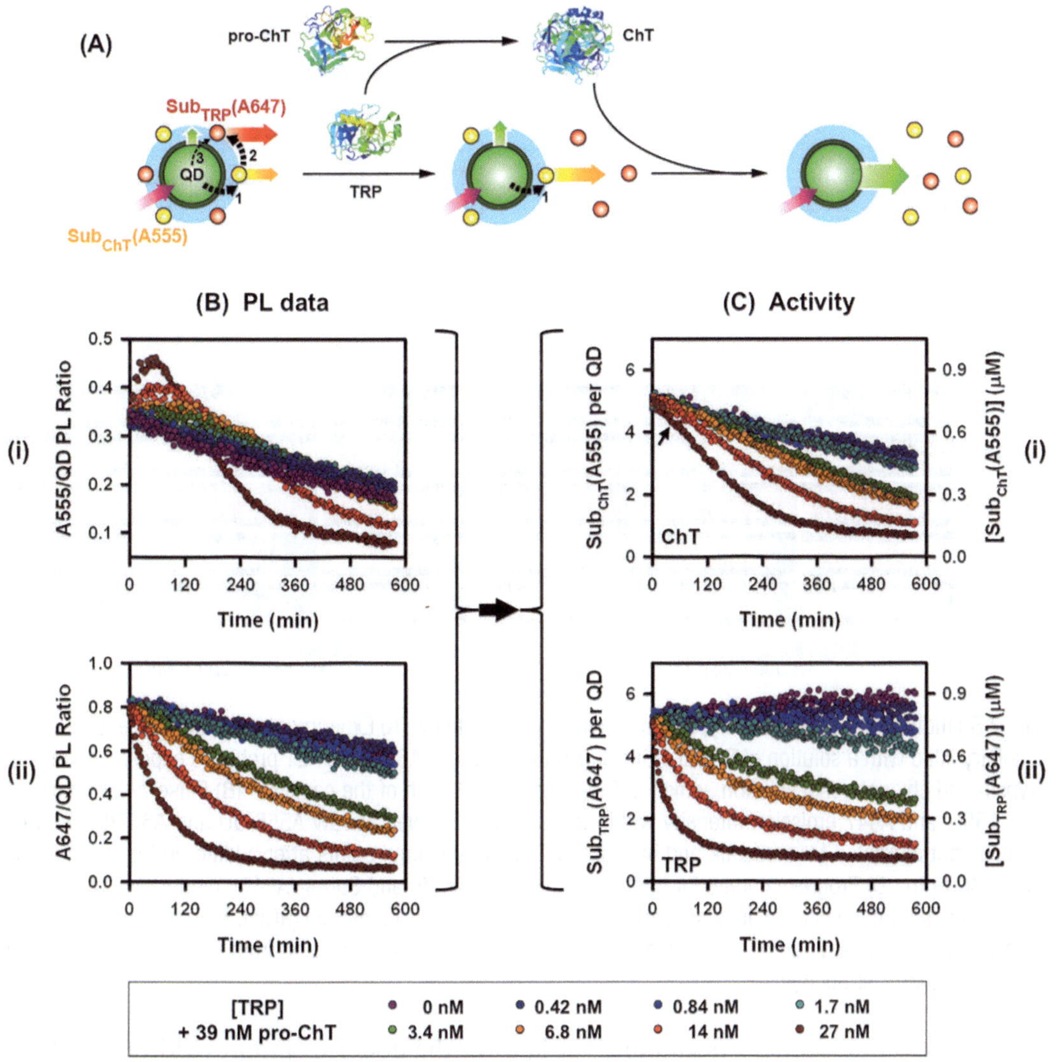

Fig. 6 (**A**) Schematic of a pro-ChT activation assay with $k_{QD\text{-}A555}$, $k_{A555\text{-}A647}$, and $k_{AQD\text{-}A647}$ indicated by *1*, *2*, and *3*, respectively. (**B**) (*i*) A555/QD and (*ii*) A647/QD PL ratios and (**C**) corresponding activity data for the hydrolysis of (*i*) Sub_{ChT} and (*ii*) Sub_{TRP} in QD520-$[Sub_{ChT}(A555)]_5$-$[Sub_{TRP}(A647)]_5$ conjugates by different concentrations of trypsin with 39 nM pro-chymotrypsin. The PL ratio data (**B**, *i–ii*) is utilized to calculate the progress curves for proteolytic activity (**C**, *i–ii*). The *arrow* in (**C**, *i*) indicates an inflection point associated with activation of pro-chymotrypsin. Digestion of Sub_{ChT}(A555) did not reach completion within the duration of the experiment. Note that the calibration data for this experiment is different than in Fig. 4. Reprinted with permission from ref. 38. Copyright 2012 American Chemical Society

numerically using the trapezoidal approximation. The value of the denominator integral in Eq. 3 can also be evaluated numerically. Dividing the value of one integral by the other yields J.

4. The Förster distance, R_0, is typically calculated by assuming that the orientation factor takes on a value of $\kappa^2 = 2/3$ and that the refractive index is $n = 1.33$–1.34 for an aqueous

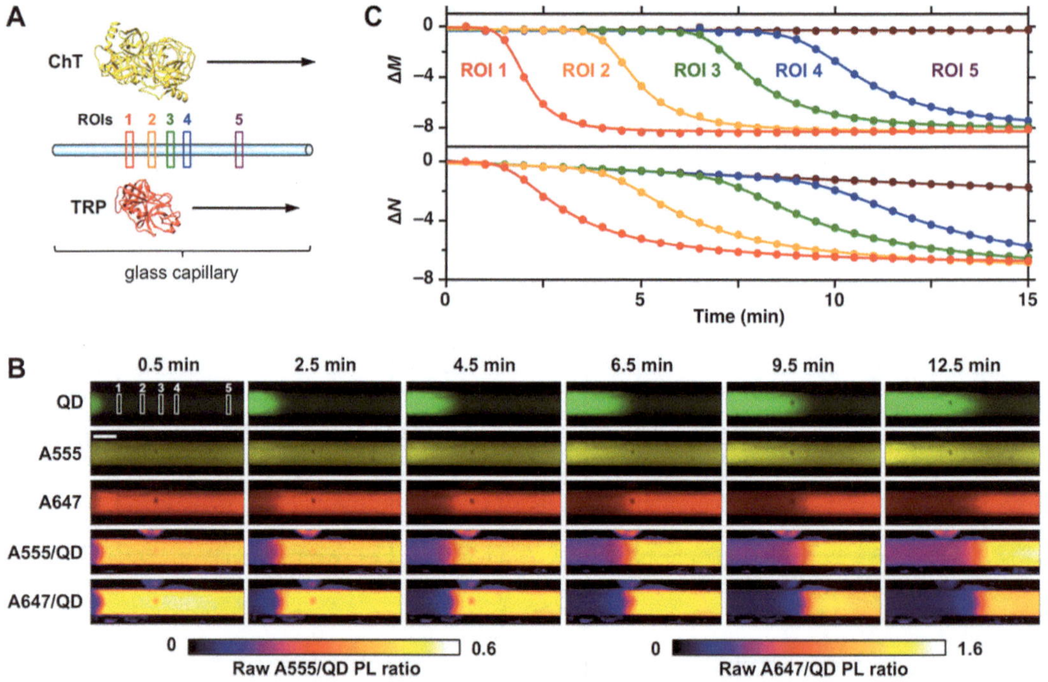

Fig. 7 Spatiotemporally resolved trypsin and chymotrypsin activity. (**A**) Experimental design: one end of a glass capillary filled with a solution of QD520-[Sub_{ChT}(A555)]$_7$-[Sub_{TRP}(A647)]$_7$ cFRET probes is exposed to a mixed trypsin and chymotrypsin solution, which diffuses along the length of the capillary. (**B**) False-color images of QD, A555, and A647 emission intensity within the capillary, as well as raw A555/QD and A647/QD PL ratio images (not corrected for crosstalk and background), at various time points after adding protease. The scale bar is 400 μm. (**C**) Progress curves for hydrolysis of Sub_{ChT}(A555) and Sub_{TRP}(A647), plotted as ΔM and ΔN (the changes from the initial values of M and N) for different regions of interest (ROIs). Note the calibration data for this experiment is different than in Figs. 4 and 6. Reprinted with permission from ref. 39. Copyright 2015 American Chemical Society

solution. If unknown, the donor quantum yield can be determined by comparison to a quantum yield standard [41–43].

5. The trend in the A1-A2 FRET efficiency has appeared to follow Eq. 11 in a pair of recent studies [36, 37]. The form of Eq. 11 is analogous to Eq. 8 and treats the multiple A2 acceptors as equivalent from the perspective of an A1 donor. The apparent suitability of this equation may reflect averaging of A1-A2 FRET across the ensemble, but otherwise remains to be elucidated at a fundamental level in relation to the photophysics and structure of the cFRET assembly.
6. Methods for the synthesis of high-quality CdSe/ZnS QDs have been published [44–48]. These procedures generally require suitable training in handling of air- and moisture-sensitive reagents and should not be undertaken by novices. Hydrophobic CdSe/ZnS QDs and related CdSeS/ZnS QDs in nonpolar solvents (e.g. toluene) are available from commercial

suppliers and are suitable for ligand exchange and transfer to aqueous media. Examples of suppliers at the time of writing include, but are not limited to, Thermo-Fisher Scientific (Carlsbad, CA, USA), Cytodiagnostics (Burlington, ON, Canada), CrystalPlex (Pittsburgh, PA, USA), and NN-Labs (Fayetteville, AR, USA).

7. Ligand exchange procedures have been published [49–52], including the glutathione (GSH) ligand exchange procedure that we utilized for preparing the QDs for the cFRET probes in this chapter [53]. Non-experts can replicate many of these procedures. Common ligands that are commercially available include 3-mercaptopropionic acid (MPA) and GSH. Lipoic acid is also available commercially and can be converted to a dihydrolipoic acid (DHLA) ligand for QDs through a one-step reduction reaction and simple purification procedure [52]. More complex DHLA-based ligands can be synthesized when suitable chemistry expertise is available [49–51]. QDs coated with DHLA and DHLA-PEG ligands have also been used to prepare cFRET probes [38].
8. To minimize aggregation over time, store ligand-exchanged aqueous QD stock solutions at 4 °C in borate buffer with pH 8.5–9.5 and low ionic strength ($\leq$100 mM). The concentration should be 5 μM or higher as dilute solutions often aggregate more quickly. Do not freeze QD solutions.
9. Aqueous QDs with ligand coatings (e.g., GSH, DHLA) are needed to permit the self-assembly of polyhistidine peptides to the ZnS shell of the QDs. The polyhistidine binds with high affinity to the ZnS shell on QDs (K_d^{-1} = 0.1–100 nM) [54, 55] and equilibrium binding is usually reached in less than 1 h. QDs transferred into aqueous media using polymer or lipid coatings may prevent this self-assembly from occurring. Most commercially available aqueous QDs have polymer or lipid coatings.
10. Detailed methods for the labeling and subsequent purification of peptides with an N-/C-terminal hexahistidine sequence and a C-/N-terminal cysteine residue with a thiol-reactive maleimide dye have been published [56, 57]. Dye-labeled peptides can also be purchased from commercial vendors such as AnaSpec (Fremont, CA, USA), BioSynthesis (Lewisville, TX, USA), JPT (Acton, MA, USA), and New England Peptide (Gardner, MA, USA).
11. The ideal acceptor dyes, A1 and A2, for the QD in a cFRET probe will meet the following criteria: (1) the peak PL wavelengths of the QD, A1, and A2 are resolved from one another, where the QD PL peak has the shortest wavelength and the A2 PL peak has the longest wavelength; (2) there is overlap

between the PL spectrum of the QD and the absorption spectra of A1 and A2 (larger overlap for A1 and smaller overlap for A2); (3) A1 and A2 have molar absorption coefficients $\geq 10^5$ M^{-1} cm^{-1} and quantum yields ≥ 0.10 (higher is better); (4) A1 and A2 have a common PL excitation minimum in the blue-UV region of the spectrum (so dye excitation can be minimized while efficiently exciting the QD); (5) A1 and A2 have good aqueous solubilities and a net negative charge (to minimize interactions with the anionic ligands on GSH-coated QDs); (6) A1 and A2 are stable in aqueous buffer; and (7) A1 and A2 are available as maleimide or, less ideally, succinimidyl ester derivatives. In our experience, A555, A647, and related Cy3 and Cy5 dyes are among the best at satisfying these cumulative criteria, although other dyes may better meet individual criteria.

12. We use the following general design strategy for peptide substrates, which are organized into functional modules in the order (1)-(2)-(3)-(4)-(5)-(6): (1) a hexahistidine sequence at one terminus (either C- or N-terminus) to bind to the ZnS shell of the QDs; (2) a spacer sequence with helical propensity (e.g., polyproline or 2-aminoisobutyric acid/alanine) following the hexahistidine sequence to help extend the peptide away from the surface of the QD; (3) a short series of primarily hydrophilic amino acid residues that are not recognized by the target protease and are unreactive with the acceptor dye labeling chemistry (*vide infra*); (4) an amino acid residue or series of amino acid residues recognized and hydrolyzed by the target protease; (5) another module analogous to (3); and (6) a terminal residue that can be selectively labeled with an acceptor dye (e.g., cysteine for maleimide derivatives of dyes, or a lysine residue or an N-terminal glycine for succinimidyl ester derivatives of dyes).
13. Borate buffer is preferred when working with QDs coated with GSH or similar anionic ligands (e.g., DHLA). The useful pH range is 8–10. Typical boric acid/borate concentrations are 10–100 mM with sodium chloride concentrations between 0 and 50 mM. If this buffer composition or pH range is unsuitable for a particular protease of interest, it can be substituted by buffers with similar pH and ionic strength. For example, Tris-borate buffer can be used to lower the pH to 7.5. Phosphate buffered saline (PBS) and buffers with pH < 7.5 are not recommended without PEG or zwitterionic ligand coatings on the QD to confer greater colloidal stability [58–64].
14. The nonbinding surface modification of the 96-well microtiter plate is advantageous when working with proteins but is not required. The methodology can also be adapted to other sizes of microtiter plate (e.g., 384-well, 1536-well).

15. The clear, UV-transparent, flat-bottom microtiter plates are convenient for calibration of the microscope imaging format. The clear bottom is required with an inverted microscope. We have used 96-well, 384-well, and 1536-well microtiter plates with clear bottoms. Multi-well/multi-chamber microscope slides can also be used.
16. The Infinite M1000 Pro plate reader (Tecan US, Inc., Morrisville, NC, USA) is a monochromator-based spectrofluorimetric plate reader equipped with a broad-spectrum xenon flash lamp source and photomultipler tube detector. For calibration samples with the prototypical QD-$(\mathrm{A555})_{M}$-$(\mathrm{A647})_{N}$ cFRET configuration, we often measure full PL emission spectra between 450 and 750 nm with 2 nm steps and 5 nm bandwidth. For real-time assays, we measure PL emission between 520 and 670 nm with 50 nm steps and 5 nm bandwidth (i.e., intensity measured at 520, 570, 620, and 670 nm, where the data for 620 nm is discarded for the analysis). This four-point method decreases the time required for PL measurements, which is an important consideration in the real-time assays. The four-point method can also be used to measure the calibration samples. Other instruments with similar spectrofluorimetric capability and specifications should be capable of similar measurements. If using a filter-based fluorescence plate reader, the technical requirements will be similar to those for a fluorescence microscope (*see* **Note 17**).
17. A fluorescence microscope has two main requirements for cFRET imaging. The first requirement is the ability to set up excitation and emission wavelengths comparable to those specified by the optical filters noted in Subheading 2.2. Relatively narrow bandpass filters are needed to satisfactorily resolve the QD and A1 (e.g., A555) emission. Either a longpass or bandpass filter can be used to resolve the emission from A2 (e.g., A647). While we use a broadband lamp with a violet bandpass filter as an excitation source, a violet laser source (e.g., 405 nm) or high power violet light-emitting diode (LED) light source can be substituted. Many models of camera will be satisfactory, although we recommend cameras with good efficiency in the red region of the spectrum. For real-time measurements, a second requirement is a mechanism of fast and automated switching between the three different emission filters and acquiring corresponding images. We achieve this switching with an automated emission filter wheel with software control. The dichroic mirror and excitation filter are mounted and controlled separately from the emission filters. A possible alternative configuration is an automated filter cube turret with a cube for each emission filter, albeit that this format requires triplication of the excitation filter and dichroic mirror.

A commercially available multichannel imaging system (e.g., QV2, Photometrics, Tucson, AZ, USA) equipped with similar filters is a third option.

18. An example of an alternative instrument to the plate reader and microscope systems is an array-based spectrometer. Vendors such as Ocean Optics (Dunedin, FL, USA) and StellarNet (Tampa, FL, USA) sell low-cost, fiber-optic, USB-connected spectrometers suitable for this type of PL measurement. The free end of a fiber-optic patch cable connected to the spectrometer can be positioned to collect PL from cFRET probes in a cuvette, microtiter plate well, or another type of sample cell or holder. A violet laser, violet LED, or suitably filtered broad-spectrum light source can be used for excitation. The potential disadvantages of such an apparatus are low throughput (versus a plate reader) and lack of imaging capability (versus a microscope). Potential advantages include the comparatively low cost, flexibility, and rapid acquisition of full spectra.
19. When multiple data sets are to be fit with the same mathematical function, the variables in that function can be classified as global variables, meaning that all data sets are fit with the same value for that variable (i.e., optimization over all data sets), or local variables, meaning that each data set is fit with a unique value of the variable (i.e., optimization within individual data sets). Although cFRET calibration data can be analyzed without global fitting, the use of global fitting can simplify the process and produce more reliable results.
20. A more complex calibration method utilizes mixtures of pre-digested peptide substrates and native peptide substrates. The pre-hydrolyzed peptides are prepared by proteolysis and the proteases are subsequently inhibited. In some cases, this method can better approximate the nonspecific adsorption of hydrolyzed dye-labeled peptide fragments on the QDs. We have previously described this calibration method in detail for nonconcentric QD-FRET probes for proteolysis [53], and we have used this method to calibrate cFRET imaging probes [39]. For the basic calibration in Subheading 3.1, the samples are prepared with M and N equivalents of A1-labeled peptide-1 and A2-labeled peptide-2, respectively, per QD. For the modified calibration, samples are prepared with M and N equivalents of A1-labeled peptide-1 and A2-labeled peptide-2 per QD, as well as $M_{max}-M$ and $N_{max}-N$ equivalents of the corresponding pre-hydrolyzed peptides, where $M \leq M_{max}$ and $N \leq N_{max}$. The cFRET probes subsequently used for enzyme assays have $M = M_{max}$ and $N = N_{max}$. Refer to refs. 39, 53 for more details.

21. The quantities in Subheading 3.1 and Fig. 2 are recommendations for 96-well microtiter plates. Volumes and concentrations can be varied to accommodate other microtiter plate sizes (e.g., 384-well, 1536-well) or other varieties of sample cell. The quantities can also be scaled back if more limited amounts of material are available. We recommend QD concentrations of at least 0.050 µM, but volumes can be varied as needed.

22. The amounts of the stock and substock solutions in Subheading 3.1 provide some excess in case a need arises to re-make a calibration sample. This excess is sufficient for at least three remade calibration samples, but does not include sufficient volume to prepare control samples with only dye-labeled peptide substrates (*see* **Note 23**). The *stock* solution is the parent solution that is used to prepare further dilutions or *substock* solutions. In turn, these substock solutions are used for preparation of samples for calibration and enzyme assays.

23. It is good practice to run a calibration experiment that also includes samples with only dye-labeled peptide substrates dissolved in buffer. Figure 8 is an addendum to Fig. 2 that summarizes the preparation of these samples. These samples

[Sub_{ChT}(A555)] Sub-Stock Solution

M	0 A555	2 A555	4 A555	6 A555	8 A555	10 A555
Sub-stock		1.0 µM	1.0 µM	2.0 µM	2.0 µM	2.0 µM
A555	0	20	40	30	40	50
QD	0	0	0	0	0	0
A647	0	0	0	0	0	0
Buffer	100	80	60	70	60	50

[Sub_{TRP}(A647)] Sub-Stock Solution

N	0 A647	2 A647	4 A647	6 A647	9 A647	12 A647
Sub-stock		1.0 µM	2.0 µM	2.0 µM	4.0 µM	4.0 µM
A555	0	0	0	0	0	0
QD	0	0	0	0	0	0
A647	0	20	20	30	23	30
Buffer	100	80	80	70	77	70

Volumes (µL): QD A555 A647 Buffer

Fig. 8 Addendum to the calibration sample matrix in Fig. 2 to include control samples with different amounts of dye-labeled peptide only (no QDs). These samples can be used to estimate the proportion of the dye PL from the samples in Fig. 2 that is due to direct excitation of the dyes versus FRET from the QD donor

are used to estimate the amount of dye PL that is a result of direct excitation of the dyes (with FRET-sensitized PL accounting for the difference in the total dye PL intensity between these control samples and the calibration samples in Fig. 2). If the control samples in Fig. 8 are to be prepared, the volumes of the Sub_{ChT}(A555) and Sub_{TRP}(A647) stock and substock solutions in Subheading 3.1 should be increased by 15 % (for the same concentrations).

24. We recommend pipetting a minimum volume of 5 μL of substock solutions to prepare samples. Larger volumes (e.g., 20 μL in Fig. 2) are preferred for greater accuracy and precision in preparing the calibration samples.

25. Although the QDs and A555 are quite resistant to photobleaching, the A647 photobleaches much more readily [36]. It is therefore good practice to incubate the samples in darkness. A covering of aluminum foil or a closed drawer is sufficient.

26. We have found that direct excitation of the A555 and A647 is negligible with a ~400 nm excitation wavelength or 405/20 excitation filter. If using different instrumentation or different instrument settings, it is advisable to confirm that direct excitation of the A555 and A647 remains negligible. Alternatively, if A1 and A2 are not A555 and A647, then an experiment to evaluate direct excitation of dye PL is recommended. Refer to **Note 23** in both cases. For plate reader assays, a moderate level of direct excitation is acceptable as the empirical calibration accounts for directly excited dye PL. In imaging assays where hydrolyzed dye-labeled peptide fragments could diffuse out of the region-of-interest (ROI), it is important to have negligible PL from direct excitation of the A1 and A2 dyes.

27. For plate reader measurements (also *see* **Note 16**), the 520, 570, and 670 nm measurement wavelengths approximately correspond to the spectral positions of the peak QD, A555, and A647 PL. If using a cFRET configuration other than the prototypical QD-$(A555)_M$-$(A647)_N$ configuration, then the wavelengths will need to change to match the PL wavelengths of the new QD, A1, and A2.

28. For plate reader measurements, all three peak PL wavelength measurements are usually made at the same settings by default. That is, the measurements are made with the same excitation intensity (controlled by lamp output and excitation monochromator bandwidth) and the same collection efficiency and sensitivity toward PL (controlled by optics, emission monochromator bandwidth, and detector gain). We have not found it necessary to change these parameters between the three PL wavelengths, although individual optimization of

the measurement settings for the three PL wavelengths is acceptable provided that the same settings are used for both calibration and enzyme assays.

29. For microscope imaging (also *see* **Note 17**), the 520/40, 565/30, and 665LP filters predominantly transmit PL from the QD, A555, and A647, respectively. Crosstalk is greater with the imaging filters than with the plate reader (monochromator bandwidth ~5 nm). If using a cFRET configuration other than the prototypical QD-$(A555)_M$-$(A647)_N$ configuration, then the filters will need to change to match the PL wavelengths of the new QD, A1, and A2.

30. With our microscope system, it is possible to change the excitation intensity (lamp output power) and camera exposure time between measurements in the three filter channels. We have found it beneficial to optimize the camera exposure time for each emitter (but to maintain a constant excitation intensity), and have found that PL ratios varied predictably with changes in camera settings [39]. The individual optimization of the three measurement channel settings is acceptable as long as the same settings are used for both calibration and enzyme assays.

31. We typically load the diagonal samples in the calibration matrix in Fig. 2 in an agarose gel. There is a consistent increase in the number of peptides per QD between these samples, and most gel combs will accommodate this number of samples. Using the same samples for gels that were used for the calibration PL measurements helps to ensure consistency and decreases consumption of materials.

32. The maximum loading of the QD with peptides can be estimated from agarose gels. When the fluorescent dye label on the peptide can be directly excited and visualized in a gel imaging system, the appearance of a new band corresponding to unbound dye-labeled peptide can indicate that the maximum peptide loading capacity of the QD has been reached. Our experience to date suggests that this type of experiment will provide a conservative estimate. Another indicator can be the number of peptides per QD at which the electrophoretic mobility of the QD no longer decreases; however, it must be noted that the magnitude of the change in mobility with each added peptide decreases as the total number of peptides increases, and a clear saturation point may not be apparent.

33. The purpose of the glycerol is to sink the sample to the bottom of the gel well. While we typically use 10 % v/v glycerol in the final sample, we have also had success with glycerol percentages between 6–20 % v/v.

34. The field strength is the applied voltage divided by the distance between the electrodes in the gel tank. For many "mini" gel systems, the applied voltage for this field strength will be close to 100 V.
35. Both the GSH-coated QDs and corresponding QD-peptide conjugates should migrate as discrete bands. The bands for the peptide conjugates may appear tighter than for the QDs alone. Any streaking should be faint compared to the main band. If streaking is significant, it may indicate a pending problem with the colloidal stability of the QDs. Significant residue in the sample wells of the gel indicates that aggregation has occurred. In both cases, a new preparation of GSH-coated QDs is recommended.
36. High-quality images of gels can be acquired with a suitable gel imaging system. Simple visual confirmation is possible by eye when the gel is illuminated under longwave UV in a viewing cabinet. In many cases, the QD and/or dye PL will be bright enough for a digital camera or smartphone to acquire an image using the viewing cabinet (or a hand-held UV lamp and suitable UV-blocking filter).
37. Blank ROIs for background correction can be dark areas in the calibration sample images themselves or separate images of buffer solution. If the latter, the blank images should be acquired under the same microscope settings as the calibration sample images.
38. For the prototypical QD-$(A555)_{M}$$(A647)_{N}$ cFRET system, the A555 PL at 520 nm is negligible compared to that of the QD. Selection of a cFRET system with a different QD or dye may require consideration of crosstalk. In this case, crosstalk can potentially be corrected through a system of simultaneous equations or through formal spectral deconvolution. Very high QD quenching efficiencies leading to dye/QD PL ratios >2 may also require that the dye PL crosstalk at the peak QD PL wavelength be considered.
39. The crosstalk of A555 PL in the A647 channel can also be calculated from a sample of A555-labeled peptide alone, directly excited at 520 nm. The crosstalk coefficient remains the ratio of the PL intensity at 670 nm over the PL intensity at 570 nm, as defined in Eq. 19. This procedure is analogous to how the crosstalk is determined for the QD. It is equivalent to the method in Subheading 3.5.1 and often simpler and more convenient, especially if the procedure in **Note 23** is used.
40. The mathematical functions suggested for fitting are empirical functions that often provide a good fit to the data and are not necessarily theoretical expectations. The ideal empirical function will fit the trend in the data well and will be as

mathematically simple as possible without compromising the quality of the fit. In our experience, functions that are monotonic over the range of *M* and *N* values are preferred. Linear functions, exponential rise-to-maximum functions, exponential decay functions, and quadratic functions are good candidates, but we generally avoid higher order polynomials.

41. The simplest mathematical function that fits the data is recommended. If the data is monotonic, then a function that is monotonic over the range of the data should be used. Linear, quadratic, and exponential decay or exponential rise-to-maximum functions are good candidate functions.

42. To assay samples in *r* rows, multiply the volumes in **steps 1–4** of Subheading 3.6 by a factor of *r*. The volume of QD stock solution will also need to increase by $(r - 1)30$ % and the volumes of the Sub_{ChT}(A555) and Sub_{TRP}(A647) stock solution will need to increase by $(r - 1)42$ %. Similarly, for *s* individual samples, mix $12.5(s + 2)$ μL of 8.0 μM Sub_{ChT}(A555), and $15(s + 2)$ μL of 8.0 μM Sub_{TRP}(A647), $12.5(s + 2)$ μL of BB2, and $10(s + 2)$ μL of 1.0 μM QDs. Aliquot 50 μL portions into *s* wells of a microtiter plate (*see* **Note 44** for an explanation of $s + 2$). The volumes of the QD, Sub_{ChT}(A555), Sub_{TRP}(A647) stock solutions will also need increase.

43. A useful test system for imaging assays is a glass capillary (~400 μm inner diameter, ~1 cm length) filled with a solution of cFRET probes. The capillary is placed on a microscope slide and a 0.5 μL droplet of protease solution is placed at one end of the capillary. Hydrolysis of the cFRET probes will be observed as the protease(s) diffuses down the capillary. *See* ref. 39 for further details. This format is only one of a multitude of possible imaging formats where a protease solution is added to the cFRET probes.

44. **Step 4** of Subheading 3.6 provides a small excess of the cFRET probe solution. If assaying *s* samples, it is advisable to prepare sufficient volume for $s + 2$ samples. This excess provides contingency if one of the assay samples needs to be re-measured and ensures that exactly 50 μL can be added to each of the 12 wells in the row of the microtiter plate.

45. The batch preparation of cFRET probes for enzyme assays is a scale-up of the same recipe used for preparation of the corresponding calibration sample. We sometimes observe that the apparent values of *M* and *N* measured from the PL ratios of the batch preparation are larger than expected. Instead of using the maximum numbers of Sub_{ChT}(A555) and Sub_{TRP}(A647) per QD from Fig. 2 (i.e., $M = 10$, $N = 12$) for enzyme assays, it can be useful to use slightly smaller numbers of these peptides (e.g., $M = 8$, $N = 9$). This variation is not applicable if

utilizing the alternative calibration from **Note 20**. Another option is to analyze the data in terms of the change in the values of M and N rather than their absolute values (*see* **Note 47**).

46. The Solver function in Excel is one method of solving the system of nonlinear equations. In some cases it may also be possible to use iterative calculations (i.e., allow "circular references" in Excel). Other software packages such as MatLab will also have built-in functions for solving a system of nonlinear equations.

47. The values of M and N will often give useful quantitative data. However, when scaling up or scaling down the preparation of cFRET probes, or preparing the conjugates for enzyme assays at a different time than the calibration samples, some variation in the absolute values of M and N can be observed. In these cases, the *change* in the values of M and N may be more effective. For example, values of M might vary between 0 and M_{max} for an initial calibration, but data from subsequent enzyme assays may yield a result that M decreases from $M = M_{max} + 1.5$ to $M = 1.5$ over the course of the assay (and similar for N). In this case, ΔM, the change in the value of M, is a more robust parameter. If large discrepancies are noted (e.g., $M_{measured} > M_{expected} + 2$) or if a new batch of QDs or peptides is prepared, then calibration should be repeated. Also note that if $M_{initial} = M_{max}$ in an enzyme assay but M does not reach zero (under conditions consistent with complete hydrolysis), it may suggest nonspecific adsorption of the hydrolyzed dye-labeled peptide fragments on the QD. *See* **Note 20** for a possible calibration method.

Acknowledgments

The authors thank the Natural Sciences and Engineering Research Council of Canada (NSERC), the Canada Foundation for Innovation (CFI), and the University of British Columbia for support of their research. W.R.A. is also grateful for support through a Canada Research Chair (Tier 2) and a Michael Smith Foundation for Health Research Scholar Award.

References

1. Chapman HA, Riese RJ, Shi GP (1997) Emerging roles for cysteine proteases in human biology. Annu Rev Physiol 59:63–88
2. Fortini ME (2002) Gamma-secretase-mediated proteolysis in cell-surface-receptor signalling. Nat Rev Mol Cell Biol 3:673–684
3. Neurath H, Walsh KA (1976) Role of proteolytic-enzymes in biological regulation. Proc Natl Acad Sci U S A 73:3825–3832
4. Ossovskaya VS, Bunnett NW (2004) Protease-activated receptors: contribution to physiology and disease. Physiol Rev 84:579–621

5. Mason SD, Joyce JA (2011) Proteolytic networks in cancer. Trends Cell Biol 21:228–237
6. Cory S, Adams JM (2002) The BCL2 family: regulators of the cellular life-or-death switch. Nat Rev Cancer 2:647–656
7. Gyrd-Hansen M, Meier P (2010) IAPs: from caspase inhibitors to modulators of NF-kappa B, inflammation and cancer. Nat Rev Cancer 10:561–574
8. Egeblad M, Werb Z (2002) New functions for the matrix metalloproteinases in cancer progression. Nat Rev Cancer 2:161–174
9. Kessenbrock K, Plaks V, Werb Z (2010) Matrix metalloproteinases: regulators of the tumor microenvironment. Cell 141:52–67
10. Koblinski JE, Ahram M, Sloane BF (2000) Unraveling the role of proteases in cancer. Clin Chim Acta 291:113–135
11. Friedl P, Alexander S (2011) Cancer invasion and the microenvironment: plasticity and reciprocity. Cell 147:992–1009
12. Ludewig S, Kossner M, Schiller M, Baumann K, Schirmeister T (2010) Enzyme kinetics and hit validation in fluorimetric protease assays. Curr Top Med Chem 10:368–382
13. Wysocka M, Lesner A (2013) Future of protease activity assays. Curr Pharm Des 19:1062–1067
14. Drag M, Salvesen GS (2010) Emerging principles in protease-based drug discovery. Nat Rev Drug Discov 9:690–701
15. Jedinak A, Maliar T (2005) Inhibitors of proteases as anticancer drugs—minireview. Neoplasma 52:185–192
16. Turk B (2006) Targeting proteases: successes, failures and future prospects. Nat Rev Drug Discov 5:785–799
17. Eggeling C, Jager S, Winkler D, Kask P (2005) Comparison of different fluorescence fluctuation methods for their use in FRET assays: monitoring a protease reaction. Curr Pharm Biotechnol 6:351–371
18. Hu H-Y, Gehrig S, Reither G, Subramanian D, Mall MA, Plettenburg O, Schultz C (2014) FRET-based and other fluorescent proteinase probes. Biotechnol J 9:266–281
19. Lee H, Kim Y-P (2015) Fluorescent and bioluminescent nanoprobes for in vitro and in vivo detection of matrix metalloproteinase activity. BMB Rep 48:313–318
20. Kim GB, Kim Y-P (2012) Analysis of protease activity using quantum dots and resonance energy transfer. Theranostics 2:127–138
21. Welser K, Adsley R, Moore BM, Chan WC, Aylott JW (2011) Protease sensing with nanoparticle based platforms. Analyst 136:29–41
22. Algar WR, Susumu K, Delehanty JB, Medintz IL (2011) Semiconductor quantum dots in bioanalysis: crossing the valley of death. Anal Chem 83:8826–8837
23. Resch-Genger U, Grabolle M, Cavaliere-Jaricot S, Nitschke R, Nann T (2008) Quantum dots versus organic dyes as fluorescent labels. Nat Methods 5:763–775
24. Blanco-Canosa JB, Wu M, Susumu K, Petryayeva E, Jennings TL, Dawson PE, Algar WR, Medintz IL (2014) Recent progress in the bioconjugation of quantum dots. Coord Chem Rev 263–264:101–137
25. Bradburne CE, Delehanty JB, Gemmill KB, Mei BC, Mattoussi H, Susumu K, Blanco-Canosa JB, Dawson PE, Medintz IL (2013) Cytotoxicity of quantum dots used for in vitro cellular labeling: role of QD surface ligand, delivery modality, cell type, and direct comparison to organic fluorophores. Bioconjug Chem 24:1570–1583
26. Tsoi KM, Dai Q, Alman BA, Chan WCW (2013) Are quantum dots toxic? Exploring the discrepancy between cell culture and animal studies. Acc Chem Res 46:662–671
27. Yong K-T, Law W-C, Hu R, Ye L, Liu L, Swihart MT, Prasad PN (2013) Nanotoxicity assessment of quantum dots: from cellular to primate studies. Chem Soc Rev 42:1236–1250
28. Petryayeva E, Algar WR, Medintz IL (2013) Quantum dots in bioanalysis: A review of applications across various platforms for fluorescence spectroscopy and imaging. Appl Spectrosc 67:215–252
29. Mattoussi H, Palui G, Na HB (2012) Luminescent quantum dots as platforms for probing in vitro and in vivo biological processes. Adv Drug Deliv Rev 64:138–166
30. Wegner KD, Hildebrandt N (2015) Quantum dots: bright and versatile in vitro and in vivo fluorescence imaging biosensors. Chem Soc Rev 44:4792–4834
31. Algar WR, Kim H, Medintz IL, Hildebrandt N (2014) Emerging non-traditional Förster resonance energy transfer configurations with semiconductor quantum dots: investigations and applications. Coord Chem Rev 263–264:65–85
32. Medintz IL, Mattoussi H (2009) Quantum dot-based resonance energy transfer and its growing application in biology. Phys Chem Chem Phys 11:17–45
33. Algar WR, Tavares AJ, Krull UJ (2010) Beyond labels: a review of the application of quantum

dots as integrated components of assays, bioprobes, and biosensors utilizing optical transduction. Anal Chim Acta 673:1–25

34. Cheung HC (2002) Resonance energy transfer. In: Lakowicz JR (ed) Topics in fluorescence spectroscopy: principles, vol 2. Kluwer, New York, pp 127–176
35. Lakowicz JR (2006) Principles of fluorescence spectroscopy, 3rd edn. Springer Science + Business Media, New York
36. Wu M, Massey M, Petryayeva E, Algar WR (2015) Energy transfer pathways in a quantum dot-based concentric FRET configuration. J Phys Chem C 119:26183–26195
37. Kim H, Ng CYW, Algar WR (2014) Quantum dot-based multidonor concentric FRET system and its application to biosensing using an excitation ratio. Langmuir 30:5676–5685
38. Algar WR, Ancona MG, Malanoski AP, Susumu K, Medintz IL (2012) Assembly of a concentric Förster resonance energy transfer relay on a quantum dot scaffold: characterization and application to multiplexed protease sensing. ACS Nano 6:11044–11058
39. Wu M, Algar WR (2015) Concentric Förster resonance energy transfer imaging. Anal Chem 87:8078–8083
40. Wu M, Petryayeva E, Algar WR (2014) Quantum dot-based concentric FRET configuration for the parallel detection of protease activity and concentration. Anal Chem 86:11181–11188
41. Wurth C, Grabolle M, Pauli J, Spieles M, Resch-Genger U (2013) Relative and absolute determination of fluorescence quantum yields of transparent samples. Nat Protoc 8:1535–1550
42. Grabolle M, Spieles M, Lesnyak V, Gaponik N, Eychmuller A, Resch-Genger U (2009) Determination of the fluorescence quantum yield of quantum dots: suitable procedures and achievable uncertainties. Anal Chem 81:6285–6294
43. Demas JN, Crosby GA (1971) Measurement of photoluminescence quantum yields—review. J Phys Chem 75:991–1024
44. Dabbousi BO, Rodriguez-Viejo J, Mikulec FV, Heine JR, Mattoussi H, Ober R, Jensen KF, Bawendi MG (1997) (CdSe)ZnS core-shell quantum dots: synthesis and characterization of a size series of highly luminescent nanocrystallites. J Phys Chem B 101:9463–9475
45. Peng ZA, Peng XG (2001) Formation of high-quality CdTe, CdSe, and CdS nanocrystals using CdO as precursor. J Am Chem Soc 123:183–184
46. Hines MA, Guyot-Sionnest P (1996) Synthesis and characterization of strongly luminescing ZnS-capped CdSe nanocrystals. J Phys Chem 100:468–471
47. Talapin DV, Rogach AL, Kornowski A, Haase M, Weller H (2001) Highly luminescent monodisperse CdSe and CdSe/ZnS nanocrystals synthesized in a hexadecylamine-trioctylphosphine oxide-trioctylphospine mixture. Nano Lett 1:207–211
48. Li JJ, Wang YA, Guo WZ, Keay JC, Mishima TD, Johnson MB, Peng XG (2003) Large-scale synthesis of nearly monodisperse CdSe/CdS core/shell nanocrystals using air-stable reagents via successive ion layer adsorption and reaction. J Am Chem Soc 125:12567–12575
49. Zhan NQ, Palui G, Mattoussi H (2015) Preparation of compact biocompatible quantum dots using multicoordinating molecular-scale ligands based on a zwitterionic hydrophilic motif and lipoic acid anchors. Nat Protoc 10:859–874
50. Susumu K, Mei BC, Mattoussi H (2009) Multifunctional ligands based on dihydrolipoic acid and polyethylene glycol to promote biocompatibility of quantum dots. Nat Protoc 4:424–436
51. Mei BC, Susumu K, Medintz IL, Mattoussi H (2009) Polyethylene glycol-based bidentate ligands to enhance quantum dot and gold nanoparticle stability in biological media. Nat Protoc 4:412–423
52. Clapp AR, Goldman ER, Mattoussi H (2006) Capping of CdSe-ZnS quantum dots with DHLA and subsequent conjugation with proteins. Nat Protoc 1:1258–1266
53. Wu M, Petryayeva E, Medintz IL, Algar WR (2014) Quantitative measurement of proteolytic rates with quantum dot-peptide substrate conjugates and Förster resonance energy transfer. Methods Mol Biol 1199:215–239
54. Sapsford KE, Pons T, Medintz IL, Higashiya S, Brunel FM, Dawson PE, Mattoussi H (2007) Kinetics of metal-affinity driven self-assembly between proteins or peptides and CdSe-ZnS quantum dots. J Phys Chem C 111:11528–11538
55. Aldeek F, Safi M, Zhan NQ, Palui G, Mattoussi H (2013) Understanding the self-assembly of proteins onto gold nanoparticles and quantum dots driven by metal-histidine coordination. ACS Nano 7:10197–10210
56. Algar WR, Blanco-Canosa JB, Manthe RL, Susumu K, Stewart MH, Dawson PE, Medintz IL (2013) Synthesizing and modifying peptides for chemoselective ligation and assembly

into quantum dot-peptide bioconjugates. Methods Mol Biol 1025:47–73

57. Sapsford KE, Farrell D, Sun S, Rasooly A, Mattoussi H, Medintz IL (2009) Monitoring of enzymatic proteolysis on a electroluminescent-CCD microchip platform using quantum dot-peptide substrates. Sens Actuators B 139:13–21
58. Zhan NQ, Palui G, Safi M, Ji X, Mattoussi H (2013) Multidentate zwitterionic ligands provide compact and highly biocompatible quantum dots. J Am Chem Soc 135:13786–13795
59. Gravel E, Tanguy C, Cassette E, Pons T, Knittel F, Bernards N, Garofalakis A, Duconge F, Dubertret B, Doris E (2013) Compact tridentate ligands for enhanced aqueous stability of quantum dots and in vivo imaging. Chem Sci 4:411–417
60. Palui G, Na HB, Mattoussi H (2012) Poly (ethylene glycol)-based multidentate oligomers for biocompatible semiconductor and gold nanocrystals. Langmuir 28:2761–2772
61. Susumu K, Oh E, Delehanty JB, Blanco-Canosa JB, Johnson BJ, Jain V, Hervey WJ, Algar WR, Boeneman K, Dawson PE, Medintz IL (2011) Multifunctional compact zwitterionic ligands for preparing robust biocompatible semiconductor quantum dots and gold nanoparticles. J Am Chem Soc 133:9480–9496
62. Stewart MH, Susumu K, Mei BC, Medintz IL, Delehanty JB, Blanco-Canosa JB, Dawson PE, Mattoussi H (2010) Multidentate poly(ethylene glycol) ligands provide colloidal stability to semiconductor and metallic nanocrystals in extreme conditions. J Am Chem Soc 132:9804–9813
63. Muro E, Pons T, Lequeux N, Fragola A, Sanson N, Lenkei Z, Dubertret B (2010) Small and stable sulfobetaine zwitterionic quantum dots for functional live-cell imaging. J Am Chem Soc 132:4556–4557
64. Mei BC, Susumu K, Medintz IL, Delehanty JB, Mountziaris TJ, Mattoussi H (2008) Modular poly(ethylene glycol) ligands for biocompatible semiconductor and gold nanocrystals with extended pH and ionic stability. J Mater Chem 18:4949–4958

Chapter 5

Preparation and Characterization of Magnetic Nano-in-Microparticles for Pulmonary Delivery

Amber A. McBride*, Dominique N. Price*, and Pavan Muttil

Abstract

The purpose of this chapter is to detail the formulation and characterization of a magnetically-targeted drug delivery vehicle, termed nano-in-microparticles (NIMs), for pulmonary drug delivery. Currently, chemotherapeutics and antibiotics are delivered systemically and result in whole body side-effects. NIMs are formulated with superparamagnetic iron oxide nanoparticles, termed SPIONs, making these particles targetable to specific lung regions using a strong external magnet. Additionally, these particles can be formulated to contain any drug or therapeutic agent, such that a therapeutic dose can be delivered to a specific tissue location using the SPIONs-magnet interaction. Finally, these particles are in the appropriate size range for pulmonary delivery, making NIMs therapeutics feasibly inhalable.

To generate these particles a solution containing lactose, SPIONs, and a microsphere dye (used as a drug surrogate) is spray-dried using a laboratory-scale spray dryer. The resulting dry powder microparticles (NIMs) can be characterized for their size and morphological properties by various techniques that are presented in this chapter.

The utility of NIMs as a magnetic field-dependent targeting delivery platform in an in vivo mouse model has been demonstrated, and a protocol detailing the intratracheal delivery of NIMs dry powder is included as a separate chapter in this book.

Key words Spray drying, Iron oxide nanoparticles, Nano-in-microparticles, Dry powders, Pulmonary delivery

1 Introduction

1.1 Spray Drying for Dry Powder Manufacturing

Spray drying in simplest terms, is a method of converting liquid solutions/ suspensions into solid dry powders. The technique originated in the food manufacturing industry, giving perishable foods like milk a longer shelf-life. However, since the 1990s spray drying has become a well-recognized laboratory technique to create pharmaceutical dry powders compatible for pulmonary delivery [1].

*These authors contributed equally to this work.

Reema Zeineldin (ed.), *Cancer Nanotechnology: Methods and Protocols*, Methods in Molecular Biology, vol. 1530, DOI 10.1007/978-1-4939-6646-2_5,

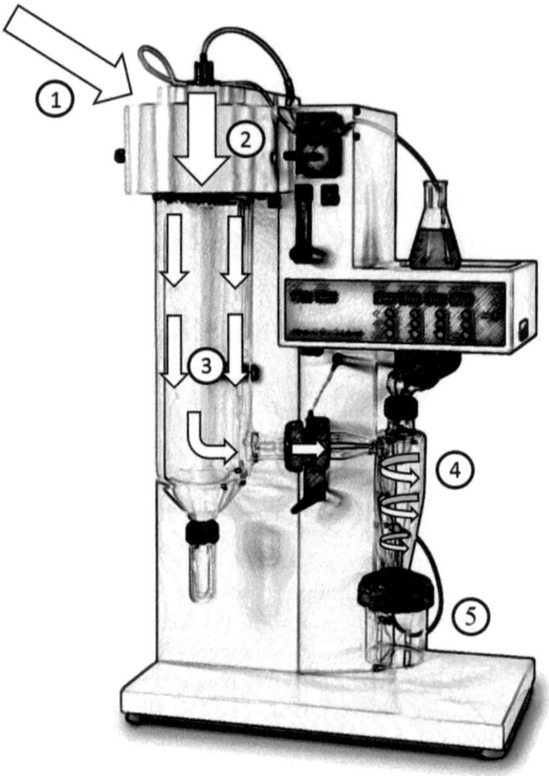

Fig. 1 A stepwise mechanism of the spray drying process. Nitrogen gas is heated to temperatures of 50–220 °C, depending on the sample that is being spray-dried (*circle 1*). The sample solution/suspension is sprayed into droplets by the nozzle of the spray drier (*circle 2*), and these droplets are dried into powders as they fall through the drying chamber (*circle 3*). The powders are separated based on inertial forces as they move through the cyclone (*circle 4*) and are collected in the collecting chamber (*circle 5*)

Spray drying is a visible process, meaning a significant portion of the spray drier consists of glassware making the entire procedure observable. The drying process begins at the nozzle, with the atomization of a feed solution, and culminates with the production of dried powders collected in the lower collection vessel. Figure 1 shows a schematic of a typical spray dryer. First, the inlet air of the spray dryer is heated to temperatures ranging between 50 °C and 220 °C (maximum) depending on the materials being spray-dried (Fig. 1—circle 1). Next, the nozzle sprays fine droplets formed from the spray drying solution/suspension (Fig. 1—circle 2). Conductive heat is exchanged between the spray gas (compressed nitrogen required to disperse the solution/ suspension) and the sample droplets in the drying chamber (Fig. 1—circle 3). The dry powders are collected in the particle collection chamber attached to the cyclone, which separates the powders from the drying medium based on its inertial forces (Fig. 1—circle 4 & 5).

Compared to other methods of powder manufacturing like milling or lyophilization, spray drying yields dry powders with good aerodynamic properties (e.g., flow, dispersibility, and particle size) and offers more control over their physicochemical properties because variables like droplet atomization, drying dynamics, and liquid properties can be optimized. Operation variables can be manipulated through interrelated parameters such as the inlet air temperature, the drying air flow rate (aspirator), the liquid feed rate, the spray flow rate (nitrogen gas), as well as percent solids in the solution/ suspension [2]. In addition, spray drying can be easily scaled up to produce large batches of powders. Volumes between 20 and 1000 mL can be spray-dried in approximately 1 h.

Lastly, dry powders can be formulated with various excipients (polymers, sugars, and/ or amino acids) for either controlled release or as a stabilizing agent to the encapsulated materials [3, 4]. Spray drying of excipients such as L-leucine or polymorphic forms of drugs could result in corrugated particles that have improved dispersion behavior [5–7].

1.2 Brief History of Therapeutic Targeting in the Lung

Inhaled aerosols have emerged as an area of interest for the administration of chemotherapeutic agents to the lung [8–10]. Otterson et al. administered inhaled doxorubicin in a phase I clinical study and later in a phase I/II clinical study; however, pulmonary dose-limiting toxicity was observed due to the delivery of a cytotoxic agent directly into the lung [8, 9]. Magnetic targeting has the potential to make aerosolized chemotherapy administered by the pulmonary route more effective by concentrating the inhaled drug at a target site within the respiratory tract. This has been shown through various in vitro and numerical models and in vivo magnetic targeting studies in efforts to limit exposure of healthy lung and airway tissue to the drug [11]. Magnetic field-dependent targeted delivery of drug-containing or surrogate vehicles to specific regions of the model airways in vitro has been demonstrated previously by us and others [11–15]. Dames et al. and Rudolph et al. targeted nebulized micron-sized magnetic droplets containing iron oxide nanoparticles and plasmid DNA, a therapeutic mimic, to specific regions in a mouse lung [11, 16]. Although significant deposition was shown in the magnetized lung lobe, separation of plasmid DNA from the iron oxide nanoparticles was observed during the delivery process.

1.3 Superparamagnetic Iron Oxide Nanoparticles (SPIONs)

SPIONs are small synthetic Fe_3O_4 particles with core sizes ranging between 5 and 99 nm in diameter. SPIONs consist of a single (individual) magnetic domain of elements that can be aligned in the presence of an external magnetic field allowing for magnetic field-dependent targeting, hyperthermia-induced cancer cell death, or MRI resonance imaging. The single domain nature of SPIONs causes demagnetization immediately after the removal of the magnetic field. SPIONs have unique physical and chemical features such as a large surface area to mass ratio, which make them ideal for ligand attachment or for the delivery of cargo payload [17].

1.4 Nano-in-Microparticle (NIMs) Characterization

To verify that dry powder NIMs are of the appropriate size, aerodynamic diameter, and morphology for deep lung delivery, we have compiled a list of the various characterization methods. Although protocols for the characterization methods listed below are merely mentioned and not detailed at length, we thought it was important to mention their use and importance. Examples of characterization data for NIMs size and size distribution are listed in detail later in this chapter.

1. *Size and size distribution*: NIMs size (micrometer) based on volume equivalent diameter can be characterized using a laser diffraction particle sizer. This instrument determines the particle size of dry powders based on laser obscuration and scattering. SPIONs size (nanometer) can be measured by dynamic light scattering (DLS) instruments.
2. *Aerodynamic sizing*: The determination of the mass median aerodynamic diameter (MMAD) is one of the most important characterization parameters in terms of particle deposition in the lung. MMAD and geometric standard deviation (GSD; the spread of the particle size distribution) for particles are determined in vitro by cascade impaction studies. Fine particle fraction (FPF) is also determined using the impactor and is defined as the percentage of particles in the respirable size range of 1–5 μm [18].
3. *Moisture uptake*: Hygroscopicity is the intrinsic tendency of a dry powder to absorb moisture from its surroundings [18]. Moisture uptake can result in local dissolution and recrystallization, leading to irreversible aggregation through solid bridge formation, which can adversely affect powder deagglomeration during aerosol generation and ultimately lung deposition [19]. Moisture uptake can be quantified using a Karl Fischer (KF) coulometric titration. Dynamic Vapor Sorption (DVS) can also be used to determine moisture uptake in dry powder formulations.
4. *Glass transition temperature (T_g):* Differential scanning calorimetry (DSC) is used to measure the T_g of the excipients. An excipient with a high T_g will remain amorphous during the spray drying process. Furthermore, if these powders are stored at a temperature lower than its T_g, it slows the transitioning into the crystalline form.
5. *Drug release and dissolution properties*: Drug release profiles are critical for inhaled drugs in order to evaluate the pharmacokinetic profile and hence the bioavailability of the drug.

6. *Surface characteristics*: Scanning electron microscopy (SEM) is used to determine particle size and surface morphology of dry powders.
7. *X-ray diffraction (XRD)*: XRD can be used to determine bond lengths and bond angles defined by intermolecular spacing, which is directly related to crystalline properties of the material. Therefore, XRD is used to measure the crystalline or amorphous state of excipients after spray drying.
8. *Determination of metal content*: Inductively Coupled Plasma—Atomic Emission Spectroscopy (ICP-AES) is an analytical technique that can be used for the detection of metal, for example the SPIONs (Fe_3O_4), in the NIMs drug delivery vehicle.
9. *Superconducting Quantum Interference Device (SQUID) analysis*: SQUID analysis can be used to measure the magnetic properties of NIMs. These measurements allow the user to calculate the magnetic moment of the SPIONs as well as the concentration of SPIONs in the NIMs.

This chapter details methodologies involved in the preparation of NIMs dry powders, a novel therapeutic targeting platform. The dry powders are created using unique excipients that are spray-dried, resulting in powders that are respirable, magnetically-targetable, and temperature-stable. The implications of this technology are broad, with potential use in lung cancer therapeutics, and the treatment of other respiratory illnesses.

2 Materials

Prepare all solutions/ suspensions using ultrapure water and store all reagents and solutions/ suspensions at 4 °C unless otherwise noted. Diligently follow all waste disposal regulations when disposing of iron oxide nanoparticles and waste materials.

1. 2% solids (w/v) FluoroSpheres® fluorescent microsphere far red dye, nominal bead size: 0.02 μm, dark red fluorescent (λ 660 nm excitation, λ 680 nm emission).
2. 50 mg/mL SPIONs, 50 nm diameter.
3. 3 % (w/v) Lactose.
4. Mini Spray Dryer.
5. Laser diffraction particle sizer.
6. Dynamic light scattering nanoparticle sizer.

3 Methods

3.1 "Control Powder" Feed Solution Preparation

The control solution [20 mL of 3.0 % (w/v) lactose] is intended for feasibility studies to formulate dry powders for control purposes before formulating dry powder NIMs. Three grams of lactose is dissolved in 100 mL ultrapure water to make a 3 % (w/v) lactose feed solution. Spray drying 20 mL of this solution yields approximately 375 mg of dry powders (*see* **Note 1**).

1. Weigh 3 g lactose and add to a 100 mL volumetric flask.
2. Add ultrapure water to the fill line of the 100 mL volumetric flask.
3. Heat solution with stir bar at 50 °C or lowest setting for 5 min to aid lactose dissolution (*see* **Note 2**).
4. Aliquot 20 mL of lactose solution into a new 50 mL beaker. Cover with Parafilm.

   $20\ \text{mL of}\ [30\ \text{mg/mL}]$ lactose solution theoretically yields $=$ $600\ \text{mg}$ lactose solids

3.2 "Control Powder" Spray Drying Parameters

Set up the spray dryer in the chemical fume hood and spray dry according to the conditions listed in Table 1 (*see* **Notes 3–4**). While spray drying, take note of how much the actual spray drying parameters deviate from the input parameters of the spray dryer.

3.3 Powder Yield Calculation

1. Determine weight of collecting vial + cap before spray drying, for example:

   $\text{Vial\&capweight} = 161611\ \text{mg}$
2. Determine weight of collecting vial + cap + powder after spray drying, for example:

   $\text{Vial\&cap\&powderweight} = 161998\text{mg}$
3. Determine weight of powder by subtracting the weight determined in 2 from 1:

Table 1
Parameter settings for spray-drying

Parameter type	Input parameters	Actual parameters (example)
Inlet temperature	190 °C	190 ± 2 °C
Outlet temperature	50 °C°	50 ± 2 °C (*see* **Note 3**)
Aspirator	90 %	90 %
Feed rate	10 %	10 %
Filter pressure gauge	−50 mbar	−62 mbar
Nitrogen Q flow	63 mmbar	63 mmbar (742 L/h)
Filter used	PTFE (Teflon)	

Table 2
Example laser diffraction measurements for particle sizing

Sizing measurements analysis type	Example measurements (in triplicate)		
$D_{v,50}$	2.66μm	2.73 μm	2.73 μm
$D_{v,90}$	6.75 μm	7.00 μm	6.77 μm
Diameter span = $[(D_{v,90}-D_{v,10})/D_{v,50}]$	2.24 μm	2.29 μm	2.21 μm
$D_{[3,2]}$	1.56 μm	1.52 μm	1.51 μm
$D_{v,10}$	0.78 μm	0.75 μm	0.74 μm

$$\text{Powderweight} = 161998 \text{ mg} - 161611 \text{ mg} = 387 \text{ mg}$$

4. Calculate percent yield using the formula:

$$\frac{\text{Weight of powder}}{\text{Weight of solids in original solution}} \times 100$$

$$\frac{387 \text{ mg final powder weight}}{600 \text{ mg starting solution solids weight}} \times 100 = 64.5\%$$

3.4 Microparticle Size Characterization

Characterize microparticle (control powder) size using a laser diffraction system. Microparticle size measurements should be performed in triplicates. *See* example measurements in Table 2.

3.5 NIMs Feed Solution Calculation

The NIMs suspension [20 mL containing a dye (drug surrogate)] is used to make dry powder NIMs. The suspension is comprised of 20.0 % (w/w) SPIONs, 10.0 % (w/w) fluorospheres far red dye, and 70.0 % (w/w) lactose for a total of 500 mg total solids or 2.5 % w/v spray drying suspension. Total solids are calculated below:

1. Calculate total solids weight first:

$$20 \text{ mL suspension } \times 2.5\ \% \left(\frac{w}{v}\right) = 20 \text{ mL } \times \frac{25 \text{ mg}}{\text{mL}}$$
$$= 500 \text{ mg total solids}$$

2. Lactose

$$\frac{350 \text{ mg of lactose}}{500 \text{ mg total solids}} \left(\frac{w}{w}\right) = 70\% \text{ Lactose}$$

3. SPIONs

$$2\text{mL of SPIONs}\left[\frac{50\text{mg}}{\text{mL}}\right] = 100\text{mg} = \frac{100 \text{ mg SPIONs}}{500 \text{ mg total solids}} \left(\frac{w}{w}\right)$$
$$= 20\% \text{ SPIONs}$$

4. Dye

$$2.5\text{mL of dye}\left[\frac{20\text{mg}}{\text{mL}}\right] = 50\text{mg} = \frac{50\text{ mg of dye}}{500\text{ mg total solids}}\left(\frac{w}{w}\right)$$
$$= 10\%\text{ Dye}$$

3.6 NIMs Feed Solution Preparation

1. Weigh 350 mg lactose and add to 5.0 mL ultrapure water in 50 mL beaker.
2. Mix using a vortex—mixer and a sonication bath 2.5 mL of the dye solution and add it to the solution from **step 1**. The resulting total volume is 7.5 mL.
3. Add 2 mL SPIONs to the lactose solution, resulting in 9.5 mL total volume.
4. Add another 10.5 mL of water to bring the final volume up to 20 mL. Cover with parafilm and label the flask.
5. Weigh a collecting vial and note its weight.

3.7 NIMs Spray Drying Protocol

1. Use the same spray dryer parameters that were used to prepare the control powder, shown in Table 1 (*see* **Notes 3–5**). While spray drying take note of how much the actual spray drying parameters deviate from the input parameters.
2. Note powder characteristics: Particles that collect on the sides of the cyclone could be agglomerates.
3. Calculate powder yield percentage as performed before with control powder and described in Subheading 3.3.

3.8 Microparticle Size Characterization

Characterize NIMs size using a laser diffraction system as done previously with control dry powder. Microparticle size measurements should be performed in triplicates. See example measurements in Table 2 (*see* **Notes 6–8**).

3.9 Spray Dryer Cleaning Protocol

1. Wear necessary personal protective equipment.
2. Run soapy water solution through spray dryer (three drops soap + 1 gal water).
3. Spray dry soapy water solution for 15–20 min.
4. Spray dry water solution for 15–20 min.
5. Spray dry 70 % ethanol for 15–20 min.
6. Clean walls and floor of chemical fume hood with soapy water and disposable towels.
7. Wipe walls, chemical fume hood ledge, and floor with dry disposable towel.

4 Notes

1. Many parameters affect actual powder yield. Generally between 50–70% of solids are recovered in the collection chamber. The spray drying process is quick; on average the time to spray dry 20 mLs of a solution/ suspension is about 10–15 minutes.
2. The solubility of alpha-monohydrate lactose in water is 21.9 g in 100 mL in water (21 % w/v). The saturation solubility of the excipient needs to be taken into account when making a spray drying solution/ suspension.
3. Water condenses inside the spray drying chamber at outlet temperatures $\leq$ 35 °C when spray drying an aqueous solution/suspension. This can introduce moisture into the final dry powder product. Therefore, the spray dryer needs to be completely dry and run at outlet temperatures > 35 °C before formulating any dry powders.
4. The exhaust hose of the chemical hood, that houses the spray dryer, can be connected to a modified HEPA filter that is exhausted to outside air.
5. During the spray drying process, some solids are inherently trapped in the filter causing a decrease in the powder yield. In the case of dry powder NIMs, SPIONs were visibly trapped in the filter.
6. Laser diffraction particle sizing SOP notes: Assume non-spherical particle geometry and make sure to input lactose density, absorptivity, and refractive index (1.52 g/cm^3, 0.010, and 1.347, respectively), SPION density (1.55 g/cm^3), and dye density (1.05 g/cm^3) into the analysis software to insure correct sizing calculations.
7. Larger particle size obtained using the laser diffraction technique is due to the agglomeration of the microparticles. Dispersive energy (0–4 bar) is applied during dry powder particle sizing (when using a powder disperser attachment to the laser diffraction particle sizer) to break particle agglomerates. However, dry dispersion may sometimes not be suitable for sizing microparticles due to the strong particle–particle cohesive attraction that may be difficult to overcome. Care should also be taken that sufficient dispersive energy is applied to the microparticles to obtain particle deagglomeration, while not breaking the microparticles into smaller particles. In cases where particles are difficult to deagglomerate, wet dispersion method could be used.
8. More information about the preparation and characterization of NIMs can be found in our 2013 American Chemical Society (ACS) Molecular Pharmaceutics publication [12].

Acknowledgment

This research was supported by the University of New Mexico Health Science Center Research and Allocations Committee (RAC) grant. AAM was supported by NSF-IGERT Integrating Nanotechnology with Cell Biology and Neuroscience Fellowship (DGE-0549500) and the NCI Alliance for Nanotechnology in Cancer New Mexico CNTC Training Center. DNP was supported by the Bill and Melinda Gates Grand Challenge Exploration (No OPP1061393) and UNM IDIP T32 training grant (T32-A1007538, P.I. – M. Ozbun).

References

1. Chan HK, Chew NYK (2003) Novel alternative methods for the delivery of drugs for the treatment of asthma. Adv Drug Deliv Rev 55:793–805
2. Cal K, Sollohub K (2010) Spray drying technique: I: hardware and process parameters. J Pharm Sci 99:575–586. doi:10.1002/jps.21886
3. O'Hagan DT, Rahman D, McGee JP et al (1991) Biodegradable microparticles as controlled release antigen delivery systems. Immunology 73:239–242
4. O'Hagan DT, Rappuoli R (2004) Novel approaches to vaccine delivery. Pharm Res 21:1519–1530. doi:10.1023/B:PHAM.0000041443.17935.33
5. Hoppentocht M, Hagedoorn P, Frijlink HW, de Boer AH (2014) Technological and practical challenges of dry powder inhalers and formulations. Adv Drug Deliv Rev 75:18–31. doi:10.1016/j.addr.2014.04.004
6. Son Y-J, McConville JT (2011) A new respirable form of rifampicin. Eur J Pharm Biopharm 78:366–376. doi:10.1016/j.ejpb.2011.02.004
7. Son Y-J, McConville JT (2012) Preparation of sustained release rifampicin microparticles for inhalation. J Pharm Pharmacol 64:1291–1302. doi:10.1111/j.2042-7158.2012.01531.x
8. Otterson GA, Villalona-Calero MA, Sharma S et al (2007) Phase I study of inhaled doxorubicin for patients with metastatic tumors to the lungs. Clin Cancer Res 13:1246–1252. doi:10.1158/1078-0432.CCR-06-1096
9. Otterson GA, Villalona-Calero MA, Hicks W et al (2010) Phase I/II study of inhaled doxorubicin combined with platinum-based therapy for advanced non-small cell lung cancer. Clin Cancer Res 16:2466–2473. doi:10.1158/1078-0432.CCR-09-3015
10. Rao R, Markovic S, Anderson P (2003) Aerosol therapy for malignancy involving the lungs. Curr Cancer Drug Targets 3:239–250. doi:10.2174/1568009033481895
11. Dames P, Gleich B, Flemmer A et al (2007) Targeted delivery of magnetic aerosol droplets to the lung. Nat Nanotechnol 2:495–499. doi:10.1038/nnano.2007.217
12. McBride AA, Price DN, Lamoureux LR et al (2013) Preparation and characterization of novel magnetic nano-in-microparticles for site-specific pulmonary drug delivery. Mol Pharm 10:3574–3581. doi:10.1021/mp3007264
13. Tewes F, Ehrhardt C, Healy AM (2014) Superparamagnetic iron oxide nanoparticles (SPIONs)-loaded Trojan microparticles for targeted aerosol delivery to the lung. Eur J Pharm Biopharm 86:98–104. doi:10.1016/j.ejpb.2013.09.004
14. Ally J, Martin B, Behrad Khamesee M et al (2005) Magnetic targeting of aerosol particles for cancer therapy. J Magn Magn Mater 293:442–449. doi:10.1016/j.jmmm.2005.02.038
15. Xie Y, Longest PW, Xu YH et al (2010) In vitro and in vivo lung deposition of coated magnetic aerosol particles. J Pharm Sci 99:4658–4668. doi:10.1002/jps.22168
16. Rudolph C, Gleich B, Flemmer AW (2010) Magnetic aerosol targeting of nanoparticles to cancer: nanomagnetosols. Methods Mol Biol 624:267–280. doi:10.1007/978-1-60761-609-2_18
17. De Jong WH, Borm PJA (2008) Drug delivery and nanoparticles: applications and hazards. Int J Nanomedicine 3:133–149
18. Telko MJ, Hickey AJ (2005) Dry powder inhaler formulation. Respir Care 50:1209–1227
19. Braun M (1996) Influence of excipients and storage humidity on the deposition of disodium cromoglycate (DSCG) in the twin impinger. Int J Pharm 135:53–62. doi:10.1016/0378-5173(95)04337-3

Chapter 6

Multifunctionalization of Gold Nanoshells

Sandra W. Bishnoi and Yujen Lin

Abstract

Gold silica nanoshells have found many applications within the field of molecular biology, including as nanoscale sensors, the detection of biomarkers, and in the treatment of solid tumors using photothermal ablation. In order for them to be targeted to specific biomarkers while also remaining stable in biological media, it is often necessary to modify their surfaces with more than one functional group. Here, we describe how to create multifunctional gold nanoshells that can be used to either target specific tumor types in vivo or for the detection of biomarkers using biological specimen.

Key words Gold nanoshells, Raman spectroscopy, Polyethylene glycol, Biomarker detection, Cancer targeting, Nitrocellulose membrane

1 Introduction

It is well accepted that gold nanoshells can be used in the treatment of solid tumors [1–5] or in the detection of many different chemical species [6, 7] due to their unique optical properties. The excitement of surface plasmons by electromagnetic radiation within the near infrared region has shown specific applicability for biological applications due to the "water window" that limits the undesirable absorption by proteins and other biomolecules within the vicinity of the nanoshells [1, 8–10]. The excitement of these surface plasmons can be used to deliver cargo off of the nanoparticle surface [11, 12], provide localized thermal ablation to tumors [4, 13, 14], or be used for surface enhanced Raman scattering (SERS) detection of biomarkers [6, 15]. For any of these applications to be successful, you must modify the nanoparticle surface to improve its compatibility in biological media (buffers, blood, etc.). The most common type of surface modification is the grafting of polyethylene glycol (PEG) [16, 17] to the surface of the nanoparticle through the formation of a gold-sulfur (Au-S) covalent bond using thiolated PEGs. PEG allows the particles to remain in circulation for longer

Reema Zeineldin (ed.), *Cancer Nanotechnology: Methods and Protocols*, Methods in Molecular Biology, vol. 1530,
DOI 10.1007/978-1-4939-6646-2_6, © Springer Science+Business Media New York 2017

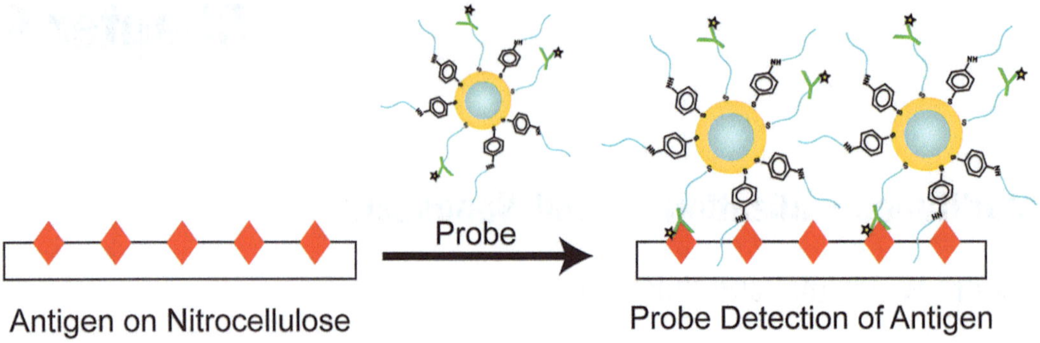

Fig. 1 Schematic of multifunctional gold nanoshells using a mixed monolayer of Raman-active polyethylene glycol and an immobilized recognition antibody bound to the particle surface. The particle's activity is then tested using a half-sandwich assay of antigen immobilized on nitrocellulose membranes

periods of time in vivo and prevents their flocculation in buffers to improve their shelf stability.

Gold nanoshells can also be modified with targeting agents (proteins, antibodies, peptides, etc.) that will allow specific delivery to a tumor or the detection of biomarkers of interest [2, 17]. In order to obtain successful targeting while maintaining their solution stability, it is often critical to control the ratio of PEG to targeting agent on the nanoparticle surface. In this chapter, we describe the surface modification of gold nanoshells, including the synthesis of a Raman active PEG [6, 16] and biofunctionalization of an antibody with a thiol that can be used to bind to the gold surface [6]. The surface of the gold nanoshell is then modified with a targeting agent (secondary antibody), as well as a Raman-active PEG that can be used to detect the presence of biomarkers in biological media (tears, sweat, blood, and urine) using Raman microscopy. Raman microscopy is used to verify the grafting of the Raman-active PEG to the nanoparticle surface by monitoring the ring breathing mode at 1090 cm^{-1}. By creating a half-sandwich assay on a nitrocellulose membrane (Fig. 1), we can determine the success of antibody conjugation to the nanoshells surface by visual inspection (at high concentrations of antigen) and through SERS (at low concentrations of antigen).

2 Materials

Prepare all solutions using ultrapure water (prepared by deionizing water to have a resistance of 18 MΩ at room temperature). Store reagents and products at 4 °C, unless otherwise specified.

1. 100 mM Phosphate buffer (PB), pH 8.0: 0.462 g of monosodium phosphate monohydrate and 0.462 g of monosodium

phosphate monohydrate in 500 mL water. Adjust pH to 8.0 using either 1 M HCl or 1 M NaOH.

2. 1.8 mM carbonate buffer: 50 mg of potassium carbonate in 200 mL of water.
3. Commercial nanoshells or in-house nanoshells that may be synthesized according to published procedures [8].
4. Tris buffer saline (TBS): 3.0 g Tris(hydroxymethyl)aminomethane (Tris) and 4.4 g NaCl in 400 mL of water. Adjust pH to 7.5 with 1 M HCl and make volume up to 500 mL with water.
5. TBS Tween-20 (TBST): 5 mL of Tween-20 into 500 mL TBS. Store solution at 4 °C for up to 3 months.
6. Blocking buffer: 5 % (w/v) bovine serum albumin (BSA) in TBST.
7. Dimethyl sulfoxide (DMSO).
8. *Para*-mercapto aniline (pMA).
9. Orthopyridyl disulfide-polyethylene glycol 5000-*n*-hydroxysuccinimide (OPSS-PEG5000-NHS).
10. Nitrocellulose membranes (0.2 μm pore size).
11. 11.3 mg/mL Whole molecule Rabbit IgG.
12. 2.2 mg/mL Fluorescein (FITC)-conjugated AffiniPure Goat Anti-Rabbit IgG.

3 Methods

3.1 Synthesis of Raman Active PEG

1. Dissolve 5 mg of *p*-mercaptoaniline (125.19 MW, 0.04 mmol) in 50 mL of DMSO in a round-bottom flask.
2. To synthesize the Raman active PEG *para*-mecrcapto aniline-polyethylene glycol (pMA-PEG), methoxypolyethylene glycol succinate *N*-hydroxysuccinimide (NHS-PEG(5000), 5000 MW, dissolve 65 mg, 0.013 mmol) in 50 μL of dimethyl sulfoxide (DMSO), then add it slowly to the *p*-mercaptoaniline prepared in **step 1**.
3. Close the flask tightly to prevent evaporation and stir overnight at room temperature.
4. The next day, place the resulting product into a 2K molecular weight cut-off (MWCO) dialysis cartridge.
5. Place the dialysis cartridge into a clean 250 mL beaker containing 200 mL of 100 mM, pH 8.0 PB and a magnetic stir bar and dialyze overnight (*see* **Note 1**).

6. The next day, remove the purified product from the dialysis cartridge using a clean needle and syringe and place it into a 50 mL conical disposable centrifuge tube.

Store aliquots of the purified product at −20 °C until needed. Product remains stable for up to 6 months.

3.2 Synthesis of Thiol-PEG-2° Antibody Conjugate

1. Warm orthopyridyl disulfide-PEG-*n*-hydroxysuccinimide (OPSS-PEG-NHS) 5K to room temperature.
2. Carefully weigh 1.5 mg of OPSS-PEG-NHS into a disposable microcentrifuge tube.
3. Add 1 mL of potassium carbonate buffer to achieve a final OPSS-PEG-NHS concentration of 1.5 mg/mL.
4. Mix the solution completely using a vortex.
5. Add 10 μL of this solution immediately to 490 μL of recognition antibody (Goat Anti-Rabbit IgG) dissolved in potassium carbonate buffer (450 μg total antibody) (*see* **Note 2**).
6. Gently mix the solution and then react overnight on ice.
7. The next day, remove excess OPSS-PEG-NHS by placing the antibody conjugate in a Nanosep 100k Omega spin column.
8. Centrifuge the column at 5000 RCF for 5–10 min.
9. Discard flow-through.
10. Resuspend the conjugate (OPSS-PEG-Goat-anti-Rabbit IgG) to a final volume of 500 μL to make a final concentration of 0.9 mg/mL.
11. Aliquot the conjugate and store at −20 °C until needed. The conjugate is stable for up to 6 months.

3.3 Characterization of Gold Nanoshells

1. Characterize the nanoshells using dynamic light scattering to determine their average hydrodynamic diameter and polydispersity.
2. Measure UV–Vis spectrophotometry between 500 and 1000 nm to ensure that the wavelength of maximum absorption (extinction) is near that of the excitation laser on the Raman spectrometer (785 nm) (*see* **Notes 3** and **4**).

3.4 Multi-functionalization of Nanoshells

1. Add 6 μL of antibody conjugate (0.9 mg/mL) to 1 mL of nanoshell solution (λ_{max} ~ 780 nm, Abs = 1.5, ~3 × 10^9 NS/mL) and incubate overnight on ice to allow sufficient antibody coverage on the nanoshell surface.

2. To this solution, add 30 μL of Raman-active PEG (*see* **Note 5**) at a concentration of 1×10^{-4} M to obtain a final Raman chromophore concentration of 3×10^{-6} M.
3. Incubate this solution for 25 min on ice prior to purification by centrifugation.
4. Centrifuge the nanoshell-containing solution at 605 RCF for 6 min and then resuspended in MQ water.

3.5 Testing of PEG Attachment

1. Confirm the Raman activity of each probe synthesized by spotting 10 μL of the probe onto a quartz slide and testing the Raman intensity in a Raman microscope with a 785 nm laser at 1078 cm^{-1}, corresponding to the ring breathing mode of pMA-PEG.
2. The intensity of this peak is dependent on the coverage of pMA on the particle surface (*see* **Note 6**).

3.6 Testing of Antibody Attachment to the Gold Nanoshells

1. Create antigen (Rabbit IgG) spots on a nitrocellulose membrane (NC) by depositing 2 μL of diluted antigen (Rabbit IgG) onto a NC membrane stacked onto filter paper (*see* **Notes 7** and **8**).
2. Dry spots on the bench for 15 min. Draw a circle around the spot with pencil to indicate where the antigen has been immobilized.
3. Immerse the NC membrane in blocking buffer and agitate for 45 min.
4. Remove membranes and immediately place in a solution containing the multifunctional gold NS (3×10^{9} NS/mL).
5. Rock membranes in the probe solution for 35 min to prevent probe sedimentation and then wash using a soft stream of room temperature water to remove excess probe.
6. Immerse membranes in cold TBST and agitate on an orbital shaker for 15 min to remove nonspecifically bound nanoshell probe. Repeat the washing process as necessary. Store membranes at 4 °C until spectral analysis (*see* **Notes 9** and **10**).

4 Notes

1. Several vendors now sell gold nanoshells that absorb in the near IR. Though the exact wavelength is not always critical for all applications, if you are coupling them with a laser you want the plasmon resonance to be near the laser wavelength.

2. Be sure to use your gold nanoshells when they are fresh (<1 week old) or if you are using commercially available particles obtain samples that have been certified to be free of endotoxins and in which excess reactants have been removed because they will be easier to functionalize. The best things to do before using your gold nanoshells are to verify that they are stable using zeta potential (should have a surface charge of ~−40 mV) and that their shell is complete using scanning electron microscopy. Incomplete shells will not be stable for very long and have a tendency to aggregate over time.
3. The dialysis serves two functions: (1) remove excess pMA from the product that will compete for surface sites on the nanoshell surface and (2) transfer the product into phosphate buffer from the original DMSO solvent.
4. When working with NHS-functionalized groups, care should be taken in measuring out the NHS containing compounds. NHS can easily undergo hydrolysis, so be sure to warm vials up to room temperature before opening to prevent condensation of water. In addition, measure masses quickly to limit exposure to water.
5. Alternatively, a commercially available Poly(ethylene glycol) methyl ether thiol (mPEG-thiol) can be used instead of the Raman-active PEG.
6. To determine ideal surface coverage of pMA-PEG on the nanoshell surface, standards can be created by adding different amounts of pMA to the nanoshells to get a peak intensity standard curve. This will allow you to estimate the total amount of pMA on the particle surface [18].
7. Several different nitrocellulose membranes were tested. The best results were obtained with membranes with a 200 nm pore size.
8. Antigen dilutions ranged from 10 ng/mL to 1 μg/mL.
9. At higher antigen concentrations (over 100 ng/mL), the positive spot is visible to the eye and appears a faint green dot within the penciled circle.
10. Spectral mapping can be conducted with a Raman microscope equipped with a 785 nm laser. Spectra of the antigen spot are collected within the range of 1070–1090 cm^{-1} every 250 μm across the spot. The intensities are converted to a heat map of the spot to determine analyte detection (Fig. 2).

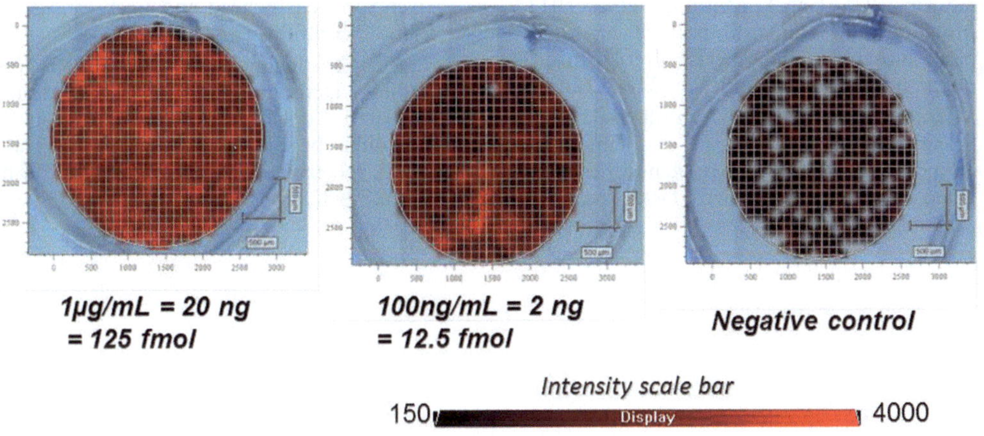

Fig. 2 Results of Half-Sandwich Assays. Raman microscopy imaging of nitrocellulose membrane containing two concentrations of rabbit IgG (1 μg/mL and 100 ng/mL) and a negative control spot (PBS). 20 μL of sample is applied to each spot in 2 μL increments. Spectra are collected in a backscattered geometry through a 20× (Numerical aperture is 0.40) microscope objective. The excitation source is a 785 nm diode laser (8 mW laser power at sample) with a spot size of 8 μm. The spectrometer is routinely calibrated with a silicon wafer. Data is collected using 100 % laser power, 1 s integration time, 20× objective, step size = 250 μm, for a total of 501 data points. Signal between 1070 and 1090 cm^{-1} is integrated and plotted as an intensity map

References

1. Bardhan R, Lal S, Joshi A et al (2011) Theranostic nanoshells: from probe design to imaging and treatment of cancer. Acc Chem Res 44:936–946
2. Chen W, Bardhan R, Bartels M et al (2010) A molecularly targeted theranostic probe for ovarian cancer. Mol Cancer Ther 9:1028–1038
3. Ayala-Orozco C, Urban C, Knight MW et al (2014) Au nanomatryoshkas as efficient near-infrared photothermal transducers for cancer treatment: benchmarking against nanoshells. ACS Nano 8:6372–6381
4. Hirsch LR, Stafford RJ, Bankson JA et al (2003) Nanoshell-mediated near-infrared thermal therapy of tumors under magnetic resonance guidance. Proc Natl Acad Sci U S A 100:13549–13554
5. O'Neal DP, Hirsch LR, Halas NJ et al (2004) Photo-thermal tumor ablation in mice using near infrared-absorbing nanoparticles. Cancer Lett 209:171–176
6. Bishnoi SW, Lin YJ, Tibudan M et al (2011) SERS biodetection using gold-silica nanoshells and nitrocellulose membranes. Anal Chem 83:4053–4060
7. Hirsch LR, Jackson JB, Lee A et al (2003) A whole blood immunoassay using gold nanoshells. Anal Chem 75:2377–2381
8. Oldenburg S, Averitt R, Westcott S et al (1998) Nanoengineering of optical resonances. Chem Phys Lett 288:243–247
9. Garcia MA (2012) Surface plasmons in metallic nanoparticles: fundamentals and applications. J Phys D Appl Phys 45:389501
10. Bishnoi SW, Rozell CJ, Levin CS et al (2006) All-optical nanoscale pH meter. Nano Lett 6:1687–1692
11. Huschka R, Barhoumi A, Liu Q et al (2012) Gene silencing by gold nanoshell-mediated delivery and laser-triggered release of antisense oligonucleotide and siRNA. ACS Nano 6:7681–7691
12. Huschka R, Neumann O, Barhoumi A et al (2010) Visualizing light-triggered release of molecules inside living cells. Nano Lett 10:4117–4122
13. Stern JM, Cadeddu JA (2008) Emerging use of nanoparticles for the therapeutic ablation of urologic malignancies. Urol Oncol 26:93–96
14. Chen C-L, Kuo L-R, Lee S-Y et al (2013) Photothermal cancer therapy via femtosecond-laser-excited FePt nanoparticles. Biomaterials 34:1128–1134
15. Huang Y, Swarup VP, Bishnoi SW (2009) Rapid Raman imaging of stable, functionalized nanoshells in mammalian cell cultures. Nano Lett 9:2914–2920

16. Swarup VP, Huang Y, Murillo G et al (2011) Modeling the cellular impact of nanoshell-based biosensors using mouse alveolar macrophage cultures. Metallomics 3:1218–1226
17. Melancon MP, Zhou M, Zhang R et al (2014) Selective uptake and imaging of aptamer- and antibody-conjugated hollow nanospheres targeted to epidermal growth factor receptors overexpressed in head and neck cancer. ACS Nano 8(5):4530–4538
18. Levin CS, Bishnoi SW, Grady NK et al (2006) Determining the conformation of thiolated poly(ethylene glycol) on Au nanoshells by surface-enhanced Raman scattering spectroscopic assay. Anal Chem 78:3277–3281

Chapter 7

Fabrication of Photothermal Stable Gold Nanosphere/Mesoporous Silica Hybrid Nanoparticle Responsive to Near-Infrared Light

Bei Cheng and Peisheng Xu

Abstract

Various gold nanoparticles have been explored in biomedical systems and proven to be promising in photothermal therapy and drug delivery. Among them, nanoshells were regarded as traditionally strong near infrared absorbers that have been widely used to generate photothermal effect for cancer therapy. However, the nanoshell is not photo-thermal stable and thus is not suitable for repeated irradiation. Here, we describe a novel discrete gold nanostructure by mimicking the continuous gold nanoshell—gold/mesoporous silica hybrid nanoparticle (GoMe). It possesses the best characteristics of both conventional gold nanoparticles and mesoporous silica nanoparticles, such as excellent photothermal converting ability as well as high drug loading capacity and triggerable drug release.

Key words Gold nanoparticle, Mesoporous silica nanoparticle, Redox responsive, Photothermal therapy

1 Introduction

Numerous gold nanostructures have been widely used in the biomedical field such as drug and gene delivery, disease screening and detection, treatment and response monitoring due to their excellent optical properties, high biocompatibility, and ease of surface modification [1–4]. The typical gold nanostructures include gold nanosphere (GNS), gold nanorod (GNR), gold nanoshell (GNSH), and gold nanocage (GNC). Among them, GNR, GNSH, and GNC have demonstrated a vast potential in converting the photon energy to heat. Upon irradiation, these gold nanoparticles could generate heat due to the localized surface plasmon resonance (LSPR) phenomenon [5–8].

The LSPR peak of GNR, GNSH, and GNC can be tuned toward the near-infrared (NIR) window (650–900 nm) through manipulating their physical shape, size, and geometry. The absorption in NIR window allows for a deeper penetration of various

Reema Zeineldin (ed.), *Cancer Nanotechnology: Methods and Protocols*, Methods in Molecular Biology, vol. 1530,
DOI 10.1007/978-1-4939-6646-2_7, © Springer Science+Business Media New York 2017

tissues and less blood absorbance interference [5]. The penetrated NIR radiation via gold nanoparticles can be transduced into intense local heat and can be applied for photothermal therapy. This noninvasive treatment strategy has boosted the applications in numerous systems and especially has proven to be promising in photothermal therapy and drug delivery. However, there are several inherent concerns preventing their translation from bench to clinical practice. Most importantly, their poor photothermal stability has limited the clinical application for photothermal therapy. Traditional gold nanoparticles gradually lose their photothermal converting capacity upon repetitive NIR irradiation. The shape and extinction of GNR, GNSH, and GNC get altered after repetitive NIR laser irradiation resulting in low heat generating capacity after each heating/cooling cycle if the generated heat could not be dissipated to their surrounding environment [9, 10]. Besides that, with the exception of GNCs, the majority of gold nanostructures are poor drug carriers, which is attributed to either a limited drug-loading capacity or uncontrolled drug release profile [11, 12]. Furthermore, it still remains challenging to use them to combine photothermal therapy with chemotherapy together, especially when a frequent medication is required during a full course treatment.

Similar to gold nanoparticles, mesoporous silica nanoparticles (MSNs) have attracted an increasing attention in their capability of loading vast drugs as well as their good biocompatibility [13]. MSNs have been extensively explored for biomedical applications, especially in drugs, proteins, peptides, DNAs, and siRNAs delivery. One of the most prominent challenges for these carriers is how to control the release behaviors of their payloads. Polyelectrolytes, macrocyclic organic molecules, and inorganic nanoparticles are among the broadly used gatekeepers to regulate the release kinetics [14–17]. As the function of these sensitive gatekeepers, even a slight physiological change such as pH and redox potential would trigger the delivery system and lead to the burst release of the payloads. Nevertheless, the in vivo drug release profile of MSNs is entirely counting on its fabrication process and biodistribution. In order to acquire a suitable drug carrier and a reliable photothermal converting agent, as well as to take advantage of the best of both worlds, we developed a gold/mesoporous silica hybrid nanoparticle (GoMe) through conjugating gold nanospheres (GNS) onto the surface of MSN [18]. Here, we describe a protocol about how to prepare a novel photothermal stable gold/mesoporous silica hybrid nanoparticle [19], which exhibits an excellent photothermal converting ability, high drug-loading capacity, and triggerable release.

2 Materials

All solutions are to be prepared using ultrapure water (prepared by deionizing water to attain a resistance of 18 MΩ cm).

The glassware is to be cleaned with base bath made by mixing 4 L isopropyl alcohol, 1 L H_2O, and 200 g KOH. Submerge the glassware in the bath for 24 h and rinse with deionized (DI) water before drying in an oven.

1. 0.54 % (w/v) Cysteamine hydrochloride solution.
2. 2 M Sodium hydroxide (NaOH) solution.
3. 0.2 % (w/v) Ethanoic solution of ammonium nitrate: dissolve NH_4NO_3 in ethanol solution at 2 mg/mL, sonicate the solution if necessary.
4. Aqua regia (hydrochloric acid:nitric acid = 3:1, V/V).

3 Methods

Conduct the following procedure at room temperature (r.t.) if not specified.

3.1 Synthesis MSN

1. Mix in a 100 mL round-bottom flask 50 mg of cetyl trimethylammonium bromide (CTAB) with 40 mg of Pluronic® F 127. Transfer 24 mL DI water to it.
2. Transfer 175 μL of 2 M NaOH to the above round-bottom flask. Heat the flask in oil-bath at 80 °C. Stir the solution at 1000 rpm for 30 min until the mixture become transparent (*see* **Note 1**).
3. Add 200 μL TEOS solution using a 1 mL syringe dropwise to the above flask while stirring at 1000 rpm. Immediately follow that by adding 20 μL MPTMS. A white precipitant will be formed within a few minutes upon addition. Heat and stir the mixture for 2 h at 80 °C (*see* **Note 2**).
4. Centrifuge the mixture at 16,000 rcf for 15 min. Remove the supernatant and resuspend the pellet in 20 mL DI water. Add 40 mg NH_4NO_3 to the suspension (so the concentration of NH_4NO_3 becomes 2 mg/mL). Stir the mixture at 500 rpm and incubate it at 50 °C for 2 h. Centrifuge the mixture at 16,000 rcf for 15 min and resuspend the pellet in ethanoic solution of NH_4NO_3. Repeat the washing process for three times to completely remove surfactant.
5. Collect the pellet and resuspend it in 20 mL ethanol. Centrifuge the mixture at 16,000 rcf for 15 min and remove the supernatant. Resuspend the pellet in DI water and collect the pellet. Wash the pellet with H_2O followed by ethanol for three

times. Centrifuge the mixture and collect the pellet. Suspend the pellet product in 2–3 mL ethanol and store at 4 °C prior to use (*see* **Note 3**).

3.2 Synthesis of Poly (ethylene glycol) Stabilized Gold Nanosphere (PEG-GNS)

1. Dissolve 12 mg gold(III) chloride trihydrate in 18 mL isopropyl alcohol. Add 0.2 mL acetic acid to the above solution (*see* **Note 4**).
2. Weight out 15.24 mg thiolated polyethylene glycol (Mw = 2000 Da) and disperse it in 2 mL isopropyl alcohol. Sonicate the poly(ethylene glycol) methyl ether thiol (PEG-SH) in the water bath sonicator until it is dispersed well. Add PEG-SH solution to the above solution from **step 1** and stir for 1 h.
3. Weight out 37.84 mg of sodium borohydride and dissolve it in 1.5 mL methanol. A lot of bubbles will be generated during dissolution. Pour the sodium borohydride solution to the mixture from **step 2** and leave to react for 24 h while preventing from light (*see* **Note 5**).
4. Separate the gold nanoparticle by precipitation in 80 mL cold hexane. Centrifuge at 2500 rcf for 30 min. Collect the pellets and disperse them in DI water. Wash the product with 20 mL DI H_2O for three times using a Millipore centricon (MWCO-10,000 Da). Each time the volume is concentrated from 20 mL to less than 1 mL. Disperse the final product in 10 mL DI water.

3.3 Synthesis of 2-(Pyridin-2-yldisulfanyl)Ethyl Acrylate Modified GNS (PDA-GNS)

1. Transfer 5 mL of PEG-GNS obtained from Subheading 3.2 in a 20 mL glass vial, and dilute with 5 mL H_2O. Transfer 40 μL of cysteamine hydrochloride solution to the above gold PEG-GNS. Stir the mixture for 24 h at room temperature.
2. Remove the unreacted cysteamine by washing three times with 10 mL DI water through a Millipore centricon (MWCO-10,000 Da) at the speed of 3000 rcf for 30 min. The final product is to be concentrated to around 100 μL through the centricon.
3. Dilute the gold nanoparticles at **step 2** with 500 μL DMSO. Dilute triethylamine with DMSO at a ratio of 1/100 (V/V) and transfer 26.5 μL of trimethylamine solution to the gold DMSO solution. Weight out monomer 2-(pyridin-2-yldisulfanyl)ethyl acrylate (PDA) and dissolve it in DMSO at a concentration of 0.918 mg/mL and add 50 μL of it to the above gold mixture.
4. Purge the whole mixture with pure N_2 for 20 min and stir at 50 °C for 24 h.
5. Add 1–2 mL isopropyl alcohol to dissolve the product. Sonicate the product in a water bath sonicator if any gold nanoparticle is attached on the wall. Add the isopropyl alcohol solution

to cold diethyl ether. GNS-PEG will precipitate out of diethyl ether and the pellet is to be collected. Repeat the precipitation for three times and resuspend the final product in 2 mL DI water (*see* **Note 6**).

3.4 Encapsulation of Doxorubicin (DOX) into MSN

1. Dissolve 10 mg of DOX·HCl in 200 μL DMSO and add with 50 μL trimethylamine. Incubate the mixture at r.t. for 30 min.
2. Suspend 18.6 mg MSN in 1 mL DMSO. Centrifuge the MSN solution at 12,000 rcf for 10 min. Remove the supernatant and resuspend the pellet in 1 mL DMSO solution.
3. Add DOX solution to MSN suspension and sonicate the mixture for 30 min to obtain a uniform dispersion. Stir the mixture for 24 h at r.t.
4. Separate unreacted DOX by centrifugation at 12,000 rcf for 10 min. Collect the pellet and wash with DI water twice. Redisperse the final product in DI water at the concentration of 1 mg/mL and the product is to be denoted as MSN@DOX.

3.5 Fabrication of GNS Decorated MSN (GoMe)

1. Add 200 μL of MSN@DOX (solid concentration 1 mg/mL) to 2 mL PDA-GNS solution. Adjust the reaction ratio between MSN@DOX to PDA-GNS so that 800 μg of MSN reacts with 3.2 nmol PDA-GNS solution.
2. Stir for 24 h at room temperature and separate unreacted PDA-GNS by three cycles of washing and centrifugation using water.
3. Resuspend the final pellet in DI water at 1 mg/mL (*see* **Note 7**).

4 Notes

1. Sodium hydroxylate is used to adjust the pH of the solution to around 11.0–11.5 when forming mesoporous silica nanoparticles. A too low or too high pH may require a different reaction time or result in different nanoparticle shapes.
2. Before adding TEOS solution, the mixture of all the other ingredients should be completely dissolved. To ensure that, stir with heat.
3. The morphology of MSN can be examined by transmission electron microscopy. If adhesion is observed, repeat the ethanoic washing with ammonium nitrate several times to completely remove surfactant. To determine the free thiol group on the surface of MSN, Ellmans' reagent may be employed. Serial dilutions of cysteine ranging from 0.1 to 1 mM are used to generate a linear standard concentration curve after incubation with Ellman's reagent for 20 min at 37 °C.

4. All the glassware used to synthesize the gold nanoparticle has to be presoaked overnight and completely cleaned with fresh prepared aqua regia ($HCl:HNO_3 = 3:1, V/V$), rinsed with DI water, and then dried in the oven prior to use. When handling with aqua regia, always conduct the work in a chemical fume hood and avoid inhaling the vapor. Neutralize the aqua regia with NaOH pellet. Be careful about the heat generated.
5. Sodium borohydride has to be freshly prepared in methanol solution and poured into the gold solution immediately. The color of the gold solution would turn from faint yellow immediately into wine-red.
6. At the step of final conjugation of PDSA, the monomer has to be completely removed of residual organic solvents. The final product should remain deep red. If it turns purple or black, it indicates that irreversible aggregation has occurred. The successful conjugation of PEG to gold nanoparticle is to be confirmed by the ^{1}H-NMR with signature chemical shift of PEG at 3.6 ppm (parts per million). The confirmation of PDSA on the surface of AU-PEG is evidenced by co-incubation with DTT, in which it can generate pyridinethiol with UV absorbance at 375 nm.
7. The size of GoMe is to be determined by TEM. In this chapter, it is expected that the particle size will have an average of 54.71 nm ± 9.63 nm.

Acknowledgment

The authors want to thank the ASPIRE award from the Office of the Vice President for Research of The University of South Carolina, the National Cancer Institute (1R15CA188847-01A1 and CCSG P30 CA44579), and the Center for Targeted Therapeutics (1P20GM109091-01) for financial support.

References

1. Khan MS, Vishakante GD, Siddaramaiah H (2013) Gold nanoparticles: a paradigm shift in biomedical applications. Adv Colloid Interface Sci 44:199–200
2. Skrabalak SE, Au L, Lu X, Li X, Xia Y (2007) Gold nanocages for cancer detection and treatment. Nanomedicine 2:657
3. Alkilany AM, Thompson LB, Boulos SP, Sisco PN, Murphy CJ (2012) Gold nanorods: their potential for photothermal therapeutics and drug delivery, tempered by the complexity of their biological interactions. Adv Drug Deliv Rev 64:190–199
4. Stern JM, Stanfield J, Lotan Y, Park S, Hsieh JT, Cadeddu JA (2007) Efficacy of laser-activated gold nanoshells in ablating prostate cancer cells in vitro. J Endourol 21:939–943
5. Huang X, El-Sayed MA (2011) Plasmonic photo-thermal therapy (PPTT). Alexandria J Med 47:1–9
6. Kwon KC, Ryu JH, Lee JH, Lee EJ, Kwon IC, Kim K, Lee J (2014) Proteinticle/gold core/shell nanoparticles for targeted cancer therapy without nanotoxicity. Adv Mater 26:6436–6441

7. Skrabalak SE, Chen J, Au L, Lu X, Li X, Xia Y (2007) Gold nanocages for biomedical applications. Adv Mater 19:3177
8. Dickerson EB, Dreaden EC, Huang X, El-Sayed IH, Chu H, Pushpanketh S, McDonald JF, El-Sayed MA (2008) Gold nanorod assisted near-infrared plasmonic photothermal therapy (PPTT) of squamous cell carcinoma in mice. Cancer Lett 269:57
9. Chen J, Wiley B, Li ZY, Campbell D, Saeki F, Cang H, Au L, Lee J, Li X, Xia Y (2005) Gold nanocages: engineering their structure for biomedical application. Adv Mater 17:2255–2261
10. Aguirre CM, Moran CE, Young JF, Halas NJ (2004) Laser-induced reshaping of metallodielectric nanoshells under femtosecond and nanosecond plasmon resonant illumination. J Phys Chem B 108:7040–7045
11. Xiao Y, Hong H, Matson VZ, Javadi A, Xu W, Yang Y, Zhang Y, Engle JW, Nickles RJ, Cai W, Steeber DA, Gong S (2012) Gold nanorods conjugated with doxorubicin and cRGD for combined anticancer drug delivery and PET imaging. Theranostics 2:757–768
12. Wu C, Yu C, Chu M (2011) A gold nanoshell with a silica inner shell synthesized using liposome templates for doxorubicin loading and near-infrared photothermal therapy. Int J Nanomedicine 6:807–813
13. Tang F, Li L, Chen D (2012) Mesoporous silica nanoparticles: synthesis, biocompatibility and drug delivery. Adv Mater 24 (12):1504–1534
14. Zhu Y, Meng W, Gao H, Hanagata N (2011) Hollow mesoporous silica/poly(l-lysine) particles for codelivery of drug and gene with enzyme-triggered release property. J Phys Chem C 115(28):13630–13636
15. Zhao LW, Zhang H, He Q, Li Y, Gu J, Li L, Li H, Shi J (2011) A glucose-responsive controlled release of insulin system based on enzyme multilayers-coated mesoporous silica particles. Chem Commun 47(33):9459–9461
16. Aznar E, Marcos MD, Martínez-Máñez R, Sancenón F, Soto J, Amorós P, Guillem C (2009) pH- and Photo-switched release of guest molecules from mesoporous silica supports. J Am Chem Soc 131(19):6833–6843
17. Vivero-Escoto JL, Slowing II, Wu C-W, Lin VSY (2009) Photoinduced intracellular controlled release drug delivery in human cells by gold-capped mesoporous silica nanosphere. J Am Chem Soc 131(10):3462–3463
18. Bahadur KCR, Xu P (2012) Multicompartment intracellular self-expanding nanogel for targeted delivery of drug cocktail. Adv Mater 24:6479–6483
19. Cheng B, He H, Huang T, Berr S, He J, Fan D, Zhang J, Xu P (2016) Gold nanosphere gated mesoporous silica nanoparticle responsive to NIR light and redox potential as a theranostic platform for cancer therapy. J Biomed Nanotechnol 12:435–449

Chapter 8

Engineering Well-Characterized PEG-Coated Nanoparticles for Elucidating Biological Barriers to Drug Delivery

Qi Yang and Samuel K. Lai

Abstract

Poly(ethylene glycol) (PEG) coatings can substantially reduce nanoparticle uptake and clearance by immune cells as well as nonspecific interactions with the biological environment, thus potentially improving nanoparticle circulation times and biodistribution in target tissues such as tumors. Naturally, the "stealth" properties of PEG coatings are critically dependent on the density and conformation of surface PEG chains. However, there are significant technical hurdles to both generating sufficiently dense PEG coatings on nanoparticles and precisely characterizing their PEG grafting densities. Here, we describe methods for preparing PEGylated polymeric nanoparticles with precisely tunable PEG coatings without the use of organic solvents, quantifying PEGylation efficiency and density using a standard fluorescence assay, and evaluating nanoparticle uptake by immune cells using flow cytometry.

Key words Nanoparticles, Poly(ethylene glycol), PEG density, PEG conformation, Macrophage uptake

1 Introduction

Because prolonged circulation times maximize nanoparticle extravasation into tumor tissue [1], the avoidance of rapid clearance by mononuclear phagocyte system (MPS) cells (e.g., Kupffer cells in the liver) is particularly important for systemically administered cancer nanotherapeutics. Poly(ethylene glycol) (PEG) is a relatively hydrophilic and flexible polymer that can reduce adsorption by proteins and other biomacromolecules and it has enjoyed considerable success in extending the circulation times of protein therapeutics [2, 3]. PEG coatings are also frequently used to reduce nonspecific cell uptake of nanoparticle drug carriers and other interactions with biological environments [4–7].

The effectiveness of stealth PEG coatings is critically dependent on the conformation adopted by its polymer chains, which in turn is determined by the PEG grafting density and molecular weight via the grafting distance (D) and Flory radius (R_F), respectively

Reema Zeineldin (ed.), *Cancer Nanotechnology: Methods and Protocols*, Methods in Molecular Biology, vol. 1530,
DOI 10.1007/978-1-4939-6646-2_8, © Springer Science+Business Media New York 2017

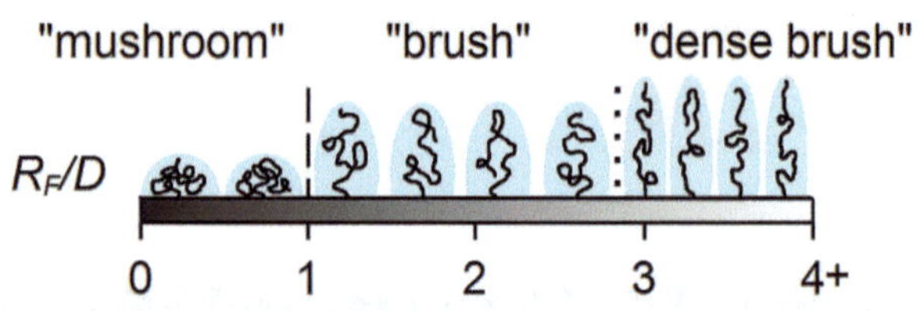

Fig. 1 PEG polymer conformation is determined by the R_F/D value. The transition between mushroom to brush and brush to dense brush conformations is indicated by the *dashed* ($R_F/D = 1.0$) and *dotted* ($R_F/D = 2.8$) *lines*, respectively. Reprinted with permission from [10], copyright 2014 American Chemical Society

(*see* **Calculation 1**). At increasing R_F/D ratios, grafted PEG chains transition from a globular "mushroom" conformation to a more extended "brush" regime, finally reaching a highly linear "dense brush" conformation at exceedingly high PEG densities (Fig. 1) [8–10]. Effective resistance to protein adsorption is frequently suggested to require complete PEG coverage of the nanoparticle surface, which presumably occurs at grafting densities resulting in overlapping PEG chains [6, 11].

Interestingly, the reported stealth properties (e.g., extended systemic circulation time) of PEGylated nanoparticles have been highly variable [6, 12–14]. These disparities likely reflect not only variations in the PEG grafting density that can be achieved by different nanoparticle formulations but also the lack of effective methods to accurately and precisely quantify the density of PEG chains present on the surface of nanoparticles [15]. PEGylated nanoparticles are typically modified with 2000 or 5000 Da PEG, but, based on the few papers reporting such values, they can possess a variety of PEG surface densities ranging from low values <0.1 PEG/nm^2 to higher ones >1 PEG/nm^2 [5, 12, 16, 17]. Nanoparticle formulation methods, composition, and physicochemical properties together control not only the optimal PEGylation strategy used but also the maximum achievable PEG density for each individual nanoparticle system. For example, the extent of liposome PEGylation is constrained by colloidal instability due to the presence of excess PEG-lipids [14, 18], whereas covalent grafting of PEG onto metallic and solid polymeric nanoparticles is limited by the density of surface reactive groups or effective reactive surface area [10, 17]. In addition to challenges in achieving comparable levels of PEG modification across different types of nanoparticles, the extent of surface PEG density is notoriously difficult to quantify for many nanoparticles without the use of complicated methodology and/or instrumentation. Direct measurements of PEG density using fluorophore-labeled PEG and indirect measurements based on detection of free PEG can interfere with the integrity of stealth

PEG coatings or are unable to differentiate between PEG present on the surface vs. in the interior of self-assembled nanoparticles. PEG shielding of charged groups can alter nanoparticle zeta potentials, but surface charge measurements are at best only an indirect and inaccurate method of gauging surface PEG density, with very poor sensitivity [6, 10, 15].

Here, we describe the preparation of PEGylated polystyrene (PS-PEG) nanoparticles using commercially available polystyrene (PS) nanoparticles. We also describe an assay for the quantification of surface PEG density, as well as uptake of the PS-PEG nanoparticles by immune cells. PS beads with well-controlled sizes and known surface densities of surface carboxyl (COOH) groups were modified using standard carbodiimide chemistry with amine-terminated PEG (PEG NH_2) at precise COOH-to-PEG NH_2 molar ratios to control the extent of PEGylation. By harnessing the fluorogenic properties of 1-pyrenylyldiazomethane (PDAM), which produces near-UV fluorescence upon reacting with COOH groups [19], we can quantify the number of COOH groups per PS-PEG or PS nanoparticle. The PEGylation efficiency and density of PS-PEG beads can then be indirectly determined based on the amount of residual COOH groups. This microplate-format assay is simple, requires only a small volume of sample, and avoids the need to remove unreacted reagent due to the fluorogenic nature of PDAM. The PEG densities quantified using this method correlated well with those determined using fluorophore-labeled PEG [10]. This assay could be used to characterize the PEG coatings of any solid nanoparticle modified through surface PEG grafting, as long as the number of available reactive groups and nanoparticle concentration are known (*see* **Notes 1–3**). To evaluate the ability of various PEG coatings to evade MPS clearance, we measured the uptake of PS-PEG and PS beads by human differentiated THP-1 (macrophage-like) cells using flow cytometry. Through the generation of nanoparticles with precisely tunable, well-characterized PEG coatings, we found that PEG grafting at substantially greater densities than those necessary to achieve a minimum dense brush conformation is essential for reducing MPS cell uptake in vitro and prolonging nanoparticle circulation in vivo [10].

2 Materials

1. 100 nm PS beads: yellow-green fluorescent 100 nm carboxylate-modified FluoSpheres® (Invitrogen, Carlsbad, CA, USA; 2.7×10^{13}–3.6×10^{13} particles/mL).
2. Reaction buffer: 50 mM sodium borate buffer, pH 7.8.
3. Methoxy PEG_{5000} amine (PEG NH_2).
4. Siliconized 1.5 mL microcentrifuge tubes.

5. Ultrasonic bath.
6. 15 mg/mL Pluronic F127 solution.
7. 1-Pyrenylyldiazomethane (PDAM).
8. Fluorescence microplate reader.
9. Human monocytic THP-1 cells (ATCC TIB-202).
10. Cell culture medium: RPMI 1640 supplemented with 10 % (v/v) fetal bovine serum, 100 U/mL penicillin, and 100 μg/mL streptomycin.
11. 100 μM phorbol 12-myristate 13-acetate (PMA) solution in DMSO, stored at −20 °C in the dark.

3 Methods

3.1 PS-PEG Synthesis

1. Dilute 100 μL of stock 100 nm PS beads with 1.4 mL of MilliQ water in a siliconized 1.5 mL microcentrifuge tube.
2. Centrifuge PS beads at 21,100 × *g* for 1 h to pellet the nanoparticles (*see* **Note 4**). Remove the supernatant and add 1.4 mL of MilliQ water. Repeat this step for a total of three washes.
3. Resuspend the nanoparticles in 1 mL of 50 mM borate buffer (pH 7.8) and briefly sonicate the sample for 1–2 min.
4. To generate fully PEGylated PS beads, weigh out and add PEG NH_2 at a 4× PEG NH_2-to-COOH molar ratio (*see* **Calculation 2**). To generate partially modified PS beads, add PEG NH_2 at the desired PEGylation ratio (e.g., for 50 % PEGylation use a 0.5× PEG NH_2-to-COOH molar ratio).
5. Weigh out and add 1-ethyl-3-(3-dimethylaminopropyl) carbodiimide hydrochloride (EDC) at a 5× EDC-to-PEG NH_2 molar ratio. Briefly sonicate the sample using an ultrasonic bath to ensure full dispersion of all PS beads in solution.
6. Rotate sample overnight at room temperature.
7. To quench the reaction, weigh out and add glycine at a 10× glycine-to-PEG NH_2 molar ratio, and allow the sample to rotate at room temperature for 30 min.
8. Centrifuge the PS-PEG beads at 21,100 × *g* for 1 h to pellet the nanoparticles. Remove the supernatant and add 1.4 mL of MilliQ water (*see* **Note 4**). Repeat this step for a total of five washes.
9. Resuspend the nanoparticles in 100 μL of MilliQ water and store at 4 °C (*see* **Note 5**).

3.2 Quantification of PEGylation Using PDAM Assay

1. Add PS-PEG beads (1 μL/well) in duplicate to a black 96-well half-area flat-bottom polystyrene plate (Fig. 2) (*see* **Note 6**).

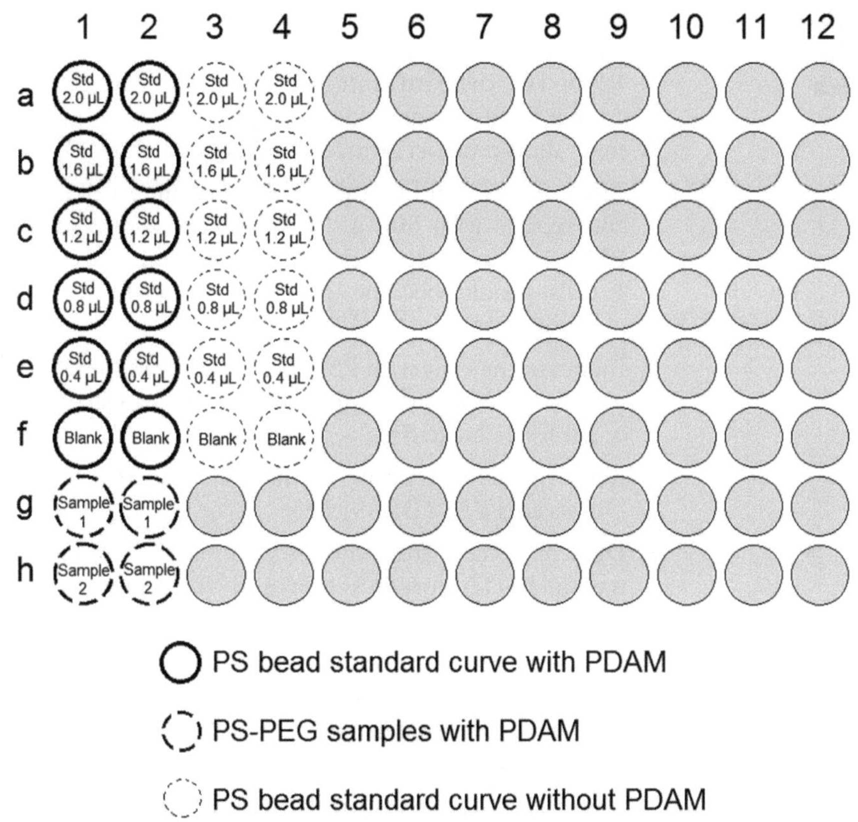

Fig. 2 Sample PDAM assay plate layout with PS bead standard curve (*thick border*), two different PS-PEG samples (*dashed border*), and PS bead standard curve without added PDAM reagent (*dotted border*)

2. Prepare a standard curve of unmodified stock PS beads in quadruplicate wells using the following volumes: 2.0, 1.6, 1.2, 0.8, 0.4, and 0 µL (Fig. 2).
3. Add 20 µL of the Pluronic F127 solution (15 mg/mL) to each well.
4. Prepare a fresh solution of 0.3 mg/mL PDAM in methanol (*see* **Note 7**).
5. Add 10 µL of methanol to half of the standard curve wells (i.e., standard curve without PDAM). Add 10 µL of the PDAM solution to the PS-PEG sample wells and to the remaining standard curve wells (Fig. 2).
6. Immediately read the PDAM fluorescence (ex/em 340/395 nm) and nanoparticle fluorescence (ex/em 480/520 nm) using a microplate reader (*see* **Calculations 2** and **3** for PEGylation efficiency, PEG density, and PEG conformation calculations).

3.3 Macrophage Cell Uptake of PS-PEG Nanoparticles

1. To differentiate human monocytic THP-1 cells into macrophage-like cells, seed 500 μL of THP-1 cells at 1.7×10^5 cells/mL into 24-well tissue culture plates in cell culture media containing 200 nM PMA. All cell incubation steps should be performed at 37 °C and 5 % CO_2.
2. After 3 days, remove the PMA-containing cell culture media and replace with 500 μL of fresh cell culture media without PMA. Upon differentiation to macrophage-like cells, the THP-1 cells should become adherent, as confirmed under light microscopy.
3. Incubate the cells with PS-PEG or PS beads at a $1{:}10^4$ cell-to-nanoparticle ratio or in the absence of nanoparticles for 4, 12, or 24 h (*see* **Note 8**).
4. Remove the cell culture media and wash the cells twice with Dulbecco's PBS (DPBS).
5. Detach the cells from the 24-well plate using 150–200 μL of trypsin-EDTA for 1–5 min and then inhibit trypsin with 1.35–1.80 mL of cell culture media.
6. Centrifuge the plate at 300 × *g* for 10 min at 4 °C. Remove the supernatant and add 500 μL of DPBS. Repeat this step for a total of three washes.
7. Gently resuspend the cells in at least 500 μL of DPBS with thorough mixing to ensure that a single-cell suspension is obtained. Transfer the cell suspension into 5 mL polystyrene round-bottom tubes.
8. Determine the cell-associated nanoparticle fluorescence using a flow cytometer with a 488-nm laser and a bandpass filter covering the 510–530 nm range. Acquire at least 10,000 viable cells per sample (*see* **Note 9**). For the nanoparticle fluorescence histogram, set a gate using untreated cells to establish the minimum gate threshold (Fig. 3). Compare the mean fluorescence intensity and % nanoparticle-containing cells (Gate 1) of

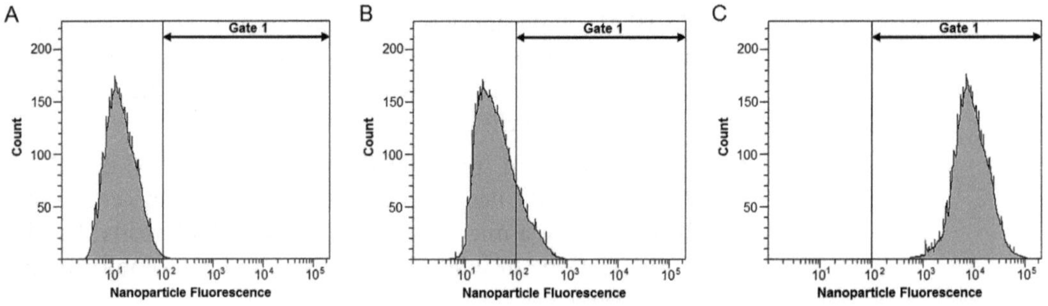

Fig. 3 Sample histograms of cell-associated nanoparticle fluorescence for (**a**) untreated, (**b**) densely PEGylated PS-PEG bead, and (**c**) control PS bead groups

each sample group to that of the PS bead group to determine the reduction in immune cell uptake of the PEGylated nanoparticles.

3.4 Calculations

1. The PEG conformational regime is dependent on the Flory radius R_F and grafting distance D between polymer chains, which can be determined using the following equations:

$$R_F = \alpha N^{3/5} \quad (1)$$

$$A = \frac{1}{P} \quad (2)$$

$$D = 2\sqrt{\frac{A}{\pi}} \quad (3)$$

where α is the monomer length of PEG (i.e., 0.35 nm), N is the number of PEG subunit repeats, A is the area occupied per PEG chain, and P is the PEG density (groups/nm^2). The mushroom and brush conformations are defined by $R_F/D \leq 1$ and $R_F/D > 1$, respectively. The dense brush conformation occurs when the thickness of the PEG layer (L) exceeds the R_F by at least twofold (i.e., when $R_F/D > 2.8$).

$$L = \frac{N\alpha^{5/3}}{D^{2/3}} \quad (4)$$

2. Use the following calculations to determine the concentration of COOH groups, number of COOH groups/nanoparticle, and COOH surface density:

$$\text{COOH concentration (mM)} = \text{Charge} \times \%\ \text{solids} \times 100\ \% \times 10 \quad (5)$$

$$\text{COOH groups/nanoparticle} = \frac{\text{COOH concentration} \times N_A}{10^6 \times \text{PS bead concentration}} \quad (6)$$

$$\text{COOH groups/nm}^2 = \frac{\text{COOH groups/nanoparticle}}{\text{SA}} \quad (7)$$

where N_A is the Avagadro constant and SA is the nanoparticle surface area in nm^2. Charge and PS bead concentration, as well as % solids, are typically reported on the certificates of analysis provided by the manufacturer and are given in mEq/g and PS beads/mL, respectively.

3. Using the ex/em 480/520 nm data, calculate the number of PS or PS-PEG beads in each well based on the PS bead standard

A

		With PDAM (in duplicate)		No PDAM (in duplicate)	
		1	2	3	4
PS bead std curve	a	51326.8	49174.2	49345.5	50538.9
	b	37287.4	36647.2	38926.2	38210.3
	c	30087.0	29838.7	29428.4	30174.7
	d	20657.0	20100.6	22355.8	20447.8
	e	11300.6	6632.8	8531.7	10164.7
	f	0.9	0.8	0.7	0.6
PS-PEG samples	g	25743.7	27490.2		
	h	24277.2	23505.3		

B

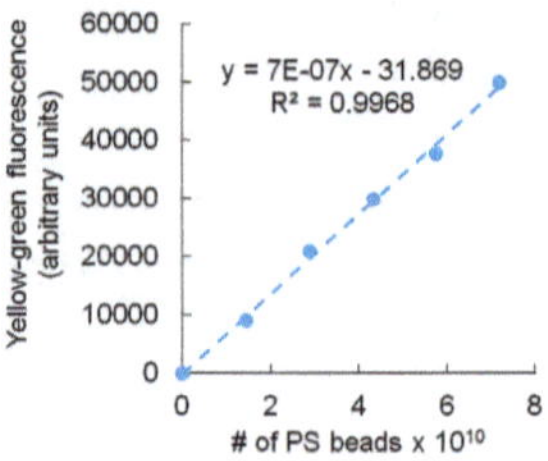

C

		With PDAM (in duplicate)		No PDAM (in duplicate)	
		1	2	3	4
PS bead std curve	a	7.5E+10	7.2E+10	7.2E+10	7.4E+10
	b	5.4E+10	5.4E+10	5.7E+10	5.6E+10
	c	4.4E+10	4.4E+10	4.3E+10	4.4E+10
	d	3.0E+10	2.9E+10	3.3E+10	3.0E+10
	e	1.7E+10	9.7E+09	1.2E+10	1.5E+10
	f				
PS-PEG samples	g	3.8E+10	4.0E+10		
	h	3.5E+10	3.4E+10		

Fig. 4 Sample data and calculated PS-PEG bead numbers. (**a**) Raw data for yellow-green bead fluorescence (ex/em 480/520 nm). (**b**) Standard curve for particle fluorescence vs. number of PS beads. (**c**) Number of PS or PS-PEG beads calculated based on the standard curve. PS bead standard curve (*thick border*), PS bead standard curve without added PDAM reagent (*dotted border*), and two different PS-PEG samples (*dashed border*)

A

		With PDAM (in duplicate)		No PDAM (in duplicate)	
		1	2	3	4
PS bead std curve	a	32939.1	33736.4	233.1	284.1
	b	26840.3	27670.8	212.5	178.5
	c	22096.8	22463.2	170.5	184.5
	d	16896.9	16220.6	146.2	169.2
	e	10295.5	9423.9	103.3	98.3
	f	3557.6	3019.6	64.8	71.7
PS-PEG samples	g	10691.7	10477.5		
	h	6941.5	6570.4		

B

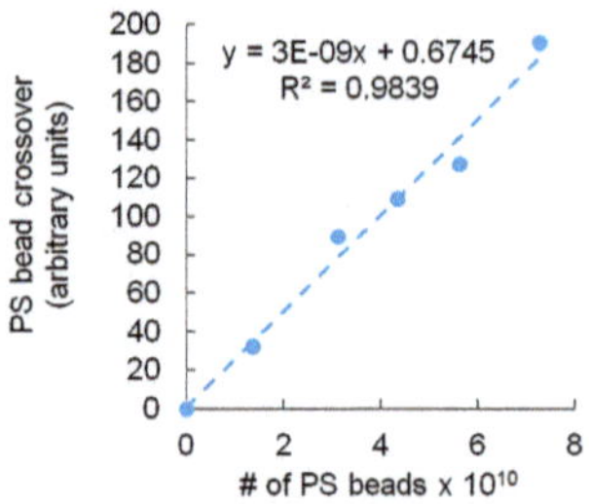

C

		With PDAM (in duplicate)	
		1	2
PS bead std curve	a	29462.3	30267.5
	b	23414.8	24247.6
	c	18697.6	19064.9
	d	13532.1	12857.8
	e	6964.9	6110.3
	f	269.0	-269.0
PS-PEG samples	g	7308.4	7087.8
	h	3563.5	3195.1

Fig. 5 Sample data and corrected PDAM fluorescence values. (**a**) Raw data for PDAM fluorescence (ex/em 340/395 nm). (**b**) Standard curve for PS bead crossover into the PDAM spectrum vs. number of PS beads. (**c**) Corrected PDAM fluorescence values calculated according to Eq. 8. PS bead standard curve (*thick border*), PS bead standard curve without added PDAM reagent (*dotted border*), and two different PS-PEG samples (*dashed border*)

curve (Fig. 4) (*see* **Note 10**). For all subsequent calculations, use the calculated number of nanoparticles per well (Fig. 4c) instead of the theoretical number of nanoparticles added to each well.

To account for the spectral crossover from the yellow-green PS beads into the PDAM fluorescence range, generate a standard curve using the ex/em 340/395 nm data for the PS bead standard curve without PDAM (Fig. 5a, b) and use the trendline equation as the crossover correction factor (cf). Calculate the corrected PDAM fluorescence values using the following equation (Fig. 5c):

$$\text{Corrected PDAM fluorescence} = \text{Raw PDAM fluorescence} - \text{bg} - \text{cf} \quad (8)$$

where bg is the average PDAM background fluorescence in the blank (0 μL PS bead) wells. The PDAM fluorescence values for

A

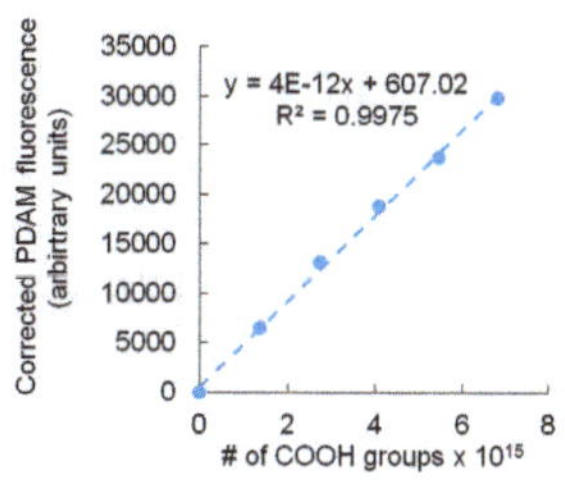

B

		With PDAM (in duplicate) 1	2
PS bead std curve	a	6.7E+15	6.9E+15
	b	5.3E+15	5.5E+15
	c	4.2E+15	4.3E+15
	d	3.0E+15	2.8E+15
	e	1.5E+15	1.3E+15
	f		
PS-PEG samples	g	1.6E+15	1.5E+15
	h	6.8E+14	6.0E+14

C

		With PDAM (in duplicate) 1	2
PS bead std curve	a	93.8%	100.6%
	b	102.0%	107.6%
	c	100.2%	103.1%
	d	104.3%	101.6%
	e	93.6%	137.8%
	f		
PS-PEG samples	g	43.4%	39.3%
	h	20.3%	18.4%

D

		With PDAM (in duplicate) 1	2
	a		
	b		
	c		
	d		
	e		
	f		
PS-PEG samples	g	56.6%	60.7%
	h	79.7%	81.6%

Fig. 6 Sample data and calculated residual COOH (%) and PEGylation (%) (**a**) Standard curve for corrected PDAM fluorescence vs. number of COOH groups. (**b**) Number of COOH groups calculated based on the standard curve. (**c**) Residual COOH (%) calculated according to Eq. 9. (**d**) PEGylation efficiency (%) calculated according to Eq. 10. PS bead standard curve (*thick border*), and two different PS-PEG samples (*dashed border*)

the blank wells only require correction for bg (i.e., do not include cf in the calculation for blank wells).

Using the corrected PDAM fluorescence values, calculate the number of COOH groups in each well based on the PS bead standard curve (Fig. 6a, b). The PEGylation efficiency (%) and PEG density (P) can be determined using the following equations (Fig. 6c, d):

$$\%\text{residual COOH} = \left(\frac{\text{Residual \# COOH groups}}{\text{\# nanoparticles} \times \text{Initial COOH groups/nanoparticle}}\right) \times 100\% \quad (9)$$

$$\%\text{PEGylation} = 100 - \%\text{residual COOH} \quad (10)$$

$$P = \%\text{PEGylation} \times \text{initial COOH groups/nm}^2 \quad (11)$$

4 Notes

1. For nanoparticles with reactive surface groups other than COOH, alternative fluorogenic compounds (e.g., amine-reactive fluorescamine) can be used.
2. If using nanoparticles other than fluorescent PS beads, the number of nanoparticles added to each well of the microplate PDAM assay should ideally be quantifiable using absorbance or fluorescence during the course of the assay to help to ensure the accuracy of the PEG density calculations. However, if such detection is not possible for a particular nanoparticle system, the concentration of PEGylated and unmodified nanoparticles could also be determined using nanoparticle tracking analysis or other methods prior to the PDAM assay [20].
3. The fluorescence intensity generated by PDAM differs between various COOH-containing reagents (e.g., 100 nm PS beads vs.

200 nm PS beads vs. glycine), so separate standard curves of corresponding unmodified nanoparticles should be prepared for each type of PEGylated nanoparticle being characterized.

4. The PEGylation procedure described here can be applied to carboxylate-modified PS beads of any size. However, the centrifugation time required to pellet PS nanoparticles will vary depending on their size. For PS beads ≥200 nm in diameter, a centrifugation time of 20 min or less is typically sufficient. PS nanoparticles smaller than ~70 nm in diameter cannot be readily pelleted using a microcentrifuge and should be washed using ultrafiltration or other methods. Due to their size, PS beads in the 70–150 nm range may not be fully pelleted even after 1 h of centrifugation with a typical benchtop microcentrifuge, resulting in partial loss of nanoparticles with each wash step. The supernatant from each wash step could be subjected to another round of centrifugation to improve sample recovery.
5. The commercially available PS beads used in this protocol are highly monodisperse with a very narrow size distribution, and PS-PEG nanoparticles also generally exhibit similar properties, with a slight increase in average nanoparticle size and distribution due to PEGylation. Aggregation is rarely observed for 100 nm PS-PEG beads fabricated using this protocol, but the size, polydispersity, and surface charge of each batch of PS-PEG beads should nevertheless be characterized to ensure that the resulting nanoparticles exhibit acceptable physicochemical properties [20], particularly because nanoparticle aggregation results in inaccurate PDAM assay results. Fully PEGylated PS beads are highly stable under storage at 4 °C.
6. The volume of PS-PEG sample used in the PDAM assay should be adjusted based on the relative concentration of the PS-PEG beads compared to the stock PS beads. The amount of PS-PEG beads added to each well should be equivalent to 1–2 μL of stock PS beads. The concentration of PS-PEG beads can be determined by comparing the PS-PEG sample fluorescence to that of stock PS beads (*see* **Calculation 3**, Fig. 4).
7. A saturated PDAM solution should be used (solubility limit ~0.3 mg/mL); the presence of a minute amount of undissolved PDAM does not appear to affect the assay results. The PDAM solution should be prepared immediately prior to its addition to the microplate wells.
8. Due to minor variations in cell growth and differentiation efficiency, an additional two to three wells should be included during the PMA-induced differentiation step for each run of the cell uptake assay. The number of viable differentiated THP-1 cells in these wells should be counted and averaged to establish the amount of particles required for a $1{:}10^4$ cell-to-nanoparticle ratio.

9. A live/dead cell stain such as propidium iodide and 7-AAD can be used to exclude dead cells from the flow cytometric analysis. However, care must be taken in selecting live/dead stains that do not exhibit spectral overlap with the yellow-green PS beads and in performing fluorescence compensation. For more detailed explanations of methods for assessing cell uptake of nanoparticles, fluorophore selection, compensation, and additional flow cytometry techniques, please refer to [21–23].

10. For the PS bead standard curve, the number of PS beads and number of COOH groups are simply a factor of the PS bead volume. Thus, the PS bead volume could be used in place of these two parameters for all of the steps in **Calculation 3**. The three standard curves depicted in Figs. 4, 5, and 6 would then be replaced with yellow-green particle fluorescence vs. PS bead volume (Fig. 7), PS bead crossover into the PDAM spectrum vs. calculated PS bead volume (Fig. 8), and corrected PDAM

A

		With PDAM (in duplicate)		No PDAM (in duplicate)	
		1	2	3	4
PS bead std curve	a	51326.8	49174.2	49345.5	50538.9
	b	37287.4	36647.2	38926.2	38210.3
	c	30087.0	29838.7	29428.4	30174.7
	d	20657.0	20100.6	22355.8	20447.8
	e	11300.6	6632.8	8531.7	10164.7
	f	0.9	0.8	0.7	0.6
PS-PEG samples	g	25743.7	27490.2		
	h	24277.2	23505.3		

B

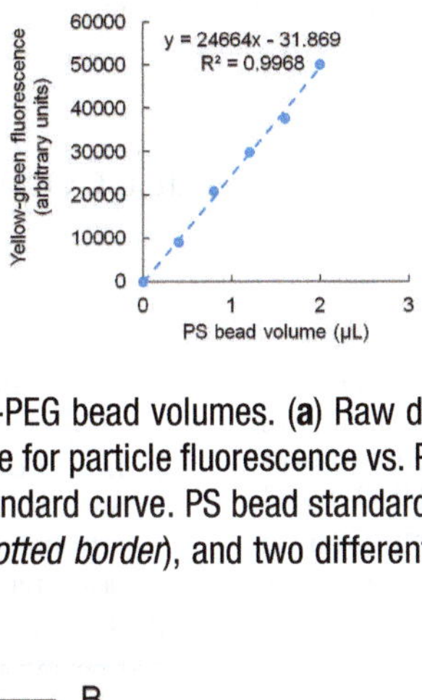

C

		With PDAM (in duplicate)		No PDAM (in duplicate)	
		1	2	3	4
PS bead std curve	a	2.08	2.00	2.00	2.05
	b	1.51	1.49	1.58	1.55
	c	1.22	1.21	1.19	1.22
	d	0.84	0.82	0.91	0.83
	e	0.46	0.27	0.35	0.41
	f				
PS-PEG samples	g	1.05	1.12		
	h	0.99	0.95		

Fig. 7 Sample data and calculated PS-PEG bead volumes. (**a**) Raw data for yellow-green bead fluorescence (ex/em 480/520 nm). (**b**) Standard curve for particle fluorescence vs. PS bead volume. (**c**) Volume of PS or PS-PEG beads calculated based on the standard curve. PS bead standard curve (*thick border*), PS bead standard curve without added PDAM reagent (*dotted border*), and two different PS-PEG samples (*dashed border*)

A

		With PDAM (in duplicate)		No PDAM (in duplicate)	
		1	2	3	4
PS bead std curve	a	32939.1	33736.4	233.1	284.1
	b	26840.3	27670.8	212.5	178.5
	c	22096.8	22463.2	170.5	184.5
	d	16896.9	16220.6	146.2	169.2
	e	10295.5	9423.9	103.3	98.3
	f	3557.6	3019.6	64.8	71.7
PS-PEG samples	g	10691.7	10477.5		
	h	6941.5	6570.4		

B

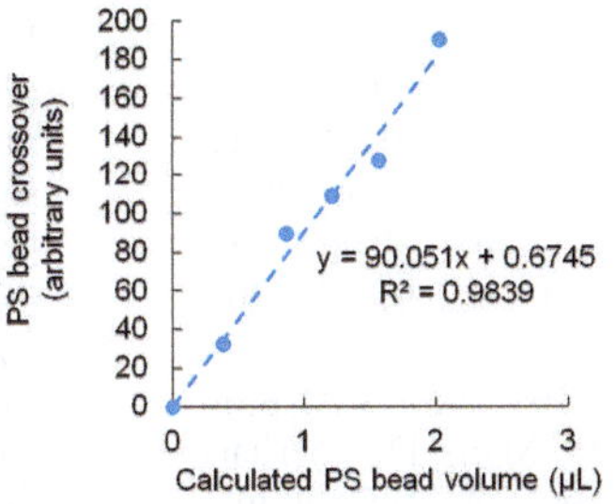

C

		With PDAM (in duplicate)	
		1	2
PS bead std curve	a	29649.8	30447.2
	b	23551.1	24381.5
	c	18807.6	19173.9
	d	13607.7	12931.3
	e	7006.3	6134.6
	f	269.0	-269.0
PS-PEG samples	g	7402.5	7188.3
	h	3652.2	3281.1

Fig. 8 Sample data and corrected PDAM fluorescence values. (**a**) Raw data for PDAM fluorescence (ex/em 340/395 nm). (**b**) Standard curve for PS bead crossover into the PDAM spectrum vs. calculated PS bead volume. (**c**) Corrected PDAM fluorescence values calculated according to Eq. 8. PS bead standard curve (*thick border*), PS bead standard curve without added PDAM reagent (*dotted border*), and two different PS-PEG samples (*dashed border*)

A

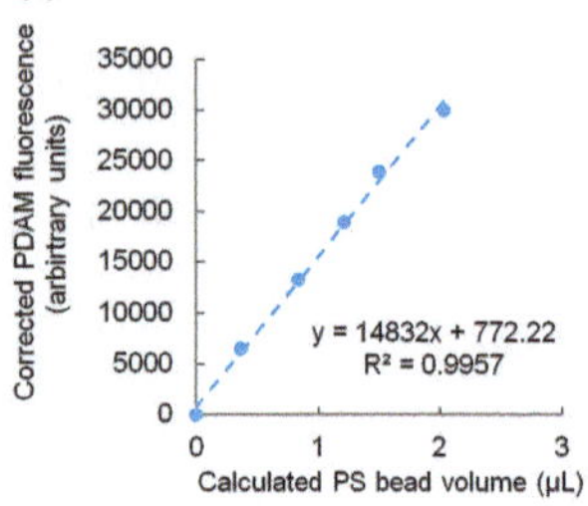

B

		With PDAM (in duplicate)	
		1	2
PS bead std curve	a	1.95	2.00
	b	1.54	1.59
	c	1.22	1.24
	d	0.87	0.82
	e	0.42	0.36
	f		
PS-PEG samples	g	0.45	0.43
	h	0.19	0.17

C

		With PDAM (in duplicate)	
		1	2
PS bead std curve	a	93.5%	100.3%
	b	101.5%	107.0%
	c	99.6%	102.4%
	d	103.2%	100.4%
	e	91.5%	133.8%
	f		
PS-PEG samples	g	42.8%	38.8%
	h	19.7%	17.7%

D

		With PDAM (in duplicate)	
		1	2
	a		
	b		
	c		
	d		
	e		
	f		
PS-PEG samples	g	57.2%	61.2%
	h	80.3%	82.3%

Fig. 9 Sample data and calculated residual COOH (%) and PEGylation (%) (**a**) Standard curve for corrected PDAM fluorescence vs. calculated PS bead volume. (**b**) Number of COOH groups calculated based on the standard curve. (**c**) Residual COOH (%) calculated according to Eq. 12. (**d**) PEGylation efficiency (%) calculated according to Eq. 10. PS bead standard curve (*thick border*), and two different PS-PEG samples (*dashed border*)

fluorescence vs. calculated PS bead volume (Fig. 9), respectively. For all samples, the calculated number of nanoparticles and number of COOH groups would be replaced by (*a*) the effective "volume" of stock PS beads calculated based on yellow-green fluorescence and (*b*) that calculated based on PDAM fluorescence, respectively. The residual COOH (%) would then be:

$$\%\text{residual COOH} = \frac{a}{b} \times 100\% \quad (12)$$

References

1. Gabizon A, Papahadjopoulos D (1988) Liposome formulations with prolonged circulation time in blood and enhanced uptake by tumors. Proc Natl Acad Sci U S A 85(18):6949–6953
2. Veronese FM, Pasut G (2005) PEGylation, successful approach to drug delivery. Drug Discov Today 10(21):1451–1458. doi:10.1016/S1359-6446(05)03575-0
3. Bailon P, Won CY (2009) PEG-modified biopharmaceuticals. Expert Opin Drug Deliv 6(1):1–16. doi:10.1517/17425240802650568
4. Lai SK, Wang YY, Hanes J (2009) Mucus-penetrating nanoparticles for drug and gene delivery to mucosal tissues. Adv Drug Deliv Rev 61(2):158–171. doi:10.1016/j.addr.2008.11.002
5. Nance EA, Woodworth GF, Sailor KA, Shih TY, Xu Q, Swaminathan G, Xiang D, Eberhart C, Hanes J (2012) A dense poly(ethylene glycol) coating improves penetration of large polymeric nanoparticles within brain tissue. Sci Transl Med 4(149):149ra119. doi:10.1126/scitranslmed.3003594
6. Jokerst JV, Lobovkina T, Zare RN, Gambhir SS (2011) Nanoparticle PEGylation for imaging and therapy. Nanomedicine (Lond) 6(4):715–728. doi:10.2217/nnm.11.19
7. Immordino ML, Dosio F, Cattel L (2006) Stealth liposomes: review of the basic science, rationale, and clinical applications, existing and potential. Int J Nanomedicine 1(3):297–315
8. de Gennes PG (1980) Conformation of polymers attached to an interface. Macromolecules 13(5):1069–1075
9. Damodaran VB, Fee CJ, Ruckh T, Popat KC (2010) Conformational studies of covalently grafted poly(ethylene glycol) on modified solid matrices using X-ray photoelectron spectroscopy. Langmuir 26(10):7299–7306. doi:10.1021/la9041502
10. Yang Q, Jones SW, Parker CL, Zamboni WC, Bear JE, Lai SK (2014) Evading immune cell uptake and clearance requires PEG grafting at densities substantially exceeding the minimum for brush conformation. Mol Pharm. doi:10.1021/mp400703d
11. Owens DE III, Peppas NA (2006) Opsonization, biodistribution, and pharmacokinetics of polymeric nanoparticles. Int J Pharm 307

(1):93–102. doi:10.1016/j.ijpharm.2005.10.010
12. Perry JL, Reuter KG, Kai MP, Herlihy KP, Jones SW, Luft JC, Napier M, Bear JE, DeSimone JM (2012) PEGylated PRINT nanoparticles: the impact of PEG density on protein binding, macrophage association, biodistribution, and pharmacokinetics. Nano Lett 12(10):5304–5310. doi:10.1021/nl302638g
13. Walkey CD, Olsen JB, Guo H, Emili A, Chan WC (2012) Nanoparticle size and surface chemistry determine serum protein adsorption and macrophage uptake. J Am Chem Soc 134 (4):2139–2147. doi:10.1021/ja2084338
14. Li SD, Huang L (2009) Nanoparticles evading the reticuloendothelial system: role of the supported bilayer. Biochim Biophys Acta 1788 (10):2259–2266. doi:10.1016/j.bbamem.2009.06.022
15. Rabanel JM, Hildgen P, Banquy X (2014) Assessment of PEG on polymeric particles surface, a key step in drug carrier translation. J Control Release 185:71–87. doi:10.1016/j.jconrel.2014.04.017
16. Budijono SJ, Russ B, Saad W, Adamson DH, Prud'homme RK (2010) Block copolymer surface coverage on nanoparticles. Colloids Surf A Physicochem Eng Asp 360(1–3):105–110. doi:10.1016/j.colsurfa.2010.02.016
17. Xia X, Yang M, Wang Y, Zheng Y, Li Q, Chen J, Xia Y (2012) Quantifying the coverage density of poly(ethylene glycol) chains on the surface of gold nanostructures. ACS Nano 6 (1):512–522. doi:10.1021/nn2038516
18. Hristova K, Kenworthy A, McIntosh TJ (1995) Effect of bilayer composition on the phase behavior of liposomal suspensions containing poly(ethylene glycol)-lipids. Macromolecules 28(23):7693–7699. doi:10.1021/ma00127a015
19. Li Y, Lander R, Manger W, Lee A (2004) Determination of lipid profile in meningococcal polysaccharide using reversed-phase liquid chromatography. J Chromatogr B Analyt Technol Biomed Life Sci 804(2):353–358. doi:10.1016/j.jchromb.2004.01.042
20. McNeil SE (2011) Characterization of nanoparticles intended for drug delivery, vol 697, Methods in molecular biology. Humana Press, New York. doi:10.1007/978-1-60327-198-1
21. Hawley TS, Hawley RG (eds) (2011) Flow cytometry protocols, vol 699, Methods in molecular biology. Humana Press, New York. doi:10.1007/978-1-61737-950-5
22. Ibuki Y, Toyooka T (2012) Nanoparticle uptake measured by flow cytometry. In: Reineke J (ed) Nanotoxicity, vol 926, Methods in molecular biology. Humana Press, New York, pp 157–166. doi:10.1007/978-1-62703-002-1_11
23. Tung JW, Heydari K, Tirouvanziam R, Sahaf B, Parks DR, Herzenberg LA, Herzenberg LA (2007) Modern flow cytometry: a practical approach. Clin Lab Med 27(3):453–468. doi:10.1016/j.cll.2007.05.001

Chapter 9

Piloting Your Nanovehicle to Overcome Biological Barriers

Steven M. Richards and Robert B. Campbell

Abstract

Designing an effective nanoparticle for selective drug transport requires careful consideration of the complex biological barriers encountered in transit to the desired target. Here, we review several of these barriers, and provide possible methods for formulating liposomal nanoparticles to overcome them. The methods include the biotinylation of an antibody, and subsequent conjugation to a PEGylated cationic lipid nanoparticle. Additionally, the incorporation of drug, and other relevant characteristics of the nanoparticle are also discussed.

Key words Nanoparticles, Liposomes, Barriers, Bevacizumab, Angiogenesis, Drug resistance, Drug carriers, Drug delivery systems

1 Introduction

The major challenge of chemotherapy is delivering clinically relevant concentrations of the agent to the desired target site. The use of conventional strategies to administer FDA approved agents is usually not sufficient to target tumors, at least not without causing significant harm to normal healthy tissues. For this reason, nanovehicle drug delivery systems have been developed to maximize the drug exposure to the target, while minimizing off-target effects. In designing a chemotherapeutic drug-loaded nanovehicle there are a number of biologic barriers that must be considered, and overcome.

Upon intravenous administration, the innate immune system represents an immediate and formidable barrier to nanoparticle drug delivery [1–3]. Following injection, serum proteins called opsonins begin adsorbing to the surface of nanoparticles, marking them for destruction by cells of the mononuclear phagocytic system (MPS) [4]. Stealth liposomes, which incorporate surface modifiers such as polyethylene glycol (PEG), have been shown to limit opsonization and subsequent recognition by the MPS. Due to reduced internalization by resident macrophages in the liver, lung, and

Reema Zeineldin (ed.), *Cancer Nanotechnology: Methods and Protocols*, Methods in Molecular Biology, vol. 1530, DOI 10.1007/978-1-4939-6646-2_9, © Springer Science+Business Media New York 2017

spleen, PEGylated liposomes have extended circulation half-lives and improved tumor targeting. This discovery has brought us a step closer to the magic bullet [5].

The unique physiology of solid tumors presents a number of additional barriers to drug delivery. Normal vasculature is hierarchical and evenly distributed, due to a tightly regulated balance of pro-angiogenic and anti-angiogenic growth factors [6]. The formation of tumor neovascular networks is driven by the overproduction of vascular growth factors such as Vascular Endothelial Growth Factor (VEGF), and the subsequent development of a highly disorganized maze of immature blood vessels [7–9]. Tumor micro vessels often display discontinuous endothelium, with open gaps and fenestra, making them more "leaky" than the normal endothelium. Additionally, the lymphatic system around the tumor is poorly developed. Taken together, there is a propensity for accumulating interstitial fluids, thus raising the interstitial fluid pressure (IFP) and disrupting the osmotic and hydrostatic pressure gradients [10, 11]. Nanoparticles must rely on diffusion to travel through tissue with elevated IFP, and cannot easily penetrate large tumors.

During the drug discovery process, pharmaceutical companies screen large compound libraries to identify lead candidates. The classic approach involves screening the library for compounds that have the highest biological activity against a given target. Many of the drugs identified with this approach are highly lipophilic. This presents a difficult challenge considering that with high lipophilicity, drugs typically exhibit greater off-target effects and higher toxicity. Over the last 15 years, pharmaceutical companies have increasingly adopted pharmacokinetic-guided screening, to predict compounds likely to succeed in clinical trials [12]. Drugs that do not conform to these properties are typically abandoned early in the drug discovery process, independent of biological activity. Nano-drug delivery is particularly well suited for drugs that display high biologic activity, but unfavorable physicochemical properties. With the nano-drug delivery approach, the physicochemical properties of the nanovehicle become the critical factor, rather than the drug itself. A wide range of materials have been utilized in the development of nano-drug delivery systems, each with unique physicochemical properties and modifiable elements [13, 14].

The following procedure describes the preparation of a liposomal nanoparticle capable of overcoming both physiological and cellular barriers. The resulting nanovehicle has a hydrodynamic size of around 100 nm, allowing it to evade both renal and hepatic elimination. The incorporation of PEG extends circulation time by limiting enzymatic degradation, and recognition by the innate immune system. Our preparation includes the conjugation of bevacizumab, an antibody inhibitor of VEGF-A, to the PEGylated liposome. The antibody selected here was chosen as part of a comprehensive antitumor approach. By exploiting known tumor features we can improve the targeting of drugs to solid tumors. The two tumor features exploited for therapeutic gain were, (1) VEGF-*vascular endothelial growth factor* production and its role in tumor growth and development, (2) and the tumor vascular supply.

A goal of our novel delivery vehicle was to first scavenge up circulating levels of soluble VEGF in blood, and to use the resulting carrier complex (that contains both conjugated and scavenged VEGF variety) to selectively target tumors. In addition, we simultaneously capitalize on the favorable interactions between a cationic nano-carrier molecule and the anionic functional groups that line tumor endothelia.

The comprehensive strategic approach was supported by a previously published study that confirmed that the conjugation of bevacizumab to the distal end of PEGylated liposomes increased their uptake not only by pancreatic tumors, but by VEGF expressing endothelial cells as well [15]. Alternative strategies have conjugated biomimetic components such as "self" peptides as a means to further elude clearance by the innate immune system [16].

2 Materials

1. Phosphate Buffered Saline, pH 7.4 (*see* **Note 1**).
2. Phospholipids and cholesterol (*see* **Note 2**).
3. 10 mM NHS-LC biotin (*see* **Note 3**).
4. 25 mg/mL Bevacizumab (*see* **Note 4**).
5. 1 mg/mL NeutrAvidin (*see* **Note 5**).
6. 13 × 100 PYREX® Culture Tubes with Teflon Liner Screw Caps.
7. Inert gas (Nitrogen or Argon) used to dry the lipid film.
8. Rotary evaporator and vacuum pump.
9. Freeze Dryer (depending on intended application).
10. Bath-type Sonicator.
11. Dialysis units for buffer exchange.

3 Methods

3.1 Biotinylation of Antibodies

1. Dialyze 4 mL of 25 mg/mL bevacizumab solution with 1× PBS, and transfer to a 10 mL centrifuge tube wrapped with aluminum foil (*see* **Note 6**).
2. Prepare a 10 mM solution of biotin reagent by dissolving 2.68 mg biotin in 1.34 mL ultrapure water.

3. Calculate the volume of biotin reagent to add to the reaction. The calculation below provides an example using a 4 mL vial of 25 mg/mL bevacizumab (MW = 149,000).

   4 mL Ab × (25 mg Ab/1 mL Ab) × (1 mmol Ab/149,000 mg Ab) = 0.00067 mmol Ab
   0.00067 mmol Ab × (30 mmol biotin/1 mmol Ab) = 0.02 mmol biotin
   0.02 mmol biotin × (1,000,000 μL/L) × (L/10 mmol biotin) = 2.01 mL biotin solution.
4. Add the biotin solution to the tube containing the PBS-antibody solution and incubate at room temperature for 30 min.
5. After 30 min, remove the unreacted biotin by dialyzing with 1× PBS.

3.2 Preparation of the Lipid Nanoparticle and Encapsulation of Drug

1. Determine the desired lipid composition (*see* Table 1).
2. Remove stock lipid solutions from the −20 °C freezer and allow them to reach room temperature either by rolling the vial in hands or placing in a warm water bath. Mix 2.5 μmol of total phospholipids in a glass tube (*see* **Note** 7).
3. Remove solvent from the lipid solution. For volumes less than 1 mL, dry the mixture under a stream of inert gas such as nitrogen or argon under a fume hood. If the volume is greater than 1 mL, place the vial inside of a round-bottom flask, and rotovap until dried lipid film can be observed without any residual visible solvent.

Table 1
Lipid composition of selected liposomal drug formulations

Liposome type	Lipid composition (Mol ratio)	Reference
Amphotericin B (AmBisome) liposomes	HSPC/Chol/DSPG (2/1/0.8)	[23]
Pegylated amphotericin B (AmB) liposomes	PEG-DSPE/HSPC/Chol (0.21/1.79/1)	[23]
Cationic, pegylated Doxorubicin liposomes	DOTAP/DOPC/Chol/DOPE-PEG/DSPE-PEG-Biotin (50/35/10/5/0.2)	[15]
Electroneutral, pegylated doxorubicin liposomes	DOPC/Chol/DOPE-PEG/DSPE-PEG-Biotin (85/10/5/0.2)	[15]
Pegylated paclitaxel loaded liposomes	EPC/Chol/MPEG (20/8/1)	[24]
Pegylated paclitaxel loaded liposomes	HEPC/Chol/MPEG (20/8/1)	[24]

4. Remove trace solvents by drying for an additional 1–2 h in a vacuum environment via a freeze drier or SpeedVac.
5. Resuspend the dried lipid film with 2.5 mL of warm 1× PBS (*see* **Note 8**).
6. Overlay the vial with an inert gas, cap, and wrap parafilm around the end of the tube.
7. Incubate at 37 °C for 1 h, mixing the tube using s vortex every 15 min, or until film is no longer observed, and the suspension is a hazy white without any visible clumping.
8. Place the lipid suspension tube on a ring stand with a test tube clamp, and lower it so that the level of water in the sonicator bath is the same as the level of liquid inside the tube.
9. Sonicate for 10 min or until the suspension is relatively clear. The suspension may need to be sonicated for longer based on the lipid composition [17].
10. The resulting suspension can be stored at 4 °C, and is usually stable for 48–72 h.

3.3 Conjugation of Biotinylated Antibody to Modified Liposomes

1. Add 2.5 mL of neutravadin to the liposomal suspension, and incubate at room temperature for 75 min.
2. Remove unbound neutravidin by dialysis with PBS overnight at 4 °C using a 300K MWCO membrane with at least two changes of the dialysis PBS.
3. Add 100 μL biotinylated bevacizumab (1 mg antibody:10 μmol lipids).
4. Remove unbound biotinylated
5. bevacizumab by dialysis with PBS overnight at 4 °C using a 300K MWCO membrane with at least two changes of PBS used for dialysis.
6. Filter liposomes through a 0.22 μM filter and begin characterization assays.

3.4 Characterizing the Nanovehicle

The size of the nanoparticle is a major determinant of targeting given its impact on pharmacokinetics and efficacy. Various techniques aimed at controlling liposome size have been described [18–21]. The surface charge and zeta potential values are important measurements used in the formulation development process and in the regulation of tissue disposition. Dynamic light scattering is one of the most frequently used approaches to attaining particle sizes and zeta potential. A particle size analyzer, such as the NanoBrook 90Plus, allows for a fast and accurate assessment of these parameters.

1. Dilute liposome suspension to 1.0 % in 2–3 mL 1× PBS.

2. Pipette dilution into acrylic square compatible with the particle size analyzer.
3. Analyze the sample. In addition to polydispersity and average diameter, The stokes–Einstein equation can be used to calculate zeta potential from the resulting data.

4 Notes

1. Tris or glycine buffers are incompatible with NHS-LC Biotin, and should be avoided.
2. Prepare standard mol% stock lipid solutions in an organic solvent such as chloroform. Glass syringes must be used when working with organic solvents, as serological pipettes will be dissolved. Lipid aliquots should be stored at −70 °C in a glass tube with a Teflon lined cap. Be sure to follow the vendors recommended storing and handling conditions to prevent unwanted degradation of the material.
3. Immediately prior to use, prepare 10 mM solution of biotin reagent by dissolving 2.68 mg biotin in 1.34 mL ultrapure water. Stock NHS-LC biotin should be stored as a solid at 4 °C.
4. Unopened vial can be stored at 2–8 °C. It can be stored at 2–8 °C for up to 8 h following dilution.
5. Immediately prior to use, reconstitute NeutrAvidin with ultrapure water and then dilute to 1 mg/mL with 1× PBS. Store the stock NeutrAvidin at 4 °C.
6. Antibody must be dissolved in an amine-free buffer at pH 7.2–8. Many commercial antibodies are not shipped in solutions that are not compatible, which necessitates the buffer exchange.
7. Consult a reference to determine the lipid in the formulation with the highest phase transition temperature (Tc). Keep the lipid preparation above this temperature from the hydration step throughout the experiment.
8. If interested in preparing a liposome with soluble drug in the aqueous core; dissolve the desired concentration of drug in 1× PBS prior to reconstitution of dry lipid film. Following the sonication step, dialyze to remove free drug. For drugs that are not readily soluble in PBS, drug entrapment can be accomplished via the pH gradient method as previously described [22].

References

1. Senior JH (1987) Fate and behavior of liposomes in vivo: a review of controlling factors. Crit Rev Ther Drug Carrier Syst 3(2):123–193
2. Drummond DC, Meyer O, Hong K et al (1999) Optimizing liposomes for delivery of chemotherapeutic agents to solid tumors. Pharmacol Rev 51(4):691–743
3. Gregoriadis G (1988) Liposomes as drug carriers: recent trends and progress. Wiley, Chichester
4. Patel HM, Moghimi SM (1998) Serum-mediated recognition of liposomes by phagocytic cells of the reticuloendothelial system—the concept of tissue specificity. Adv Drug Deliv Rev 32 (1–2):45–60, S0169-409X(97)00131-2 [pii]
5. Papahadjopoulos D, Allen TM, Gabizon A et al (1991) Sterically stabilized liposomes: improvements in pharmacokinetics and antitumor therapeutic efficacy. Proc Natl Acad Sci U S A 88(24):11460–11464
6. Folkman J (1995) Angiogenesis in cancer, vascular, rheumatoid and other disease. Nat Med 1(1):27–30
7. Yuan F, Dellian M, Fukumura D et al (1995) Vascular permeability in a human tumor xenograft: molecular size dependence and cutoff size. Cancer Res 55(17):3752–3756
8. Seymour LW (1992) Passive tumor targeting of soluble macromolecules and drug conjugates. Crit Rev Ther Drug Carrier Syst 9 (2):135–187
9. Huang SK, Mayhew E, Gilani S et al (1992) Pharmacokinetics and therapeutics of sterically stabilized liposomes in mice bearing C-26 colon carcinoma. Cancer Res 52 (24):6774–6781
10. Jain RK (1989) Delivery of novel therapeutic agents in tumors: physiological barriers and strategies. J Natl Cancer Inst 81(8):570–576
11. Jain RK (1990) Physiological barriers to delivery of monoclonal antibodies and other macromolecules in tumors. Cancer Res 50(3 Suppl):814–819
12. Lipinski CA, Lombardo F, Dominy BW et al (2012) Experimental and computational approaches to estimate solubility and permeability in drug discovery and development settings. Adv Drug Deliv Rev 64:4–17
13. Laouini A, Jaafar-Maalej C, Limayem-Blouza I et al (2012) Preparation, characterization and applications of liposomes: state of the art. J Colloid Sci Biotechnol 1(2):147–168
14. Blanco E, Shen H, Ferrari M (2015) Principles of nanoparticle design for overcoming biological barriers to drug delivery. Nat Biotechnol 33(9):941–951
15. Kuesters GM, Campbell RB (2010) Conjugation of bevacizumab to cationic liposomes enhances their tumor-targeting potential. Nanomedicine 5(2):181–192
16. Rodriguez PL, Harada T, Christian DA et al (2013) Minimal "Self" peptides that inhibit phagocytic clearance and enhance delivery of nanoparticles. Science 339(6122):971–975. doi:10.1126/science.1229568
17. Caffrey M (1993) LIPIDAT a database of thermo data and association information on lipid. CRC Press, Boca Raton
18. Barnadas-Rodriguez R, Sabés M (2001) Factors involved in the production of liposomes with a high-pressure homogenizer. Int J Pharm 213(1):175–186
19. de Paula Rigoletto T, Silva CL, Santana MHA et al (2012) Effects of extrusion, lipid concentration and purity on physico-chemical and biological properties of cationic liposomes for gene vaccine applications. J Microencapsul 29 (8):759–769
20. Pupo E, Padrón A, Santana E et al (2005) Preparation of plasmid DNA-containing liposomes using a high-pressure homogenization–extrusion technique. J Control Release 104 (2):379–396
21. Wagner A, Vorauer-Uhl K (2011) Liposome technology for industrial purposes. J Drug Deliv 2011:591325. doi:10.1155/2011/591325
22. Mayer LD, Tai LC, Bally MB et al (1990) Characterization of liposomal systems containing doxorubicin entrapped in response to pH gradients. Biochim Biophys Acta Biomembranes 1025(2):143–151
23. van Etten EW, ten Kate MT, Stearne LE et al (1995) Amphotericin B liposomes with prolonged circulation in blood: in vitro antifungal activity, toxicity, and efficacy in systemic candidiasis in leukopenic mice. Antimicrob Agents Chemother 39 (9):1954–1958
24. Kan P, Tsao CW, Wang AJ et al (2011) A liposomal formulation able to incorporate a high content of Paclitaxel and exert promising anticancer effect. J Drug Deliv 2011:629234. doi:10.1155/2011/629234

Chapter 10

Detecting Sonolysis of Polyethylene Glycol Upon Functionalizing Carbon Nanotubes

Ruhung Wang, Vasanth S. Murali, and Rockford Draper

Abstract

Polyethylene glycol (PEG) and related polymers are often used in the solubilization and noncovalent functionalization of carbon nanomaterials by sonication. For example, carbon nanotubes are frequently sonicated with PEG-containing surfactants of the Pluronic® series or phospholipid-PEG polymers to noncovalently functionalize the nanotubes. However, PEG is very sensitive to degradation upon sonication and the degradation products can be toxic to mammalian cells and to organisms such as zebrafish embryos. It is therefore useful to have a simple and inexpensive method to determine the extent of potential PEG sonolysis, as described in this chapter. Intact PEG polymers and degraded fragments are resolved on sodium dodecyl sulfate polyacrylamide gels by electrophoresis and visualized by staining with barium iodine (BaI_2). Digitized images of gels are acquired using a flatbed photo scanner and the intensities of BaI_2-stained PEG bands are quantified using *ImageJ* software. Degradation of PEG polymers after sonication is readily detected by the reduction of band intensities in gels compared to those of non-sonicated, intact PEG polymers. In addition, the approach can be used to rapidly screen various sonication conditions to identify those that might minimize PEG degradation to acceptable levels.

Key words Polyethylene glycol, Pluronic®, Phospholipid-PEG, Sonication, SDS-PAGE, Carbon nanotubes, Functionalization, Nanotoxicity

1 Introduction

Polyethylene glycol (PEG) and related polymers are often used as dispersants in the preparation of carbon nanotubes and other nanomaterials (NMs) for use in aqueous environments. Various PEG constructs are also used in the covalent or noncovalent functionalization of NMs, often to provide functionalities for appending specific ligands to the NMs for biomedical applications. It is well known that ultrasound sonication involved in the dispersion and functionalization processes generates cavitation bubbles that collapse, producing high local heat, pressures, and shear forces [1–3]. In addition, sonication in aqueous media is capable of splitting water into hydrogen atoms and hydroxyl radicals that combine to produce H_2O_2 and free radicals. Both sonolytic damage and free radical attacks on polymers

Reema Zeineldin (ed.), *Cancer Nanotechnology: Methods and Protocols*, Methods in Molecular Biology, vol. 1530, DOI 10.1007/978-1-4939-6646-2_10,

have been proposed to contribute to the degradation of PEG [4–6], a lipid–PEG conjugate [7], and PEG-containing block copolymers of the Pluronic® series (also known as poloxamers) [8, 9]. Results of our recent studies [10, 11] further demonstrate that the sonolysis of PEG and PEG-containing polymers, including Pluronic® F-68 and F-127 (also known as poloxamer 188 and 407) and phospholipid-PEG (PL-PEG) constructs, is greatly affected by the ultrasound power, frequencies, and sonication times. Moreover, sonolysis of Pluronic® surfactants generates degradation products that are highly toxic to cultured cells and zebrafish embryos after probe or bath sonication [10, 12]. Thus, it is crucial to monitor polymer integrity after sonication under the specific experimental conditions used to determine whether structural alterations in polymer structure have occurred and whether potentially toxic byproducts have been generated. Described here is a simple and inexpensive approach to rapidly detect sonolytic damage to PEG polymers that does not require expensive instrumentation such as a mass spectrometer. The first step in the method outlined here is to prepare a sample of sonicated PEG under conditions anticipated to degrade the polymer. The sonicated PEG provides a positive control of degraded material while non-sonicated PEG provides a negative control of intact material. The second step involves sodium dodecyl sulfate–polyacrylamide gel electrophoresis (SDS-PAGE) that is modified to resolve the intact PEG material and its degraded fragments in the gel [13]. After electrophoresis, PEG bands in the gel are stained with BaI_2 [14]. An inexpensive flat-bed photo scanner capable of producing uncompressed image files with high resolution is sufficient to convert a SDS-PAGE gel with BaI_2-stained PEG bands into a digital image file. Finally, the relative amounts of intact or degraded PEG in the gel are quantified using the free *ImageJ* software. The SDS-PAGE plus BaI_2 staining method is now routinely embedded in our studies of nanotoxicology and cancer therapy research where sonication of various types of PEG-containing polymers is used [10–12].

2 Materials

1. PEG solution: 0.2 mM PEG8000 in water. Weigh 0.16 g polyethylene glycol (average molecular weight 8000) and dissolve in 80 mL MilliQ water. Add water to 100 mL, filter through 0.22 μM membrane and store at 4 °C.
2. Resolving gel buffer: 1.5 M Tris–HCl, pH 8.8. Weigh 18.16 g Tris base and dissolve in 75 mL MilliQ water. Adjust pH to 8.8 with 1 M HCl and add water to 100 mL. Store at room temperature for up to a year.
3. Stacking gel buffer: 0.5 M Tris–HCl, pH 6.8. Weigh 7.88 g Tris–HCl and dissolve in 75 mL MilliQ water. Adjust pH to 6.8 with 1 M NaOH and add water to 100 mL. Store at 4 °C.

4. 40 % acrylamide: 40 % (w/v) acrylamide–bis-acrylamide (mix ratio 29:1). Store at 4 °C (*see* **Note 1**).
5. 10 % (w/v) sodium dodecyl sulfate (SDS) in water. Weigh 10 g SDS (*see* **Note 2**) and dissolve in 80 mL MilliQ water. Add water to 100 mL. Store at room temperature.
6. 10 % (w/v) ammonium persulfate (APS) in water. Weigh 1 g APS and dissolve in 8 mL MilliQ water. Add water to 10 mL. Store at 4 °C
7. TEMED: *N*,*N*,*N*,*N'*-tetramethyl-ethylenediamine. Store at 4 °C.
8. Isobutanol: water-saturated isobutanol. Measure 80 mL isobutanol into a bottle, add 20 mL MilliQ water. Mix vigorously, and then allow the two layers to separate without further disturbance (*see* **Note 3**).
9. 1.5 M Tris–HCl, pH 6.8, dissolved in water. Weigh 23.64 g Tris–HCl and dissolve in 75 mL MilliQ water. Adjust pH to 6.8 with 1 M NaOH, add water to 100 mL, and store at 4 °C.
10. Electrophoresis buffer: 0.025 M Tris base, 0.192 M glycine, 0.01 % (w/v) SDS in MilliQ water. Make 1 L of 10× concentrated stock buffer by dissolving 30 g Tris base, 144 g glycine, and 10 g SDS in 800 mL MilliQ water, and then add water to 1 L. Store at room temperature. Dilute 100 mL 10× stock buffer with 900 mL MilliQ water to make 1 L working buffer before use.
11. 0.1 % (w/v) bromophenol blue (BPB) dye solution: Dissolve 0.1 g BPB in 100 mL water and store at 4 °C.
12. SDS sample loading buffer (2×): 0.125 M Tris–HCl (pH 6.8), 4 % (w/v) SDS, 10 % (v/v) β-mercaptoethanol, 0.01 % (w/v) BPB, 20 % (v/v) glycerol. To make 10 mL add 0.83 mL of 1.5 M Tris–HCl (pH 6.8), 0.4 g SDS, 1 mL β-mercaptoethanol, 1 mL of 0.1 % (w/v) BPB, and 2 mL glycerol to 5 mL MilliQ water. Mix well and store in 1 mL aliquots at 4 °C.
13. Gel fixing solution: 50 % methanol, 10 % acetic acid in MilliQ water. To make 1 L, measure 100 mL acetic acid into a 1 L bottle, add 500 mL methanol and 400 mL MilliQ water, mix well and store at room temperature.
14. $BaCl_2$ solution: 5 % (w/v) barium chloride in water. Weigh 5 g $BaCl_2$ and dissolve in 80 mL MilliQ water. Add water to 100 mL and store at room temperature in an air tight bottle (*see* **Note 4**).
15. Iodine solution: 0.05 M (10 % v/v) I_2 in water. Measure 10 mL iodine stock solution (as received at 0.5 M concentration) and add to 90 mL MilliQ water in a glass bottle. Wrap the bottle with aluminum foil to protect it from light and store at room temperature.

16. *ImageJ* 1.50b (available as of September 2015, *see* **Note 5**) on a Windows 7 computer with Java 1.6.0_20 (64-bit) installed.

3 Methods

3.1 Preparation of PEG Sonolysis Positive Control Samples

The following procedures describe sonication conditions using a bath sonicator in a 4 °C cold room.

1. Rinse a glass vial and cap (27.25 × 57 mm screw thread vial with rubber lined cap) three times with MilliQ water, place in a metal autoclave basket covered loosely with aluminum foil and bake at 200 °C for 2 h to destroy potential endotoxin contaminants (*see* **Note 6**). Allow the glass vial and cap to cool down to room temperature before use.
2. Fill the glass vial halfway with 10 mL of 0.2 mM PEG solution, and chill to 4 °C prior to sonication (*see* **Note 7**).
3. Prechill the bath sonicator and the cooling coil that connects to a refrigerated water bath circulator to 4 °C in a cold room (*see* **Note 8**).
4. Fill the bath sonicator tank with 1400 mL of 4 °C distilled water, just below the maximum water level marked inside the tank. Hang the cooling coil into the tank, on the inner sidewall, such that the coil is immersed in the water bath.
5. Secure the glass vial on a rack that hangs over the sonicator tank such that the vial is suspended in a central position in the sonication bath and the PEG solution in the vial is below the water bath level (*see* **Note 9**). Use only one vial at a time and place it in the same position each time, as changing location can change the power delivered to the vial.
6. Operate the sonicator at 37 kHz frequency (*see* **Note 10**) and 100 % power output level that corresponds to 120 W specified by the manufacturer (*see* **Note 11**).
7. Collect a 100 μL aliquot of PEG sample from the vial at 15, 30, 45, 60, and 90 min of sonication. Terminate the sonication at 120 min.
8. Store all sonicated and non-sonicated PEG samples at 4 °C for later use.

3.2 Resolving PEG by SDS-PAGE

Skip to **step 9** if using pre-cast SDS-PAGE gels. The procedures described below in **steps 1–9** are for casting multiple standard 4 % stacking, 15 % resolving SDS-PAGE mini-gels using a commercial gel caster system.

1. A gel sandwich consists of a single glass plate, a single alumina plate, and the gel between them. Assemble a stack of multiple gel sandwiches using two 1.5 mm spacers flanked between one

8 cm × 10 cm glass plate and one alumina plate of the same size for each gel (*see* **Note 12**). Place gel sandwiches in gel caster (*see* **Note 13**), ensure the glass plate of each sandwich faces the front. Secure caster faceplate onto the caster using clamps on both sides (*see* **Note 14**). Insert a gel comb into the first gel sandwich facing the front; make a mark at 1 cm below the bottom of the comb teeth on the caster faceplate to help judge how much acrylamide solution to pour into the gel later, and then remove the comb.

2. Prepare 10 mL of 15 % acrylamide resolving gel solution for each gel by combining the following reagents in order in a 50-mL disposable plastic conical centrifuge tube: 3.75 mL MilliQ water, 2.5 mL of 1.5 M Tris–HCl (pH 8.8), 3.75 mL of 40 % acrylamide, and 100 μL of 10 % SDS. Mix by gentle inversions. Add 100 μL of 10 % ammonium persulfate and 5 μL of TEMED, mix by gentle inversion and immediately pour about 8 mL of the resolving gel mixture into a gel sandwich (the openings created by gaps between spacers) by draining along one side of the sandwich to avoid bubble formation. Fill the sandwich to the 1-cm mark drawn on the faceplate, gently rock the caster from side to side and tap the bottom of the caster against the bench top to allow air bubbles to rise up to the top, and gently overlay each gel with 400 μL of water-saturated isobutanol (*see* **Note 15**).
3. Let the caster stand until the resolving gel has completely polymerized, which usually takes about 30 min (*see* **Note 16**).
4. Decant the isobutanol, gently fill the caster with MilliQ water using a squirt bottle, then decant the water and invert the caster on a paper towel to drain out water (*see* **Note 17**).
5. Prepare 5 mL of 4 % acrylamide stacking gel solution for each gel by combining the following reagents in order in a 50-mL disposable plastic conical centrifuge tube: 3.15 mL water, 1.25 mL of 0.5 M Tris–HCl (pH 6.8), 0.5 mL of 40 % acrylamide, and 50 μL of 10 % SDS. Mix by gentle inversions. Add 50 μL of 10 % ammonium persulfate and 5 μL of TEMED, mix by gentle inversion as before and immediately pour onto the resolving gel, allowing excess stacking gel mixture to overfill the sandwich, scrape off bubbles on the top.
6. Quickly insert a 10-well gel comb (1.5 mm thick) into the gel sandwich, at a slight angle to prevent trapping air, and allow the comb sides to rest on the top of the spacers (*see* **Note 18**). Insert the remaining combs from back to front sandwiches in the same manner rather quickly before the gel polymerizes (*see* **Note 19**).
7. Let the stacking gel stand until polymerization is complete, which usually takes ~60 min.

8. Using a razor blade, detach the stack of gel sandwiches from the caster and separate them into individual gel sandwiches. Take care to keep the comb and spacers between the glass and alumina plates in place. Scrape excess gel from front and back of plates, spray with MilliQ water and wrap the gel sandwiches in plastic wrap, lay flat in a container with air-tight lid and store at 4 °C for later use (*see* **Note 20**).
9. Install a gel sandwich containing a 4 % stacking, 15 % resolving SDS polyacrylamide gel on a gel electrophoresis apparatus, glass plate facing the front, fill the reservoirs with electrophoresis buffer, and remove the comb (*see* **Note 21**).
10. Put 10 μL of sonicated or non-sonicated 0.2 mM PEG sample in a microcentrifuge tube. Add 10 μL of 2× concentrated SDS sample loading buffer to each tube and mix the contents.
11. Heat the sample in a water bath or a heating block at 100 °C for 3 min.
12. Centrifuge the heated samples at 1000 × *g* for 10 s to bring down any condensate on the sides and caps of the tubes.
13. Load samples into the gel well (20 μL of heated sample per lane) by using a fine-tipped long gel-loading pipette tip to layer samples onto the well underneath the buffer. Electrophorese at a constant voltage of 100 V (*see* **Note 22**) until the blue dye front (from the BPB dye in the samples) has reached 0.5–1 cm from the bottom of the gel. This will take about 2 h (*see* **Note 23**).
14. Following electrophoresis, detach the gel sandwich from the electrophoresis apparatus, gently loosen and slide away both spacers, and pry the gel plates open with a small spatula. While the gel adheres to the alumina plate, use a razor blade to cut through the gel along the interface between the stacking and resolving gels, and discard the stacking gel. Carefully lift the resolving gel and immerse it into a tray of water (*see* **Note 24**).

3.3 BaI_2 Staining of PEG Bands

1. Rinse the gel with distilled water and soak it in 100 mL of gel fixing solution for 5 min. Slosh the solution over the gel gently on a shaker.
2. Decant the fixing solution carefully; save it in a glass bottle and store at room temperature for reuse up to five times. Rinse the gel with distilled water, and soak it in 100 mL of $BaCl_2$ solution for 10 min on a shaker.
3. Decant the $BaCl_2$ solution carefully; save the $BaCl_2$ solution for reuse up to five times. The color of the blue dye near the bottom of the gel will fade with staining and a horizontal strip of the gel near the dye front will turn white while the rest of the gel remains semi-transparent. Rinse the gel again

with distilled water, and then soak it in 100 mL of 5 % iodine solution for 5 min or until dark brown bands appear in the gel (*see* **Note 25**). Longer exposure to iodine leads to darker background color.

4. Decant the iodine solution carefully back into a glass bottle (*see* **Note 26**); it can be reused multiple times until the color of the iodine solution becomes lighter. Remove excess iodine staining in the gel background by soaking the gel in distilled water while gently shaking, and replace with clean water when the water color turns brown. Repeat the de-staining with water multiple times until the PEG bands in the gel are readily visible and the rest of the gel is clear of any yellowish background stain (*see* **Note 27**). Cover the container in which the gel is soaking with a lid to protect the gel from incident light (*see* **Note 28**).

3.4 Scanning BaI_2-Stained SDS-PAGE Gels Using a Flat-Bed Photo Scanner

1. Configure the flat-bed scanner such that the gel is scanned using the highest pixel density (600 pixels per inch or greater), highest color-depth (a 16-bit Red Green Blue color palette or greater), and the image file is saved in an uncompressed TIFF (Tagged Image File Format) format (*see* **Note 29**). Also, a preview feature in the software is important to restrict scanning to only the area that contains the gel, otherwise the image files become substantially larger than a regular photo or document file.
2. Lay a clean and dry sheet of write-on transparency film on the scanner bed. Rotate and/or flip the gel in the water tray to the proper orientation before carefully lifting it out and laying it down slowly on the transparent sheet. Avoid trapping air bubbles underneath the gel. Do not push or pull the gel once it is laid flat on the sheet. Lift the sheet and rotate it slightly to position the gel straight on the scanner bed. Fill the sample loading wells with water to minimize shadows casted from the gel walls on the sides of the wells. Add a few drops of water on the gel, if necessary, to prevent dehydration. Gently lay another transparent sheet on top of the gel; from side-to-side to avoid trapping bubbles. Place a few sheets of crisp white paper over the transparent sheet and close the scanner lid before starting the scan.
3. At the preview step, crop the scan area to include only the gel or a portion of the gel of interest. Inspect the preview image to make sure air bubbles and water marks are absent. Also, rotate the preview image to match the correct orientation of the gel.
4. After scanning, preserve the gel by wrapping in plastic wrap (*see* **Note 28**), store flat at 4 °C protected from light, or discard it.

3.5 Quantifying PEG Band Intensity Using ImageJ Software

The following procedures outline only the essential steps required for quantifying BaI_2-stained PEG band intensities, as shown in Fig. 1.

1. Launch *ImageJ* software (*see* **Note 5**).
2. Open Fig. 1 image file using ***File → Open*** in *ImageJ*.
3. Crop the horizontal section of the gel marked 'Intact PEG Band' (*see* **Note 30**):
   - Choose the ***Rectangular Selections*** Tool from the *ImageJ* toolbar.
   - Draw a rectangle around the 'Intact PEG Band' section across the gel (*see* **Note 31**).
   - Crop the selected area using ***Image → Crop*** (*see* **Note 32**).
   - Save the cropped 'Intact PEG Band' gel section image using ***File → Save as → Tiff***, and give it a *File_name.tiff*, then hit ***Save***.
4. The gel analysis routine requires the image to be a grayscale image.
   - Convert the cropped RGB image to grayscale using ***Image → Type → 32-bit***.
   - Save the grayscale image using ***File → Save as → Tiff***, and give it a *File_name.tiff*, then hit ***Save***.
5. If needed, the brightness and contrast of the grayscale image can be adjusted (*see* **Note 33**).
6. To acquire the total pixel intensity of the intact PEG bands before and after sonication, a rectangular area around the band

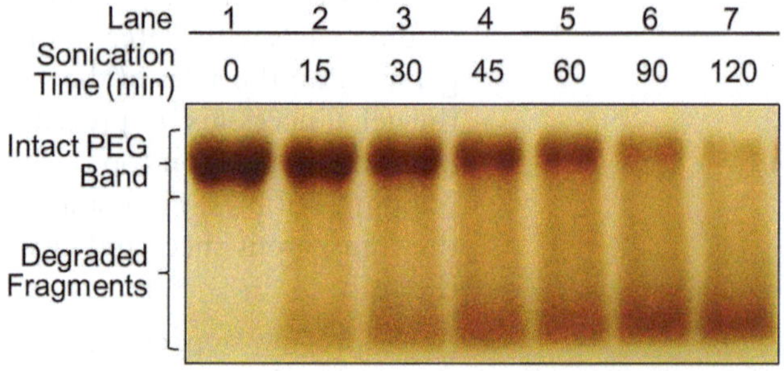

Fig. 1 Representative sonolysis of polyethylene glycol as a function of bath sonication time resolved by SDS-PAGE with BaI_2 stain. PEG 8000 at a concentration of 0.2 mM was sonicated using an ultrasonic bath operated at 37 kHz and 120 W. A representative gel was loaded with 10 μL of PEG samples acquired after bath sonication for different times. Intact PEG polymers and degradation products in the sonicated and non-sonicated PEG samples were resolved by SDS-PAGE followed by BaI_2 staining

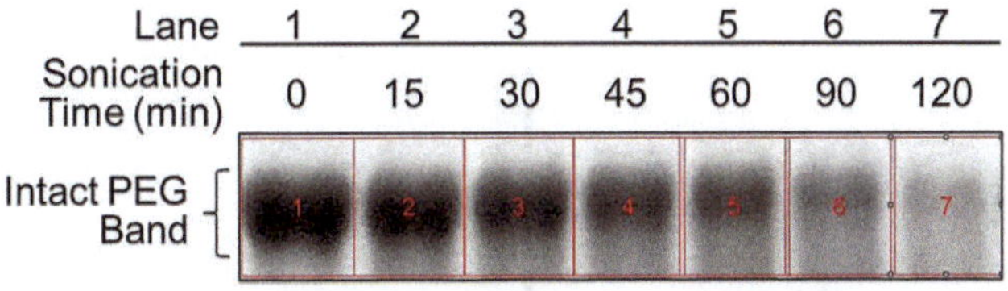

Fig. 2 Representative grayscale gel image of intact polyethylene glycol bands with BaI_2 stain. The section of the gel in Fig. 1 where intact PEG bands reside was cropped and converted to grayscale image using *ImageJ* software. The *rectangles* highlighted in *red* that enclose an intact, non-degraded PEG band in each lane define the areas where pixel intensity profile of the samples are analyzed and compared

is selected in each lane where the pixel intensity profile within a rectangle is plotted:

- Choose  the ***Rectangular Selections*** Tool from the *ImageJ* toolbar.
- Draw a rectangle around the intact, non-degraded PEG band in lane 1 on the far-left of the grayscale gel image, as shown in Fig. 2 (*see* **Note 34**).
- After drawing the rectangle over the band in first lane, press the "1" key on the keyboard or go to ***Analyze*** → ***Gels*** → ***Select First Lane*** to set the rectangle in place. The non-sonicated PEG band in lane #1 will now be highlighted and have a "1" marked in the middle of it (*see* **Note 35**).
- Use the mouse to click and hold in the middle of the "1" rectangle on the first lane and drag it over to the next lane on the right, where the 15-min sonicated sample was loaded. Center the rectangle over the lane left-to-right, but don't worry about lining it up perfectly on the same vertical axis. *ImageJ* will automatically align the rectangle on the same vertical axis as the first rectangle.
- Press the "2" key on the keyboard or go to ***Analyze*** → ***Gels*** → ***Select Next Lane*** to set the current rectangle in place. The 15-min sonicated PEG band in lane #2 will now be highlighted and have a "2" marked in the middle of it, as shown in Fig. 2.
- Repeat these steps for the rest of bands in lanes #3 to #7, in order from left to right, on the gel. Make sure to press the "2" key each time (not to press 3, 4, 5 ...) to set the rectangle in place (*see* **Note 36**).
- Save the grayscale gel image with rectangles set around the bands, shown as Fig. 2, using ***File*** → ***Save as*** → ***Tiff***, and give it a file name such as *PEG_sonolysis_bands.tiff*, then hit ***Save***.

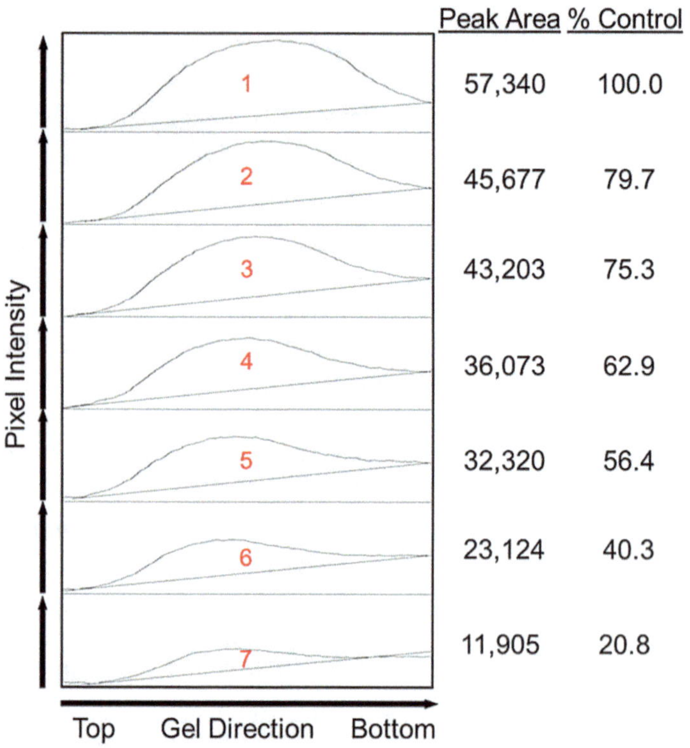

Fig. 3 Quantifying intact PEG bands in non-sonicated and sonicated samples based on pixel intensity profile plots. On the *left*, the pixel intensities of the selected areas (shown as red rectangles in Fig. 2 that enclose the intact PEG band in each lane) are plotted against gel electrophoresis direction, from *top* to *bottom*. The pixel intensity of a band is quantified as the background-corrected area under the peak in the pixel intensity profile plot. In tabulated form on the *right*, the relative abundance of intact PEG in sonicated and non-sonicated samples is presented as peak area and as % of control where the amount of intact PEG in the non-sonicated sample in *Lane 1* was set to 100 %

- After all the rectangles are set in place around every band, press the "3" key or go to ***Analyze → Gels → Plot Lanes*** to generate an intensity profile plot of each lane in the gel (*see* **Note 37**).
- Save the intensity profile plots of the gel, shown as Fig. 3, using ***File → Save as → Tiff***, and give it a file name such as *Plots_PEG_sonolysis_bands.tiff*, then hit ***Save***.

Each profile plot section in Fig. 3 represents the relative density of the contents of the band over each lane. The sections are arranged top to bottom on the profile plot, corresponding to the lanes from left to right in the gel. Because there were seven lanes selected in Fig. 2, there are seven sections in the profile plot shown in Fig. 3. Scroll the mouse wheel up-and-down to see the profile plot corresponding to each lane from left-to-right in the gel image.

The peaks in the profile plots correspond to the dark bands in the grayscale gel image. Higher peaks represent darker bands. Wider peaks represent bands that cover a wider size range (thicker bands) on the original gel.

7. Images of real gels are likely to have some background signal, so the peaks don't reach down to the baseline of the profile plot and appear to float above the baseline of the profile plot. It will be necessary to close off the peak before its size is measured:
   - Choose  the ***Straight Line*** selection Tool from the *ImageJ* toolbar.
   - For each peak you want to analyze in the profile plot, draw a line across the base of the peak to enclose the peak (*see* **Note 38**).
   - After each peak has been closed off at the base, select  the ***Wand*** Tool from the *ImageJ* toolbar.
   - Move up to the top profile plot section and click inside the peak with the  ***Wand*** Tool; the border of the selected peak area is highlighted in yellow. A "Results" window will pop up showing the measurement of the peak area. The first column in the results table shows the order of the peaks clicked with the ***Wand***, the second column (Area) shows the peak area measurement that indicates the overall pixel intensity of the peak.
   - Repeat this for each peak in order going down the profile plot (*see* **Note 39**).
8. When all of the peaks have been highlighted correctly, save the results by clicking

   File → ***Save as*** in the Results window. Give it a file name and file type such as *Results_PEG_sonolysis_peaks.txt*, in a "Text Tab delimited" format that can be opened with *Microsoft Excel* for data analysis (*see* **Note 40**).
9. Set the pixel intensity value of a control non-sonicated PEG-containing polymer as 100 % and compare the values of samples subjected to sonication for increasing time; the relative levels of sonolytic degradation that has occurred in each sample can be readily assessed.
10. A representative application of the method described above is shown in Fig. 4 where the sonolytic degradation of distearoyl phosphatidylethanolamine-PEG-COOH (DSPE-PEG-COOH) was detected and quantified in a sample that also contained single-walled carbon nanotubes (SWNTs). In the absence of sonication, the PEG portion of DSPE-PEG-COOH was evident in a single band that was near the dye front

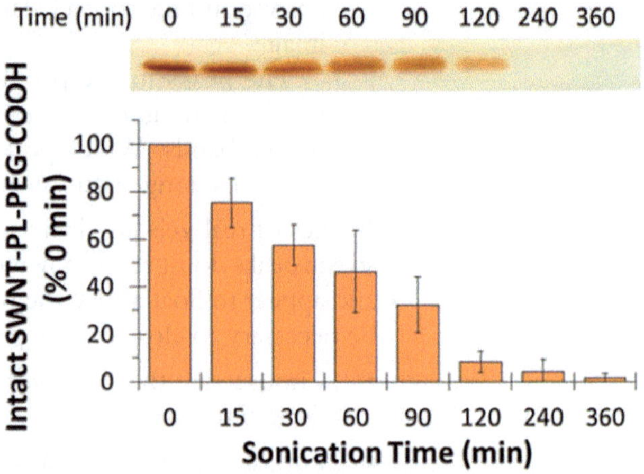

Fig. 4 Sonolytic degradation of DSPE-PEG-COOH in the presence of SWNTs. 5 mg of SWNTs were sonicated in 10 mL of 0.35 mM DSPE-PEG-COOH for the indicated times. The samples were resolved by SDS-PAGE followed by BaI_2 staining and the stained bands are shown at the *top* of the figure. The gels were then scanned and the band intensities quantified using *ImageJ* software. The data are presented as % density relative to 0 min as a function of sonication time, shown at the *bottom* of the figure. Reproduced from Murali et al. 2015 [11] with permission from SAGE Publications

after BaI_2 staining. Within 15 min of sonication the intensity of the band had visibly declined due to PEG sonolysis and continued to decline until it was almost absent by 360 min.

4 Notes

1. Unpolymerized acrylamide is a potent neurotoxin and is absorbed through the skin. The effects of acrylamide are cumulative. Wear gloves while working and avoid direct contact through bare skin.
2. SDS powder is harmful if inhaled and may cause respiratory irritation. Wear personal protective equipment, including gloves, clothing, and respiratory mask, to avoid breathing dust.
3. After the isobutanol and water layers settle, the upper layer will be isobutanol and the lower layer will be water; use the upper layer without disturbing the lower layer.
4. Barium chloride is one of the most common water-soluble barium salts. It is toxic if swallowed or inhaled. Avoid contact with skin, eyes, and clothing and avoid breathing vapors and dust.

5. The latest version of *ImageJ* software can be downloaded from the official *ImageJ* site at http://imagej.nih.gov/ij/, for initial installation or for upgrade. Extensive documentation related to *ImageJ* basic concepts, installation, tutorials and examples, macro language, and many more are all freely available [15]. In addition, *ImageJ* source code and extended plugins for specific applications are freely available in the public domain.
6. Lipopolysaccharides (LPS), also known as lipoglycans and endotoxin, are large lipid-polysaccharide molecules found in the outer membrane of gram-negative bacteria and elicit strong immune responses in animals. Inactivation of possible endotoxin contaminants is recommended when the final material is to be used with cultured cells or intact animals.
7. Sonolysis of PEG-containing polymers is concentration and temperature dependent.
8. The temperature of the sonication bath is kept below 18 °C throughout the sonication period.
9. The position of the sample vial during sonication is a key variable in bath sonication [16, 17].
10. Sonication power level and ultrasound frequency are critical factors that influence sonolytic damage [2, 18]. There is an inverse relationship between frequency and the size of cavitation bubbles because larger bubbles generated at lower frequencies generally create more extreme heat and pressure when they implode [2, 3, 19]. Pluronic® polymers were readily degraded upon bath sonication at 37 kHz or probe sonication at 20 kHz frequency, but no apparent degradation was observed when subjected to bath sonication at 80 kHz frequency with similar power level and duration [10].
11. The power delivered to the sonicator bath can be determined by measuring the change in bath temperature (starting at 22 °C) as a function of sonication time, at room temperature without a cooling coil [17]. This method uses the equation $P = (\mathrm{d}T/\mathrm{d}t) \times M \times \mathrm{Cp}$, where P is the acoustic power (W), T is the temperature (K), t is time (s), M is the mass of water (1400 g for this bath sonicator), and Cp is the specific heat capacity of water at 298 K (4.18 J/g K). The power measured by this approach was ~80 W for this sonication system [11].
12. Alumina ceramic back plates have the advantage that they transfer heat 40 times more rapidly than glass plates, which facilitates cooling. However, regular glass plates can be used instead of alumina plates. Clean away any dust and gel pieces adhering to the plates from previous use. Spray a small amount of ethanol and wipe with a clean Kimwipes to remove any watermarks.

13. When less than the maximum number of gel sandwiches is needed, place an 8 cm × 10 cm plastic or glass space-filler behind the stack of gel sandwiches to fill up the caster completely.
14. The gel sandwich should not move after the caster is clamped. Add more space-filler plastic or glass plates if needed.
15. Oxygen inhibits polymerization of PAGE gels. Usually in preparing such gels a degassing step, using vacuum, is required; however for the small size gels used here, this step is not needed. An isobutanol layer is added on the top of each gel to keep the gel levels the same and to prevent contact of the gel with oxygen in the air. Deliver the isobutanol slowly along the spacer at the side of the sandwich. Make certain the caster is level using a bubble level.
16. Do NOT pour the excess acrylamide down the sink. The mixture will polymerize in the pipes and clog them. Wait until the mixture has polymerized in the 50-mL tube, then discard in hazardous trash. This excess material is also a good indicator whether the gel has polymerized properly and is ready for the next step.
17. The polymerized resolving gel should remain in place and inside the gel sandwiches even when the caster is upside-down.
18. Instead of the standard 10-well combs, 1.5-mm thick 15-well combs can also be used. More samples can be loaded in a single gel with 15 wells and the volume of each sample loaded per lane is also reduced by half (10 μL or less needed), which conserves valuable samples.
19. If acrylamide begins to ooze out when the first comb is inserted, it has already started to polymerize and there is no need to continue with the rest of the gels. Thus, practice quickly inserting the combs before making the stacking gel solution.
20. The gels will be good for up to a month if kept wet and refrigerated. Inspect the gel before use. If there are air bubbles in the gel or the gel has separated from the glass or alumina plate, discard the gel.
21. If possible, remove the comb after the reservoir is filled with electrophoresis buffer, then work the comb out slowly by gently rocking it side to side while pulling it out. Be cautious of collapsing wells when removing the comb. If a well(s) has collapsed, use a micropipette tip to gently lift the collapsed walls back to a standing position.
22. A constant current setting at 20 mA per gel is fine to use.

23. A pilot experiment should be performed to determine the migration of a PEG-containing polymer, intact and degraded, relative to the tracking blue dye after 1 h of electrophoresis.
24. Cut a small notch on one corner to mark the orientation of the resolving gel before staining.
25. Iodine is commonly used as a starch indicator to test for the presence of starch in foods, drugs, paper, textiles, and other products where iodine dissolved in an aqueous solution reacts with starch, resulting in an intensely purple-black colored complex.
26. Wrap the iodine solution bottle with foil to protect from light. Wear gloves and a lab coat to protect skin and cloth from iodine stains.
27. Speed up the de-staining step by using larger volumes and more frequent changes of water. Also, place the container on a shaker to agitate water over the gel, which helps to de-stain the gel more evenly.
28. The iodine stain will fade over time in water. The best way to preserve the stain is to wrap the gel in plastic wrap with no excess water, place it flat in a plastic bag or container together with a sheet of wet paper towel, and store at 4 °C protected from light. If the gel is left in water too long and bands becomes too faint, the gel can be re-stained with iodine until all bands are saturated with BaI_2 stain again and then destain with water to remove background color.
29. The ability to store image data in a lossless format makes a TIFF file a useful image archive, because, unlike standard JPEG or PGN files, a TIFF file using lossless compression (or none) may be edited and re-saved without losing image quality.
30. The dominant bands in the gel shown in Fig. 1 correspond to the intact PEG band in lane 1 (the non-sonicated PEG sample on the far-left lane) and the sonicated bands in the other lanes (lanes 2–7) to the right.
31. To select the color of the rectangle go to ***Edit* → *Option* → *Colors***, make a color selection from the list, and hit "OK".
32. Instead of crop, a copy of the selected area can be created using ***Image* → *Duplicate***. The copy is named in the "Title" box. Hit "OK" and a new window will open containing a copy of the selected area of the image.
33. The brightness and Contrast of the gel image can be adjusted in *ImageJ*:
    - Choose ***Image* → *Adjust* → *Brightness/Contrast***. A new window "B&C" will appear with a histogram of pixel intensity, displaying the range of pixels with the lowest intensity on the left and the highest on the right, and

with corresponding values listed on the bottom of the graph. The current pixel intensity distribution of the image is shown in four sliders for the minimum, maximum, brightness, and contrast ranges.

- To make the bands look darker, by cutting off low-intensity pixels, slide the "Minimum" (top) slider to the right. This sets the bottom of the display range to a higher value than the previous display.
- To make the bands look brighter, by cutting off high-intensity pixels, slide the "Maximum" (second) slider to the left. This sets the top of the display range to a lower value than before.
- Adjusting the "Brightness" (third) slider changes both the top and the bottom intensity values displayed without changing the size of the range displayed.
- Adjusting the "Contrast" (fourth) slider changes both the top and bottom brightness values and the size of the display range.
- The "Auto" button chooses the best display range, based on a saturation of 0.35 % of the pixels in the image.
- The "Reset" button acts as an undo button and resets the image to its original (full) display range.
- The "Set" button allows the user to input values for the top and bottom of the display range with the option to propagate these values to all other images open in *ImageJ*.
- None of the adjustments made to the Brightness and Contrast of the image alter the histogram and the pixel intensity values of the image permanently until the "Apply" button is hit.

34. *ImageJ* assumes that the lanes run vertically (individual bands are horizontal), so the rectangle drawn should be tall and just narrow enough to enclose a single band.
35. To select the color and font of the labels go to ***Image → Overlay → Labels***. A new window "Labels" will appear, in which color, font size, and other properties of the labels can be selected. Hit the "OK" button to accept the selections.
36. If an error has been made in setting the size or the order of the rectangles, reset the rectangles using ***Analyze → Gels → Reset***, and start it over from the first lane.
37. If it is desirable to have two plots to compare side-by-side, go to ***Analyze → Gels → Re-plot Lanes*** to reset the rectangles.
38. This step requires some subjective judgment to decide where the peak ends and the background noise begins.

39. If a mistake has been made when clicking with the ***Wand*** tool, such as clicking the area outside a peak, the program still records the pixel intensity of that clicked region, and it will report that value as an entry in the Results window. A quick fix is to highlight the unwanted entry in the Results window, hit "Clear" under the "Edit" tab to erase it before clicking the next area with the ***Wand*** tool. To erase the whole set of measurements and reset the Results window counter, go to ***Analyze*** → ***Gel*** → ***Label Peaks***, go back to the top of the profile plot, and begin clicking inside the peaks again, starting with the first peak in the first section. The Results window should clear and begin showing new values.
40. The values in the Results windows can be copied to a spreadsheet program, such as *Microsoft Excel*, by clicking ***Edit*** → ***Select All*** to highlight all the values, followed by ***Edit*** → ***Copy*** in the Results window. Go to an *Excel* spreadsheet, right-click and hit ***Paste***, and the two columns of values will be transferred into *Excel* in the exact order.

Acknowledgments

The authors thank the University of Arizona SEMATECH/Semiconductor Research Corporation Engineering Research Center for Environmentally Benign Semiconductor Manufacturing (Grant ERC425-048), the National Cancer Institute (Grant R15-CA152917), and the National Institute for Environmental Health Sciences (Grant R15-ES023666) for supporting this work.

References

1. Neppiras EA (1984) Acoustic cavitation series: Part one: Acoustic cavitation: an introduction. Ultrasonics 22:25–28
2. Suslick KS (1990) Sonochemistry. Science 247:1439–1445
3. Suslick KS, Flannigan DJ (2008) Inside a collapsing bubble: sonoluminescence and the conditions during cavitation. Annu Rev Phys Chem 59:659–683
4. Vijayalakshmi SP, Madras G (2004) Effect of temperature on the ultrasonic degradation of polyacrylamide and poly(ethylene oxide). Polym Degrad Stab 84:341–344
5. Vijayalakshmi SP, Madras G (2005) Effect of initial molecular weight and solvents on the ultrasonic degradation of poly(ethylene oxide). Polym Degrad Stab 90:116–122
6. Kawasaki H, Takeda Y, Arakawa R (2007) Mass spectrometric analysis for high molecular weight synthetic polymers using ultrasonic degradation and the mechanism of degradation. Anal Chem 79:4182–4187
7. Zeineldin R, Al-Haik M, Hudson LG (2009) Role of polyethylene glycol integrity in specific receptor targeting of carbon nanotubes to cancer cells. Nano Lett 9:751–757
8. Koda S, Mori H, Matsumoto K, Nomura H (1994) Ultrasonic degradation of water-soluble polymers. Polymer 35:30–33
9. Watanabe T, Okabayashi M, Kurokawa D, Nishimoto Y, Ozawa T, Kawasaki H, Arakawa R (2010) Determination of primary bond scissions by mass spectrometric analysis of ultrasonic degradation products of poly(ethylene oxide-block-propylene oxide) copolymers. J Mass Spectrom 45:799–805
10. Wang R, Hughes T, Beck S, Vakil S, Li S, Pantano P, Draper RK (2013) Generation of

toxic degradation products by sonication of Pluronic® dispersants: implications for nanotoxicity testing. Nanotoxicology 7:1272–1281

11. Murali VS, Wang R, Mikoryak CA, Pantano P, Draper R (2015) Rapid detection of polyethylene glycol sonolysis upon functionalization of carbon nanomaterials. Exp Biol Med (Maywood) 240:1147–1151
12. Wang R, Meredith AN, Lee MJ, Miadzvedskaya L, Braun E, Pantano P, Harper S, Draper R (2016) Toxicity assessment and bioaccumulation in zebrafish embryos exposed to carbon nanotubes suspended in Pluronic® F-108. Nanotoxicology 10(6):689–698
13. Laemmli UK (1970) Cleavage of structural proteins during the assembly of the head of bacteriophage T4. Nature 227:680–685
14. Kurfürst MM (1992) Detection and molecular weight determination of polyethylene glycol-modified hirudin by staining after sodium dodecyl sulfate-polyacrylamide gel electrophoresis. Anal Biochem 200:244–248
15. Abràmoff MD, Magalhães PJ, Ram SJ (2004) Image processing with ImageJ. Biophotonics Int 11:36–42
16. Nascentes CC, Korn M, Sousa CS, Arruda MAZ (2001) Use of ultrasonic baths for analytical applications: a new approach for optimisation conditions. J Braz Chem Soc 12:57–63
17. Taurozzi JS, Hackley VA, Wiesner MR (2011) Ultrasonic dispersion of nanoparticles for environmental, health and safety assessment—issues and recommendations. Nanotoxicology 5:711–729
18. Suslick KS, Price GJ (1999) Applications of ultrasound to materials chemistry. Annu Rev Mater Sci 29:295–326
19. Sostaric JZ, Riesz P (2002) Adsorption of surfactants at the gas/solution Interface of cavitation bubbles: an ultrasound intensity-independent frequency effect in sonochemistry. J Phys Chem B 106:12537–12548

Chapter 11

Methods for Generation and Detection of Nonstationary Vapor Nanobubbles Around Plasmonic Nanoparticles

Ekaterina Y. Lukianova-Hleb and Dmitri O. Lapotko

Abstract

Laser pulse-induced vapor nanobubbles are nonstationary nanoevents that offer a broad range of applications, especially in the biomedical field. Plasmonic (usually gold) nanoparticles have the highest energy efficacy of the generation of vapor nanobubbles and such nanobubbles were historically named as plasmonic nanobubbles. Below we review methods (protocols) for generating and detecting plasmonic nanobubbles in liquids. The biomedical applications of plasmonic nanobubbles include in vivo and in vitro detection and imaging, gene transfer, micro-surgery, drug delivery, and other diagnostic, therapeutic, and theranostic applications.

Key words Laser, Vapor nanobubbles, Plasmonic nanobubble, Gold nanoparticles

1 Introduction

The increasing need in multifunctional cellular agents that support a wide range of medical functions from the diagnosis to the surgery and to the therapy resulted in a new discipline named theranostics. Historically, most of theranostic solutions were supported with materials, often nanoparticles with multiple functions. However, the reality of their biological and clinical applications posed several fundamental challenges:

- Nonspecific uptake of nanoparticles by nontarget cells and tissues creates toxicities and reduces the efficacy, and requires increasing the dose of nanoparticles to achieve a desired effect.
- Current biological functions of clinically safe nanoparticles appear to be limited and do not support a holy grail promise of nanomedicine in general.

This is why, in our search for the ideal cell level nano-agent, we came to the concept of nano-events instead of nano-materials, and introduced plasmonic nanobubbles (PNB), nonstationary

Reema Zeineldin (ed.), *Cancer Nanotechnology: Methods and Protocols*, Methods in Molecular Biology, vol. 1530,
DOI 10.1007/978-1-4939-6646-2_11, © Springer Science+Business Media New York 2017

Table 1
Applications and functions of PNBs

Field	PNB generation	PNB detection	Application
Physics, material science	Laser pulse with the fluence above PNB generation threshold	Optical via the scattering mechanism	On-demand mechanical nano-impact or optical scattering, imaging of nanoparticles
Biology	Laser pulse with the application-specific fluence	Optical via the scattering mechanism	Delivery of molecular cargo into target cell, on-demand mechanical impact in target cell, imaging of specific cells
Medicine	Near-infrared laser pulse with the application-specific fluence	Acoustic	Diagnosis Drug and gene delivery Nano-surgery Combination chemo- and radiation therapy

mechanical events at the nanoscale, nano-explosions in fact, to cover a wide spectrum of medical and nonmedical applications (Table 1). A plasmonic nanobubble is generated around light-absorbing (usually plasmonic) nanoparticle in liquid when the nanoparticle is exposed to a short laser pulse (Fig. 1a) through the chain of the physical processes: optical absorption—heating of the nanoparticle surface—heating and evaporation of adjacent liquid—vapor expansion and collapse. The Table 1 below outlines various applications and functions of PNBs, and basic requirements for their generation and detection. Next, the chapter below discusses various scientific and methodological aspects of PNB generation and detection. Finally, there is an application-specific example of the PNB generation protocol.

The absorption of optical energy by micro- and nanoparticles in liquid, and the follow-up photothermal conversion and heating of the surrounding liquid induce vapor bubbles around such particles if the incident optical fluence (laser pulse energy per unit area) exceeds a specific threshold [1–11] (Fig. 1). The energy efficacy of vapor bubble generation increases when the particle-to-liquid heat transfer is localized and the bulk heating of liquid is minimized. This thermal confinement is usually achieved by shortening the duration of the optical excitation to minimize thermal diffusion [12]. In the case of a nanoparticle, the duration of the optical excitation shortens to a nano- and pico-second range to prevent the bulk heating of the surrounding liquid [12–14]. This, in turn, makes the generation of a transient vapor nanobubble a highly nonstationary process [15, 16]. The combination of the nano-size of the optical absorber with the drastic increase in the photothermal efficacy of plasmonic nanoparticles (compared to that of any molecular absorbers) resulted in a new class of nano-events, plasmonic

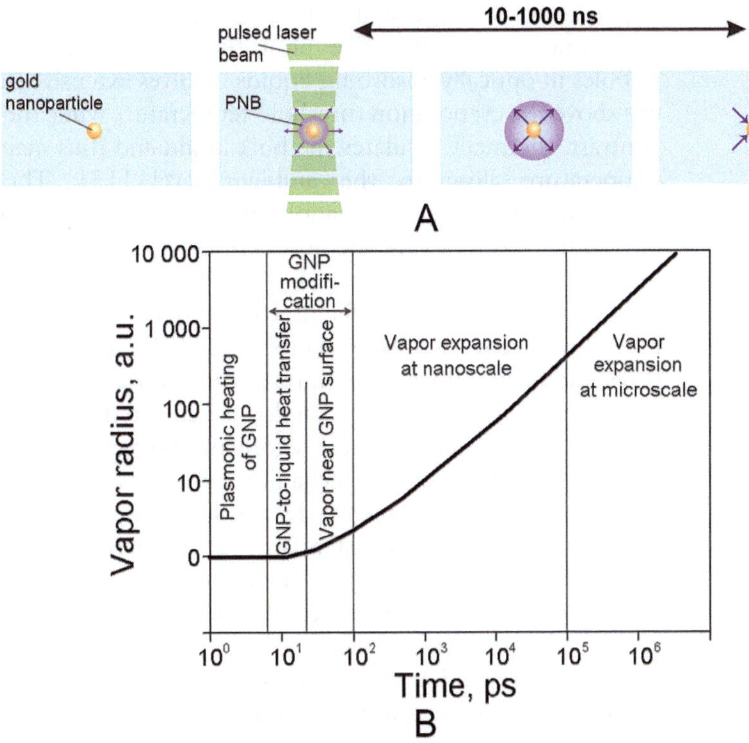

Fig. 1 (**a**) The generation of plasmonic nanobubbles (PNB): a gold nanoparticle (GNP) in liquid is exposed to a short laser pulse. Optical absorption results in rapid heating of the GNP and evaporation of adjacent liquid and a pressure build up inside a vapor. After this internal pressure in the vapor exceeds the external pressure, the vapor rapidly expands into a nanobubble, and then collapses back to the GNP. (**b**) A temporal sequence of the above-described processes involved into the generation of PNB [25]

nanobubbles (PNBs)—vapor nanobubbles, generated via the photothermal conversion around plasmonic nanoparticles [4–7, 9–11, 15–20].

The physical properties of PNBs were shown to be different both from those of the *stationary photothermal effects* of plasmonic nanoparticles under continuous optical excitation and of laser-induced vapor bubbles in liquid via the mechanisms of *optical breakdown* or homogeneous optical absorbance by liquid. The photothermal properties of nanoparticles under stationary excitation are determined by their preset properties, such as optical absorbance, which remain permanent during their optical excitation. In contrast, an intense short pulsed excitation of a metal nanoparticle during the generation of a PNB results in a rapid dynamic modification of the optical absorbance, size, structure, and phase state of the nanoparticle [21–24] and results in entirely new optical, physical, and biomedical properties of PNB compared to those of plasmonic nanoparticles [16, 22]. For example, compared to gold nanospheres with a broad excitation visible spectrum, a gold nanosphere-generated PNB yields an ultra-narrow peak in near-infrared [16, 25]. The photothermal generation of vapor bubbles in optically absorbing liquids involves extensive bulk heating above the evaporation threshold temperature while the PNB, in contrast, thermally insulates the bulk liquid and thus maintains its temperature close to the ambient level [15]. The optical breakdown-induced vapor nanobubbles do not require significant optical absorbance by the medium. However, an optical breakdown involves high local pressures and temperatures, and often shock waves, thus making it difficult to precisely control the optical breakdown-generated vapor nanobubble [26]. The relatively high threshold of laser fluence and intensity for optical breakdown limits biomedical applications of breakdown-generated nanobubbles. In contrast, PNBs demonstrated excellent biologic safety [16, 20] because of their localized mechanical, nonthermal impact and low threshold energies down to 5–15 mJ/cm^2 [27, 28], which match even the federal laser safety standards [29]. The remote on-demand generation, precise control of their mechanical impact and easy optical and acoustic detection result in promising biomedical applications of PNBs for diagnostics, therapy, and theranostics [9, 20, 26–28, 30–34] and in various industrial applications [17, 35, 36].

However, the applications of PNB are still relatively limited compared to those of plasmonic nanoparticles or laser-induced vapor bubbles in liquids. This is largely caused by the lack of the universal methodology of PNB generation in real conditions. A *PNB is not a particle but rather a transient nonstationary nano-event* which results from several transient nanoscale processes at sub-nanosecond time scale (Fig. 1b). Under excitation of a plasmonic nanoparticle with an ultra-short single laser, these processes include: photon-phonon-heat conversion, nanoparticle surface-to-liquid heat transfer, liquid evaporation, and vapor bubble expansion and collapse. The nonstationary nature of these processes, coupled with the dynamically changing optical and thermal properties of the nanoparticle under high (melting) temperatures, seriously complicates the modeling of PNBs, compared to the modeling of stationary or low temperature photothermal effects. Experimental studies of PNBs at the nanoscale usually describe their properties under the specific duration of the excitation laser pulse and for the specific nanoparticle system. Such properties are difficult to extrapolate into other laser pulse durations and nanoparticle systems. In addition, the majority of experimental models and protocols use nanoparticle ensembles, multiple laser pulses, and indirect detection of PNBs through their secondary cumulated effects. All these factors distort the understanding of the PNB's generation mechanism. As a result, the practical use of PNBs remains rather challenging for a broad community.

2 Generation of Plasmonic Vapor Nanobubbles Around Laser-Heated Gold Nanoparticles

Here, we discuss the key factor for generation of the plasmonic nanobubbles, the *duration of optical excitation*, in the range from picosecond to continuous excitation. The discussed protocols employ various nanoparticle systems—from isolated nanoparticles (solid gold nanospheres (also known as colloids) [37]) to their suspensions and to large clusters of aggregated nanoparticles.

2.1 Initial Development of PNB

To estimate how fast a vapor may develop at the surface of a 60 nm solid gold nanoparticle (GNP), the GNP's surface temperature dynamics were simulated in water in response to a single laser pulse. In simulations, the laser fluence was fixed at the level of 66 mJ/cm^2, which is well above the threshold for generation of PNB. In this model, and for the initial stage of the GNP heating, we considered that the level of the optical absorbance cross-section of the GNP remained constant during its interaction with the laser pulse (although at later stages it changed drastically due to the GNP heating and melting). We approximated the vapor onset temperature by the critical temperature for water. This relatively high threshold ensures the onset of vapor near the GNP surface under any conditions. After this temperature level was achieved, we did not model the follow-up temperature dynamics because the laser-induced temperatures rapidly reach the GNP surface melting conditions and thus the GNP optical absorbance, structure, and size undergo radical dynamic changes [21, 22]. All these dynamic changes cannot be easily incorporated into existing models.

We defined the vapor onset time t_{PNB} (Fig. 2a) as the time interval from the beginning of the laser pulse (at the laser intensity level $1/e^2$) to the time point when the GNP surface temperature reaches the vapor onset threshold. Naturally, the vapor onset time cannot be shorter than the GNP thermalization time which has been approximated by 5 ps [23, 24, 38, 39]. The vapor onset time was analyzed as a function of the laser pulse duration from 20 ps to 14 ns (black curve in Fig. 2b).

We also considered continuous excitation as a separate case (see below). The shortest pulses provided the shortest vapor onset times. Formally, vapor onset time was even shorter than the GNP thermalization time and was therefore approximated by the longer one, GNP thermalization time (Fig. 2b). The vapor onset time grew with the duration of the laser pulse. We further defined "the PNB energy" of the laser pulse as the percentage of the laser pulse energy which corresponds to the time interval from the vapor onset to the end of the laser pulse (Fig. 2a). This "PNB energy" indicates the incident optical energy that can be utilized by a PNB. We analyzed this PNB energy as a function of the pulse duration (red

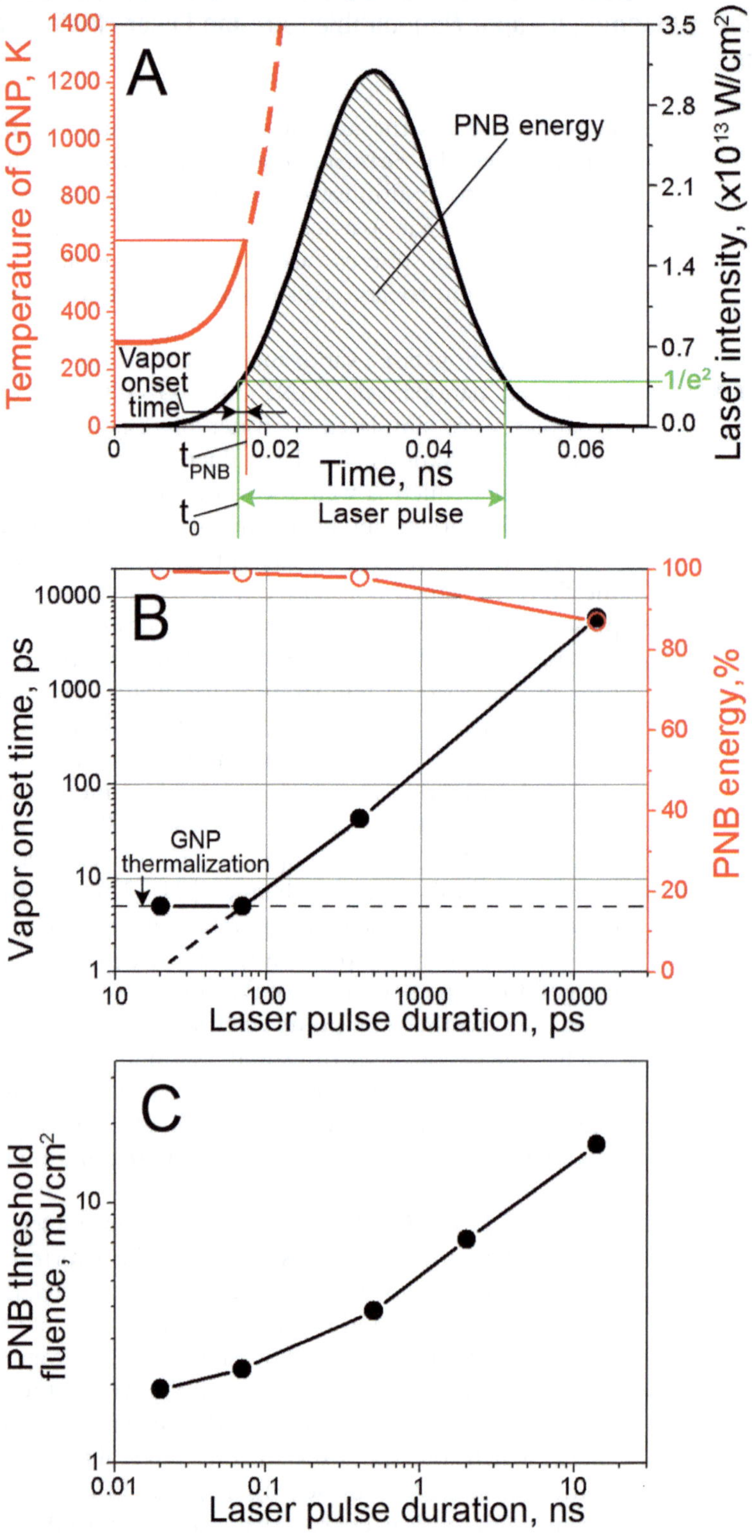

Fig. 2 (**a**) The calculated time-course of the temperature of gold 60 nm nanospheres in water (*red curve*) during the absorption of a single laser pulse at 532 nm (pulse duration 20 ps) with a Gaussian temporal profile (*black curve*) with the fluence of 66 mJ/cm^2. (**b**) The calculated vapor onset time (*black curve*) and the portion

curve in Fig. 2b). For picosecond pulses, the vapor onset time was only a small fraction of the whole pulse duration and hence the level of PNB energy was relatively high. Longer pulses showed a decrease in the PNB energy due to the increased thermal losses for the bulk heating of the surrounding water. Finally, we estimated the vapor onset threshold fluence which was defined as the fluence required to achieve the vapor onset temperature of the GNP surface (Fig. 2c). The PNB's threshold fluence increased with the pulse duration, mainly due to the increased energy losses to the bulk heating of water. Thus, the modeled vapor onset time and the laser threshold fluence were the lowest for the shortest pulses. In particular, for the picosecond pulses the pulse energy was almost totally utilized to generate the PNB. Next, we present the experimental studies of PNBs.

2.2 The Influence of the Laser Pulse Duration on the PNB Generation Around Isolated GNPs Under Resonant Optical Excitation

To study the influence of the excitation pulse duration on PNB generation, the isolated GNPs were studied in water using single laser pulses at 532 nm, which is close to the wavelength of plasmon resonance in 60 nm GNPs. Individual GNPs and PNBs were imaged via our time-resolved optical scattering method (Fig. 3a, b) [19]. The maximal diameter of the expanding and collapsing individual PNB was quantified through the duration of its optical scattering time-response (Fig. 3c) [15]. This PNB metric was applied to characterize the energy efficacy of PNB generation for a specific laser fluence. Under the fixed applied laser fluence (66 mJ/cm^2), PNBs were observed for all three picosecond pulse durations from 20 to 400 ps, but were not observed for the nanosecond pulses (Fig. 3d). The maximum PNB lifetime (and hence the maximum energy efficacy of PNB generation) was observed for the shortest pulse of 20 ps. Apparently, the applied fluence, 66 mJ/cm^2, was above the PNB generation threshold for 20 and 70 ps pulses, close to the threshold for the 400 ps pulse and below the threshold for the 14 ns pulse (Fig. 3d). We next measured the PNB generation threshold fluence as a function of the laser pulse duration (red curve in Fig. 3d).

The minimum threshold, which is less than 18 mJ/cm^2, was observed for the shortest, 20 ps pulse. The 20-fold increase in the pulse duration from 20 to 400 ps increased the threshold fluence 6.4-fold to 115 mJ/cm^2, while for the nanosecond pulse, the PNB generation threshold fluence increased by almost two orders of magnitude (red curve in Fig. 3d). Thus, the laser pulse duration

Fig. 2 (Continued) of the laser pulse energy (*red curve*) which corresponds to the portion of the pulse after the vapor onset as a function of the laser pulse duration at 532 nm wavelength and fluence of 66 mJ/cm^2. (**c**) The calculated PNB's generation threshold fluence as a function of laser pulse duration at 532 nm wavelength. Reprinted from [25]

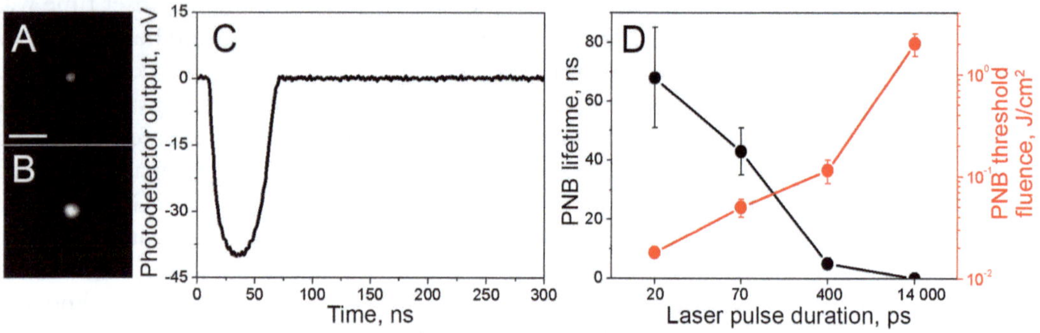

Fig. 3 Generation of PNBs around isolated GNPs in water [25]. Optical scattering time-resolved images of (**a**) an individual gold 60 nm sphere in water and (**b**) a PNB generated around the same sphere in single 20 ps pulse excitation at 532 nm. Scale bar: 2 μm. (**c**) Illustration of the typical time-response of the PNB. The lifetime is measured as the duration at the level of 0.5 of the maximum amplitude of the PNB-specific signal. (**d**) Dependences of the PNB lifetime (*black curve*) under specific excitation wavelength of 532 nm and fluence of 66 mJ/cm^2 and dependence of the PNB generation threshold fluence (*red curve*) at the excitation wavelength of 532 nm upon the excitation duration

radically influences both the energy efficacy and the threshold fluence of PNB generation.

These experimental results qualitatively agree with the above simulations. Quantitatively, the experimentally observed PNB generation thresholds were higher than the estimated values. This disagreement may be caused by several factors that were not taken into account in the theoretical model, but they reduced the efficiency of PNB generation. Namely, our model did not account for the additional energy required to (1) overcome the surface tension pressure (which is very high for isolated 60 nm GNPs), (2) evaporate a specific volume of liquid for the formation of a PNB, and (3) compensate a substantial dynamic decrease in the optical absorbance of a GNP during its interaction with the laser pulse. The latter effect is caused by (1) vapor around the GNP that significantly changes the dielectric functions of gold and, hence, reduces optical absorbance at the resonance wavelength [40], (2) extensive heating, melting and size reduction of the GNP [22, 41–46], and (3) additional scattering of the incident excitation laser beam by the vapor–water boundary [15]. All these factors were not taken into account in our model and might explain the almost one order of magnitude difference between the theoretical and experimental PNB generation threshold fluences. A more accurate theoretical prediction of the threshold fluences requires a fairly complex computational methodology that is capable, in particular, of connecting the heat and mass transfer processes in and around a GNP with the dynamic variation of its optical absorbance. So far, such models do not exist. In addition, the detection limit of an individual PNB in our experiments might have been relatively high, above 200 nm, and thus the smallest PNBs (generated under the lower fluences) might have been missed.

Nevertheless, the above experimental data were based on the direct detection of individual PNBs and therefore they correctly describe the influence of the laser pulse duration on the PNB generation threshold and energy efficacy. To summarize, short picosecond pulses provide the best energy efficacy of photothermal PNB generation, while the use of popular nanosecond lasers may require a 100-fold increase in the laser energy.

2.3 GNP Ensembles vs. Isolated Particles

The isolated GNPs studied above are not typical for real-world photothermal applications, where GNPs are used in the form of suspensions or/and aggregated clusters. For example, active bio-targeting of GNPs results in their intracellular clustering [20, 47, 48]. Many industrial applications employ suspensions of GNPs [17, 35, 36]. We therefore studied the PNB lifetimes (a metric of the energy efficacy of PNB generation) as a function of the cluster size for isolated GNP clusters (Fig. 4) and the concentration for GNP suspension (Fig. 5) under a specific level of the laser fluence, 66 mJ/cm^2, above PNB generation threshold fluence. The excitation wavelength of 532 nm was close to that of the plasmon resonance for the 60 nm solid spheres employed. Based on our previous results, we used the most efficient 20 ps pulse. GNP clusters in water were formed via the salt-driven aggregation of GNPs. The relative size of each individual GNP cluster was quantified via the pixel amplitude of its optical scattering image (Fig. 4a). The PNB lifetime was measured for individual clusters in response to a single laser pulse (Fig. 4c). The PNB lifetime increased with the GNP cluster size almost linearly and exceeded that of a single GNP

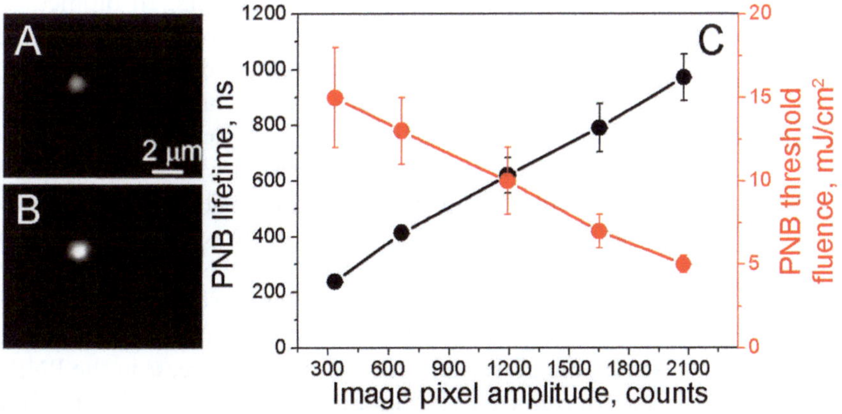

Fig. 4 Generation of PNBs around isolated GNP clusters in water under resonant excitation with 20 ps laser pulse at 532 nm [25]. (**a**) Optical scattering time-resolved images of a GNP cluster in water and (**b**) a PNB generated around the same cluster in single 20 ps pulse excitation at 532 nm. (**c**) The energy efficacy of PNB generation (measured via the lifetime of individual PNBs at 66 mJ/cm^2, *black curve*) and the PNB generation threshold fluence (*red curve*) as functions of the GNP cluster size (quantified via the pixel amplitude of the optical scattering image of a GNP cluster)

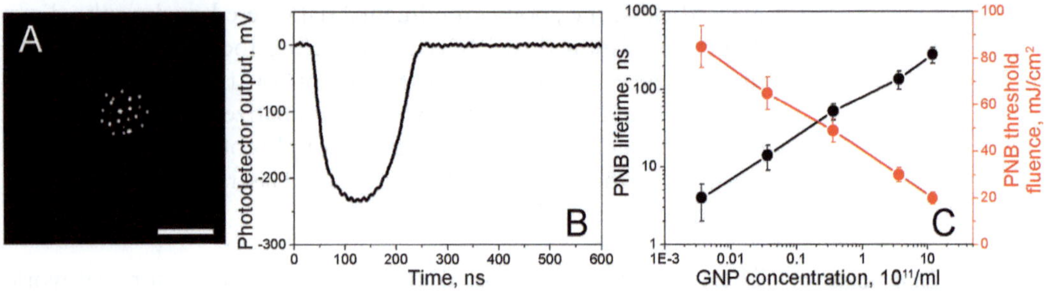

Fig. 5 Generation of PNBs in water suspension of single GNPs under resonant excitation with 20 ps laser pulse at 532 nm [25]. (**a**) Optical scattering time-resolved image of PNBs generated at laser fluence of 66 mJ/cm^2. Scale bar: 5 μm. (**b**) Illustration of the typical time-response of the PNBs. (**c**) The energy efficacy of PNB generation (measured via the lifetime of individual PNBs at 66 mJ/cm^2, *black curve*) and the PNB generation threshold fluence (*red curve*) as functions of the GNP concentration in the suspension

by approximately fivefold (black curve in Fig. 4c). This significant increase in PNB generation efficacy of the cluster vs. isolated GNP under identical laser fluence can be explained by: (1) the enhancement of plasmonic properties and the increased optical absorbance of the cluster [22], and (2) the coalescence of the initial vapors around GNPs into the joint vapor blanket around the whole cluster, which increases the bubble radius and hence reduces the surface tension pressure [15]. The clustering of GNPs also resulted in an almost fourfold decrease in the PNB threshold fluence compared to that for an isolated single GNP; from 18 to 5 mJ/cm^2 (red curve in Fig. 4c). This effect provides a unique opportunity to selectively generate PNBs only around the largest GNP clusters at the minimum laser fluence, and without generating PNBs around single unclustered GNPs or their small clusters. In biomedical applications, this cluster size effect allows a dramatic improvement in the target cell specificity of PNBs compared to that of GNPs [20].

For water suspensions of unclustered single GNPs, we observed multiple PNBs under a single pulse excitation (Fig. 5a). These multiple PNBs were generated synchronously and were analyzed through an integrated optical scattering time-response (Fig. 5b). A PNB lifetime has been averaged over ten responses obtained from ten different areas of the suspension. An increase in the GNP concentration by four orders of magnitude increased the PNB lifetime from 4 to 280 ns (black curve in Fig. 5c) and at the same time caused an almost fourfold decrease in the PNB threshold fluence (red curve in Fig. 5c). Even at the maximum GNP concentration, the PNB generation threshold in suspension (20 mJ/cm^2) was significantly higher than that for individual GNP clusters (5 mJ/cm^2). Therefore, GNP clusters provided higher energy efficacy of the PNB generation compared to that for GNP suspensions.

The effects of GNP clustering contribute to the PNB generation and detection in suspension. Firstly, in experiments with GNP suspension, the maximum GNP concentration studied corresponds to the averaged distance between individual GNPs in the order of 1 μm. This distance is comparable with the maximum size of PNBs and may cause a coalescence of several PNBs in a larger one with a longer lifetime. Secondly, an increase in GNP concentration increases the probability of a single GNP being exposed to a laser pulse. In our conditions, the probability of PNB generation in suspension at the low concentration was less than 1. This influenced the averaging of the PNB lifetime over 10 pulses that were applied to the different areas of the suspension. The increase in the GNP concentration increased the PNB generation probability and, accordingly, the average lifetime. Thirdly, at high GNP concentrations the PNB generation probability becomes equal to 1 and a further increase in the PNB lifetime is caused by the increase in the number of simultaneously generated PNBs whose integrated optical scattering effect was detected as a single time-response of a longer duration compared to that from a single PNB (in addition to the mentioned above effect of coalescence of several small PNBs into one large PNB at high GNP concentration). These three effects explain the influence of the GNP concentration upon the PNB generation energy efficacy and threshold. Therefore, the GNP suspension does not correctly describe the PNB generation mechanism for individual GNPs. Among three GNP systems studied, single GNPs, suspensions of GNPs, and clusters of tightly aggregated GNPs, the latter showed the highest PNB generation efficacy.

2.4 Continuous Optical Excitation

To model the PNB generation under continuous optical excitation, we estimated the thermal response of an isolated GNP to continuous wave (c.w.) laser excitation at 532 nm under the same optical dose (fluence) as employed above for the pulsed excitation. Under the same optical dose (fluence) as employed above for the pulsed excitation, the PNB threshold temperature could not be achieved due to intense thermal losses. In this model, the duration of optical excitation was 1 s. The estimated threshold fluence turned out to be nine orders of magnitude higher; 2×10^9 mJ/cm^2. Experimental studies of isolated GNPs in water under these conditions, which are identical to those described in second section for the pulsed excitation, resulted in no detectible PNBs in the range of the laser intensities below 2 MW/cm^2 and the duration of excitation up to 20 s (fluences of up to 4×10^7 J/cm^2).

The GNP suspensions at the highest concentration of 10^{12} GNP per mL also did not return any detectable PNBs under the c.w. excitation at this laser intensity and for a duration as long as 60 s. When the GNP suspension was replaced by individual large (microscopically visible) GNP clusters (Fig. 6a), a microscopic PNB was detected after 30 s of excitation at laser intensity of 2 MW/cm^2 (Fig. 6b). As the excitation was continued, PNBs grew from micro to almost macro size almost linearly with the time (Fig. 6c). For

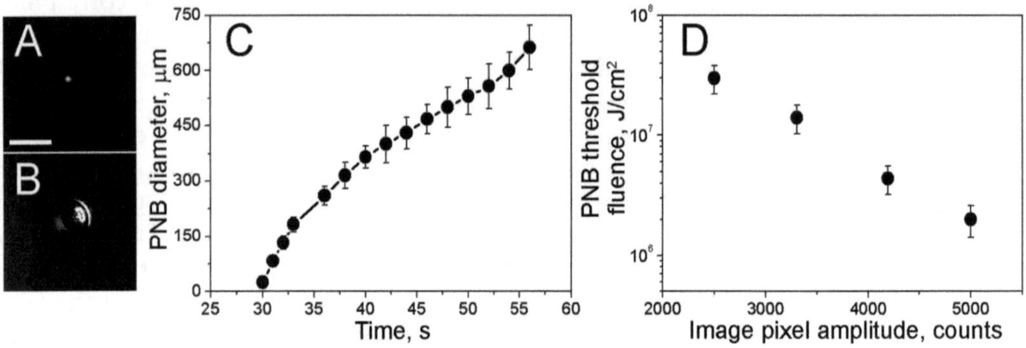

Fig. 6 Continuous excitation of PNBs [25]. (**a**) Optical scattering time-resolved image of a GNP cluster and (**b**) PNB generated around GNP cluster at the c.w. excitation (2 MW/cm^2, 532 nm). Scale bar: 25 μm. (**c**) Dependence of the PNB diameter upon continuous excitation time (532 nm), the change in the slope occurs when the bubble diameter reaches 0.12 mm, the height of the cuvette, after that, the bubble growth is basically two-dimensional. (**d**) PNB generation threshold fluence at continuous excitation of PNB upon the GNP cluster size quantified via the pixel image amplitude of the optical absorbance of a GNP cluster

isolated GNP clusters, the PNB generation threshold fluence decreased with the cluster size (Fig. 6d), which was similar to what was observed under pulsed excitation (Fig. 4c).

The above results show that the c.w. generation of PNBs requires multi-order increase in optical fluence compared to the pulsed excitation, and in many cases cannot be achieved at all. The vapor onset times under continuous excitation are associated with a thermal diffusion radius of 12 mm (for thermal diffusion from a spherical GNP [15]), which is four orders of magnitude larger than the maximum size of a GNP cluster, and more than five orders of magnitude larger than the size of an individual GNP. This spatial scale characterizes the size of the water volume heated by a GNP and clearly indicates that the c.w. laser excitation results in the bulk heating of water. In contrast, the PNB generation under short pulse excitation involves heating and evaporation of the water within several nanometers from the GNP surface and does not affect the bulk water temperature as we previously observed [15]. The PNB generation under c.w. laser excitation, therefore, is achieved through a bulk thermal impact on the surrounding media, while the pulsed nonstationary excitation results in the localized mechanical, nonthermal impact of a rapidly expanding and collapsing PNB which, in addition, thermally insulates the bulk media from the laser-heated GNP [15]. This difference makes the c.w. generation of PNBs similar to the laser-induced generation of vapor bubbles in an optically absorbing homogeneous liquid. Therefore, the advantage of plasmonic nanoparticles over optically absorbing liquids is achieved only under a short pulse excitation. In this case, the high optical absorbance of plasmonic nanoparticles efficiently supports the localized heating of the surrounding liquid above the vaporization threshold. Longer, especially continuous, optical excitation of plasmonic nanoparticles in three-dimensional liquids delocalizes the thermal effect from nano- to macro-scale. In this case, any advantage of the nanosize of optical absorbers is lost, as well as the energy efficacy, and the suspension of plasmonic nanoparticles in transparent liquids becomes almost equal to the homogenous solution of optically absorbing liquids. In a case of planar and thermally isolated surface, the continuous excitation of GNPs [49] still may provide some localization of thermal effect. However, it cannot support the generation of a PNB because the latter is a three-dimensional phenomenon.

2.5 Off-Resonant Excitation

In addition to the generation of PNBs at the wavelength near the peak of plasmon resonance, we studied PNB generation at off-resonant near-infrared wavelengths in the range of 700–800 nm, far from a stationary plasmon resonance. Colloidal gold is considered to have a poor optical absorbance in this spectral range, about 1 % of that at the resonance wavelength at 530–540 nm [16]. The off-resonant excitation of isolated GNPs with a 20 ps pulse revealed an ultra-narrow, just 3 nm wide, peak at 782 nm (Fig. 7a). For gold colloids used in this experiment, the spectral width of the optical absorption spectrum was about 100 nm. Under identical laser fluence, the PNB lifetimes at 782 and 532 nm were close, thus implying that the levels of optical absorbance of GNPs at 532 and 782 nm are similar. Interestingly, we observed a similar effect for longer pulses [16]. This effect is very unusual for gold colloids and has never been observed under c.w. excitation of gold nanoparticles. We therefore studied how this off-resonant effect depends upon the duration of the near-infrared laser pulse (Fig. 7b). At a fixed laser fluence, 66 mJ/cm^2, the PNB lifetime rapidly dropped with the pulse length and no PNBs were observed for 400 ps and 14 ns pulses. Compared to resonant excitation (Fig. 3d), this unusual near-infrared peak was limited only to short picosecond pulses. It was impossible to induce PNBs with pulses longer than 70 ps under laser fluences up to 300 mJ/cm^2.

We further theoretically estimated the GNP surface temperature dynamics at 780 nm, and determined the vapor onset times using the similar simulation approach as described above for the resonant excitation (Fig. 7c). Next, based on the published data for similar GNPs [3, 4, 7, 28, 50] we estimated that the actual expansion of a PNB does not begin simultaneously with the onset of the laser pulse (Fig. 1b) and may be delayed by at least 50 ps. We therefore used the time window from the vapor onset to the beginning of the active expansion of the PNB to estimate the percentage of the pulse energy that corresponds to this off-resonant PNB and determined the "off-resonant PNB energy" (Fig. 7c). Based upon similar calculations, this off-resonant PNB energy exceeded zero only for the short picosecond pulses of 20 and 70 ps (red curve in

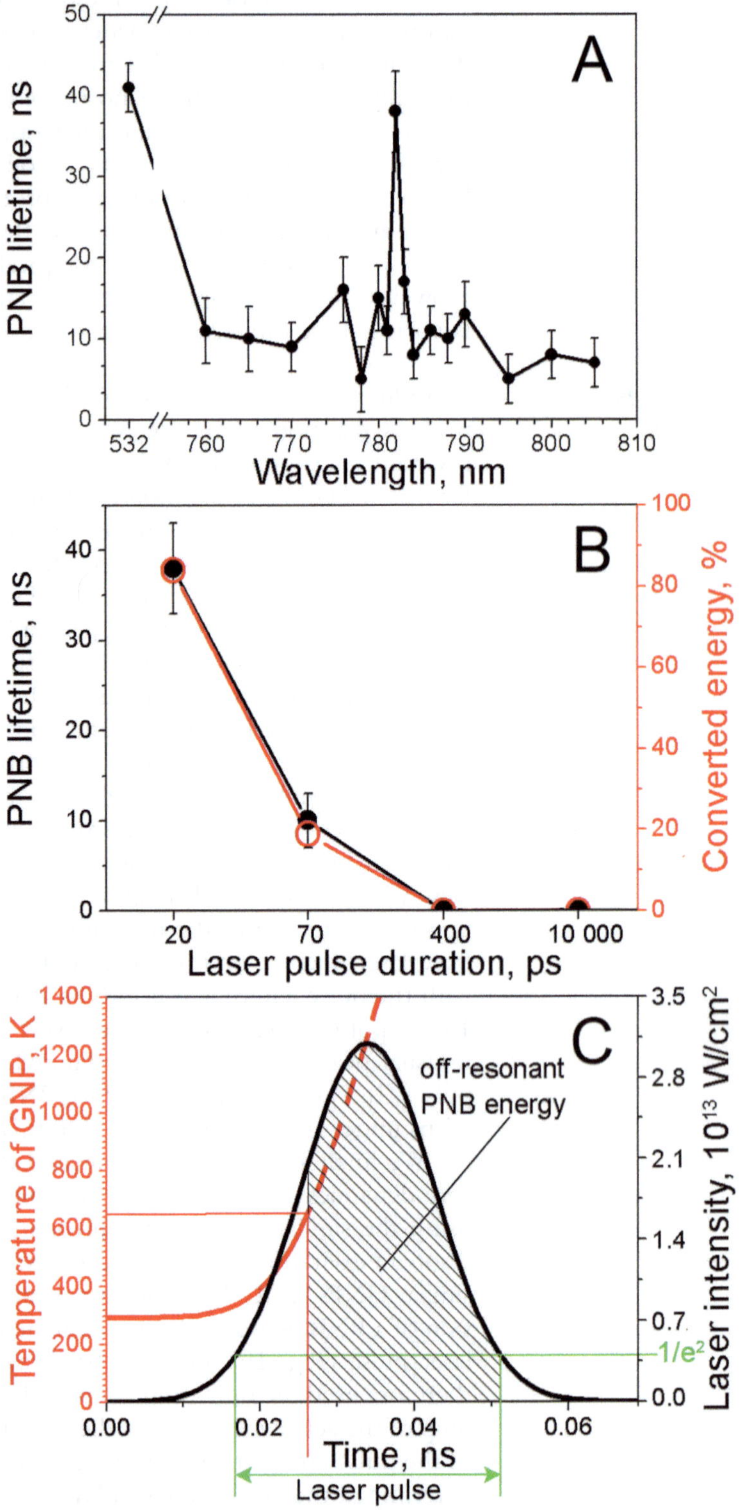

Fig. 7 Off-resonant generation of PNBs around isolated individual GNPs in water obtained for 60 nm gold spheres irradiated by the 20 ps laser pulse at fluence

Fig. 7b). Interestingly, the pulse duration functions of the estimated off-resonant PNB energy and the experimentally measured PNB lifetime were very close (Fig. 7b). To explain this high off-resonant photothermal efficacy of gold colloids under short pulse excitation, we previously hypothesized that a new transient plasmonic structure may emerge and exist during this short time window and this structure transiently develops a high and narrow peak of optical absorbance at 782 nm [16].

This hypothetical transient plasmonic structure may include hot melted gold droplets in a vapor near the surface of the parent GNP. The system of metal droplets, vapor, and the parent GNP surface may have a high optical absorbance similar to a plasmonic grating and thus efficiently convert the near-infrared pulse into a PNB. As a PNB actively expands, it mechanically destroys this structure. The coincidence of the experimental and theoretical data in Fig. 7b supports the hypothesized transient nature of such plasmonic structure. Its ultra-narrow, 3 nm wide, peak of optical absorbance has never been reported for any isolated plasmonic structures. Furthermore, this peak is practically forbidden by electrodynamic theory, which allows for narrow spectral peaks in optical absorbance only for regular arrays and layers of plasmonic materials [51–54]. This novel, nonstationary plasmonic effect requires further in-depth studies. Nevertheless, it opens new opportunities for practical applications of plasmonic nanoparticles under "nonstationary plasmonics" and radically improves the spectral selectivity and photothermal efficacy of gold colloids at wavelengths where such properties cannot be achieved under stationary plasmonic conversion.

In the generation of PNBs, there was a nine order of magnitude difference in the energy efficacy and threshold of the PNB generation with the variation of the duration of the optical excitation of plasmonic nanoparticles from picosecond pulses to continuous excitation. In addition, there was a strong dependence of the PNB generation parameters upon the nanoparticle state: isolated, suspension, or clustered. Finally, there was a nonstationary off-resonant excitation of plasmonic nanoparticles at the wavelengths where the stationary optical properties of plasmonic nanoparticles formally exclude any efficient photothermal response. Naturally, other parameters of plasmonic nanoparticles influenced the PNB generation. The influence of the GNP size on the PNB generation

Fig. 7 (Continued) 66 mJ/cm^2 [25]. (**a**) PNB lifetime spectra. (**b**) Experimentally measured PNB lifetime (*black curve*) and theoretically calculated off-resonant PNB energy (*red curve*) as functions of the duration of the excitation laser pulse at 782 nm. (**c**) The calculated time-course of the GNP surface temperature of (*red curve*) during the absorption of a single 20 ps laser pulse at 782 nm with a Gaussian temporal profile (*black curve*). The *shaded area* of the pulse shows the time window that determines the fraction of the laser pulse defined as an "off-resonant PNB energy" was extensively analyzed by us previously [15, 20]. Generally, the solid spheres of a smaller size or larger than 200 nm required more fluence to generate identical PNBs under the resonant excitation [15]. The results obtained here for 60 nm gold colloids are fairly representative of GNPs of other diameter because the variation of the nanoparticle size in a wide range from 10 to 250 nm resulted in less than one order of magnitude variation in the PNB generation energy efficacy and threshold [15, 55]. The shape and structure of the GNPs of similar size also influenced the PNB generation energy efficacy and threshold fluence by less than one order of magnitude [28, 30, 48]. Therefore, the duration of the optical excitation appeared to be the most critical factor in the photothermal generation of PNB compared to the GNP properties. PNB generation follows the several universal rules:

- A PNB can be generated around a plasmonic nanoparticle using both pulsed nonstationary and continuous stationary optical excitation.
- The maximum energy efficacy of the photothermal generation of PNB is achieved with picosecond laser pulses, while the minimum energy efficacy is associated with continuous optical excitation which requires up to nine orders of magnitude more energy to generate plasmonic nanobubble, compared to picosecond laser pulses.
- The clusters of aggregated nanoparticles provide the maximal energy efficacy of PNB generation compared to isolated nanoparticles or their suspensions.
- For short laser pulses, generation of PNBs does not cause bulk heating of surrounding liquid, while continuous optical excitation of plasmonic nanoparticles results in an opposite effect of significant bulk heating of surrounding liquid.
- Short picosecond off-resonant near-infrared optical excitation of gold colloids results in efficient generation of plasmonic nanobubbles at a specific wavelength and in a very narrow, nanometers-wide, spectral interval around 780 nm.

3 Detection of Plasmonic Vapor Nanobubbles

We analyze three protocols (techniques) that employ optical scattering and acoustic detection in identifying and quantifying individual photothermally induced plasmonic vapor nanobubbles at a wide range of excitation energies. In optically transparent media, the best quantitative detection can be achieved by measuring the duration of the optical scattering time-response, while in an opaque media, the amplitude of the acoustic time-response well describes PNBs in the absence of stress waves.

The science and the methods for the detection of inertial vapor bubbles of various origins were well developed for macro- and micro-sized bubbles and mainly employ their ability to emit pressure and to scatter the incident light [1, 15, 18, 19, 28, 55–69]. Recent developments in nanoscience reduced the spatial and temporal scale of vapor bubbles to nanometers and nanoseconds. Unlike their larger analogs, vapor nanobubbles require much higher sensitivity and resolution of the detection methods for their imaging, quantification, and identification among other phenomena such as transient heating and the generation of stress waves. Here we analyze several experimental techniques for the imaging and quantitative analysis of transient vapor nanobubbles as single events and we troubleshoot some related errors. Due to the multiple biomedical applications of PNBs and related phenomena, it should be noted that we consider the transient events, but not the materials (particles) that are often also called nanobubbles [70, 71]. We also do not consider the cavitation of preexisting bubbles that is well studied elsewhere [72].

3.1 PNB Model

While PNBs may have various sources of energy (the heating of liquid above the boiling threshold, local rarefaction, and plasma discharge), we employed an experimental model of a single PNB in water. Such a model provides maximal precision, control, and reproducibility in PNB generation through the localized transient photothermal heating of liquid above the evaporation point. This was achieved through the optical excitation of individual 60 nm gold nanospheres in water with single short laser pulses (70 ps, 532 nm) at specific fluences above the PNB generation threshold. We used the plasmonic conversion of optical energy into heat to control the maximal diameter and lifetime of the PNBs through the fluence of a single laser pulse, as described in details previously [15, 18, 19, 28, 55]. This experimental model includes an internal metal nanoparticle that acts as the source of the bubble energy during bubble generation and prevents the development of extreme temperatures and sonoluminescence (the emission of short bursts of light from imploding bubbles in a liquid when excited by sound) at the collapse stage, unlike "classical" bubbles that are generated in homogeneous media. Another important difference in the model employed is the absence of an external acoustic field that is often used alone or in combination with optical energy to generate a vapor bubble. The above conditions and the nanoscale size resulted in a single cycle of the vapor nanobubble that did not oscillate.

3.2 Methods and Protocols of PNB Detection

First, we consider imaging methods. Optical scattering phenomena allow both PNB imaging and monitoring of PNB's dynamics. Direct imaging of slower and larger macro- and micro-bubbles employed different cameras and light sources. There is the possibility of using a continuous light source and of capturing a short

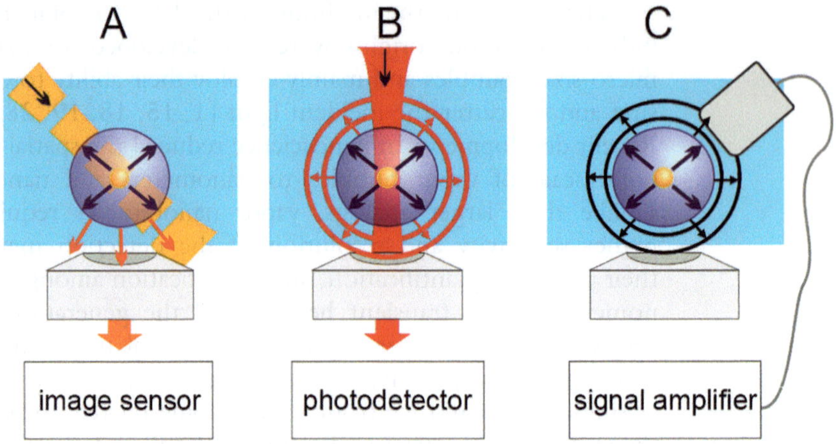

Fig. 8 Methods for detecting vapor nanobubbles in liquid [10]. (**a**) Optical time-resolved scattering imaging is obtained with a short probe laser pulse and a slow image detector; (**b**) optical scattering (extinction) time-response is obtained with a continuous focused probe laser pulse and a fast photodetector; (**c**) acoustical time-response is obtained with an ultrasound detector

transient PNB with high-speed image detectors. However, that would require a nanosecond gating speed, sub-micron spatial resolution, and the corresponding high optical sensitivity. Dynamic transmission electron microscopy and time-resolved diffraction of X-rays can even better provide direct imaging of the dynamics of a PNB. Unfortunately, the cost and technical complexity of such solutions turn them into unique tools with very limited availability.

Alternatively, the imaging of a transient PNB can also be realized with much more affordable equipment using slow cameras and pulsed light sources (Fig. 8a) providing:

1. Pulsed illumination with a shorter duration than a PNB lifetime within a nano- and pico-second range.
2. Sufficient energy of the optical pulse to compensate the very small scattering cross-section of the PNB.
3. Precise synchronization of the illuminating pulse with the PNB source.

These requirements suggest using a pulsed laser as the illumination source. The illumination angle and the numerical aperture of the collecting lens further determine the signal-to-noise ratio of this imaging scheme. Forward scattering results in the maximal scattering efficacy but cannot be fully separated from incident light that creates a high background. We achieved the best results with angled side illumination (Fig. 8a), providing that the numerical aperture of the imaging (collecting) lens is lower than the angle of incidence of the illuminating radiation. In this case, the lens collects only the light scattered by the PNB. This scheme allows the imaging of a single transient PNB with a lifetime down to 10 ns

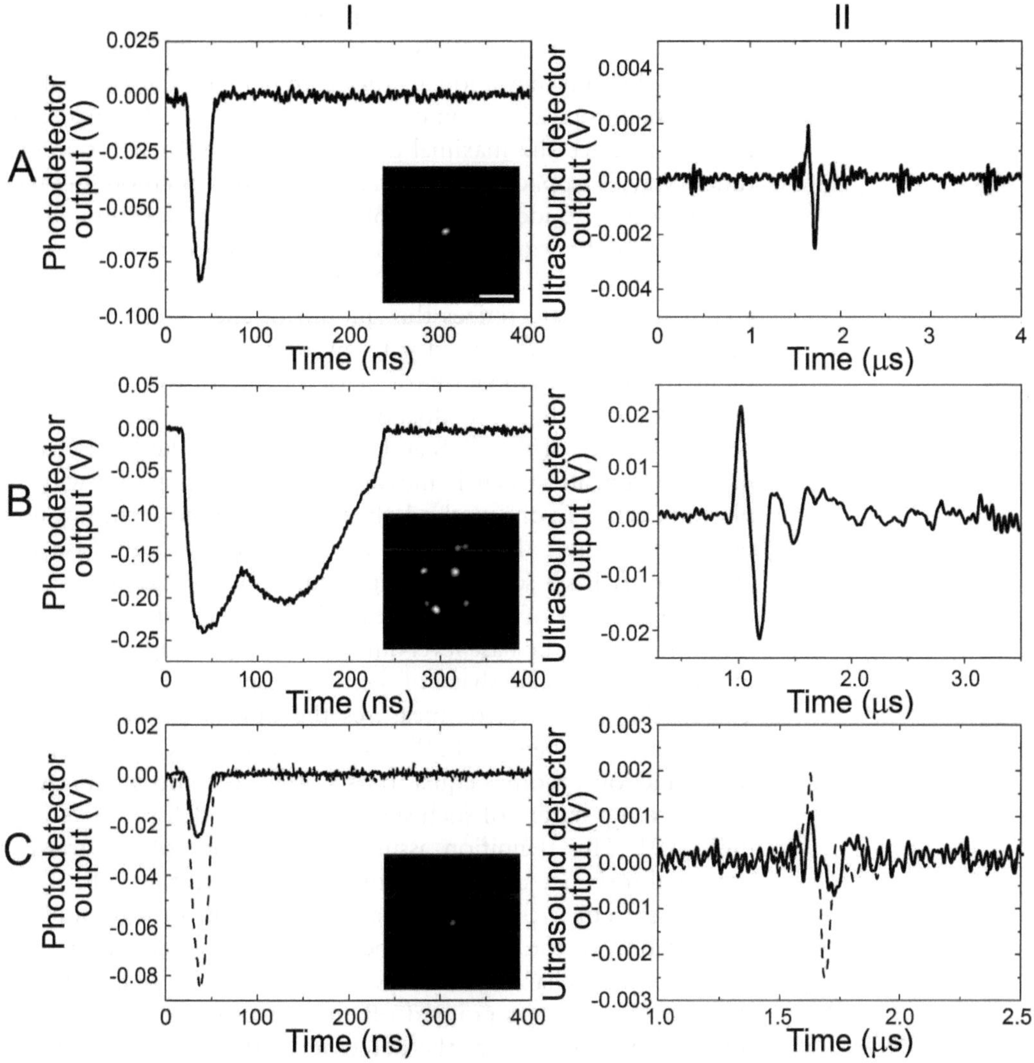

Fig. 9 (**a**) Three methods of detecting a single PNB. (*I*) Typical optical scattering (extinction) time-response obtained with continuous probe laser shows the expansion and collapse of the PNB (metrics—amplitude and duration) and time-resolved optical scattering imaging (*insert*) with a pulsed probe laser (metric—a pixel image amplitude). (*II*) Typical acoustical time-response obtained with an ultrasound sensor (metric—amplitude). (**b**) The same signals obtained for several simultaneously generated PNBs of different maximal diameter. (**c**) Influence of the experimental settings: (*I*) The diameter of the continuous probe beam is increased by 10–15 % and the angle of incidence of the pulsed probe beam increased from 45° to 135°; (*II*) The resonance frequency of the acoustic sensor is decreased from 10 to 5 MHz. Corresponding signals as shown in (**a**) are shown with *dashed lines*. Scale bar is 15 μm. Reproduced from [10]

(Fig. 9a) [10]. Most of the current CCD- and CMOS-based cameras can do such imaging. We used Andor Luka EMCCD (charged coupled device with electronic multiplication) and Cannon 50D (equipped with a CMOS sensor) stock cameras, both with long exposure times in the dark, to avoid precise synchronization with the PNB excitation laser pulse. In this method, the pixel image amplitude is used as a PNB metric, but it is not very practical because: (1) any deviation in the alignment of the probe beam would require recalibration of the system, and (2) this metric will not characterize the maximal diameter of a PNB when one fixed time delay is applied. The advantage of this method is in the relatively precise identification of a PNB and its location. It also shows the number of PNBs if multiple events occur (Fig. 9b).

The maximal diameter of a PNB is the most important parameter that also characterizes the amount of energy received by the bubble. It can be measured with another optical scattering technique that employs the monitoring of the intensity of a continuous probe beam with a broadband high-speed photodetector. The beam is focused at the PNB and its scattering by the PNB changes its axial intensity which is measured as a time-response with the photodetector. In one method, the beam is pointed at the low noise detector through the aperture and produces a high base level (Fig. 8b). A PNB scatters the light and thus increasingly reduces the axial intensity of the probe beam during its expansion stage and brings it back to the base level during its collapse stage. This results in the bubble-specific shape of the time-response (Fig. 9a panel I). Technically, the detector measures the optical extinction of the probe beam, but since a PNB does not absorb any optical energy, the extinction becomes equal to its scattering component. Due to the scattering nature of such signals they were defined as "scattering" [10]. This definition assumes the absence of any transient optical absorbance developed simultaneously with a PNB. If such absorbance emerges (due to plasma formation or any nonlinear modification of the optical properties of the media), the method (protocol) may characterize a PNB incorrectly [73, 74]. In another method, the beam is pointed off the detector aperture and produces a low base level at the detector. In this case, only the light scattered by a PNB will reach the detector and will increase its output signal, also producing a time-response with a bubble-specific shape [10].

The most precise way to measure the maximal diameter of a single PNB is to measure the duration of the PNB-specific signal (Fig. 9a panel I) which was shown to correlate to its maximal diameter [10, 15, 18, 19, 28, 55]. The amplitude of the PNB response also depends upon the maximal diameter of the PNB, but is very sensitive to experimental factors that are difficult to control. The first is the diameter and divergence of the probe beam at the PNB's plane. The smaller the beam waste, the higher the sensitivity of PNB detection. An increase in the beam's diameter by 10–15 % and/or a slight deviation of the beam axis may cause a several-fold decrease in the signal amplitude of a dip-shaped PNB signal (Fig. 9c panel I). Such conditions occur during changing the sample chamber or while scanning a heterogeneous sample across the beam. The simultaneous generation of multiple PNBs around different sources of thermal energy (for example, in suspension around optically absorbing molecules or nanoparticles) instead of a single one, increases the signal amplitude, but such an increase is just an ensemble effect (Fig. 9b panel I). The simultaneous generation of several PNBs of different maximal sizes influences not only the amplitude but also the shape of the PNB time-response (Fig. 9b panel I). Smaller PNBs form a sharp front and fewer large PNBs form a long tail of lower amplitude. While the generation of PNBs under some settings may typically involve such a multi-PNB pattern, it is still possible to estimate the lifetime of the largest PNB(s) that represent the maximal deposition of the thermal energy by measuring the duration of the time-response at the reduced level instead of at half of maximum [10]. However, the best rule is to avoid such distorted signals because they may lead to misinterpretation of the bubble parameters [73]. In all three considered cases (single PNB, single PNB with misaligned probe beam, multiple PNBs) the durations of the bubble-specific signals could be linked to the maximal diameter of the PNB (or the largest PNB as in Fig. 9b panel I), while their amplitudes differed significantly and therefore, their use as PNB metrics may lead to artifacts [74].

The third method of PNB detection employs the pressure waves generated during the bubble expansion and collapse (Fig. 8c) [10]. In the case of a single inertial bubble, the pressure and rarefaction waves produce a typical signal (Fig. 9a panel II). This is definitely the simplest and the least expensive method of the three, because it does not require expensive optical sources, optics, and sensors. In addition, it detects PNBs in optically opaque media, so it is probably the most universal of the methods. The most obvious metric of the acoustic signal is its maximal (peak-to-peak) amplitude. However, the correct identification and measurement of a PNB with a standard acoustic detector can be challenging in a single-pulse mode. Most detectors have a resonant frequency that is less than or equal to 10 MHz where their sensitivity is maximal. For small PNBs with lifetimes from 5 to 100 ns, the corresponding pressure rise times and associated frequencies seem to be higher than the resonant frequencies of most acoustic sensors. Therefore, the sensor signal does not show the real pressure, but rather represents a response function of the sensor. In this case the amplitude of the output signal of the acoustic sensor significantly depends upon its resonant frequency and may cause a significant error (Fig. 9c panel II). For a specific acoustic sensor, the amplitude of its output also depends upon the number of simultaneously generated PNBs (Fig. 9b panel II). Therefore, a reliable measurement of the PNB diameter through the amplitude of acoustic response assumes that a single PNB is generated.

The next important task is the identification of a PNB and its discrimination from other phenomena such as transient heating or

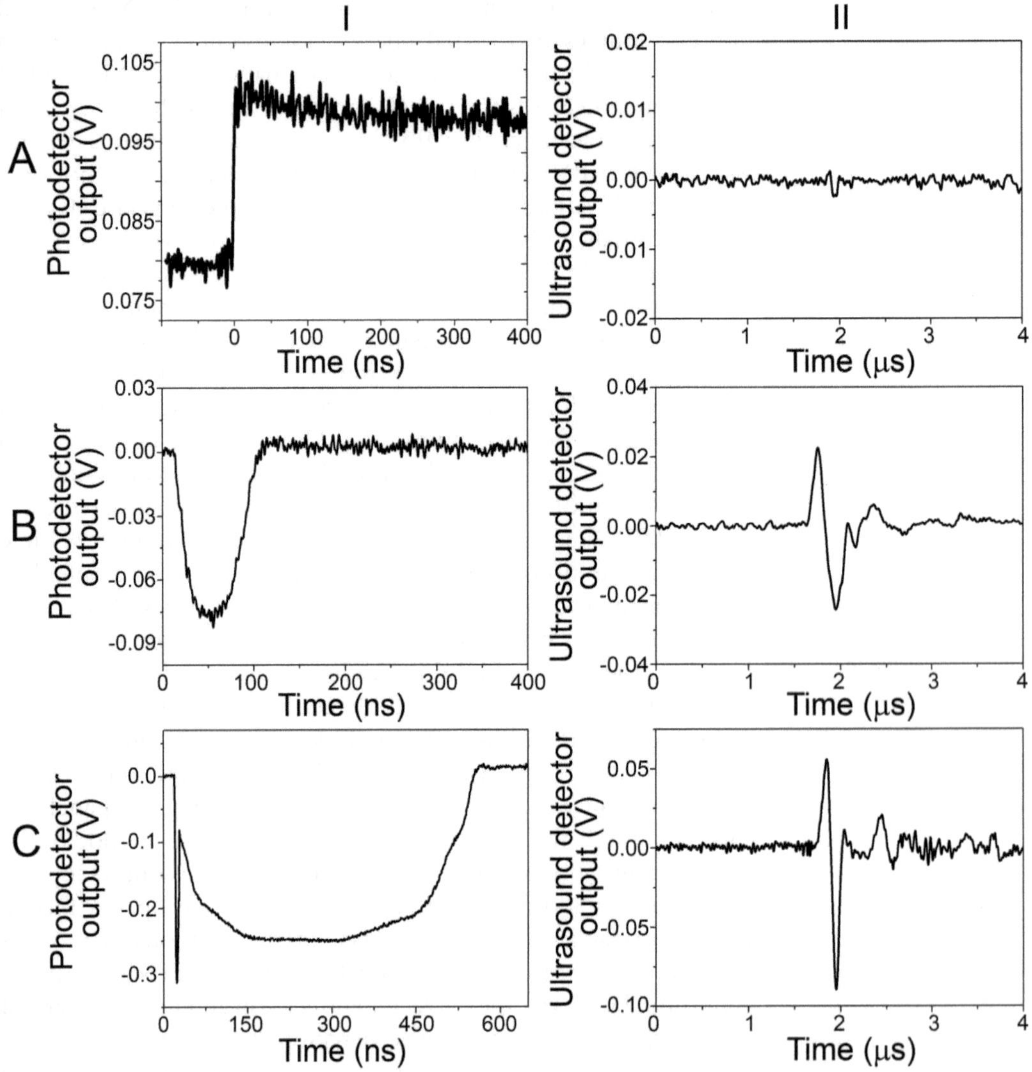

Fig. 10 Illustrations of typical optical scattering (or extinction) (*left*) and acoustic (*right*) time-responses of three different phenomena [10]: (**a**) transient heating of the gold nanoparticle and the media with a single laser pulse at a fluence below the PNB generation threshold; (**b**) single transient vapor nanobubble; (**c**) PNB accompanied by a stress wave that produces a sharp and short optical signal in the very beginning of the time-response

stress waves (Fig. 10). The optical scattering response identifies heating through a thermal lens effect that allows the detection and measurement of rapid heating and gradual cooling due to thermal diffusion (Fig. 10a) [10]. This purely refractive effect does not produce any optical scattering like a PNB does. Next, under high transient temperatures at short time scales, the generation of stress waves (and shock waves) also influences the refractive index of the media and creates a distinct short (relative to the bubble and heating time scale) signal of nanosecond duration that is determined by the speed of sound and the aperture of the probe beam (Fig. 10c). Both phenomena can be clearly distinguished from the bubble (Fig. 10b). However, all these three different phenomena do not much influence the shape of the acoustic response, but rather its amplitude (Fig. 10), which is minimal for heating, increases for a bubble and becomes the maximal for stress waves [10]. Therefore, an acoustic time-response is much less bubble-specific than an optical scattering time-response.

The above analysis compares three protocols for the detection of PNBs under fixed excitation conditions. However, in reality the generation of PNBs may occur in a wide range of excitation fluences from pulse to pulse and even within the aperture of a single pulse. These factors cause a wide variation in the maximal diameter of the PNB. Therefore, it is important to understand the range of the linear correlation between the PNB metric and its excitation conditions that determine the PNB's maximal diameter. We compared the four metrics discussed above, the pixel amplitude of the scattering image, the amplitude and duration of the optical scattering time response and the amplitude of the acoustic response, as functions of the fluence of the excitation laser pulse, the parameter that in this model, determines the maximal diameter of the PNB when the fluence exceeds the PNB generation threshold. All bubbles can be generated in water around individual identical gold nanospheres. This model provides a very precise deposition and conversion of optical energy into a bubble. Three types of signals, optical response, image, and acoustical response can be obtained simultaneously for each individual event.

For the scattering image, we observed the relatively early saturation and nonlinear behavior of the pixel image amplitude compared to the duration of the time response. Time-resolved scattering images were obtained under a fixed delay between the excitation and probe laser pulses. With an increase in the maximal PNB diameter and lifetime, the moment of illumination moved further from the moment when the PNB reaches its maximal diameter. This explains the observed nonlinear effect of the pixel image amplitude. Another technical limitation of the imaging method is the dynamic range of the image sensor. If it is less than 60 dB, a wide range of PNB diameters would cause either saturation of the images of large bubbles or low sensitivity in the detection of small bubbles.

We analyzed three detection techniques (protocols) for imaging and measuring transient vapor nanobubbles generated as single events at nanoscale around laser pulse-heated metal nanoparticles. In optically transparent media, the location of nanobubbles can be best determined with time-resolved optical scattering imaging by using a delayed short optical pulse with regular CCD or CMOS cameras. The best quantitative analysis of vapor nanobubbles in the widest range of excitation energies and bubble diameters can be achieved by measuring the duration (lifetime) of the optical scattering time-response by using a low-power continuous laser and matching photodetector. In the case of opaque media, the amplitude of the acoustical time-response provides good sensitivity and linearity in a range of excitation conditions that are limited by the onset of stress waves that additionally increase the amplitude of the nanobubble signal. The simultaneous use of two or three of these methods (protocols) provides the best results in the identification, imaging, and measuring of transient nanobubbles in a single event experiment.

3.3 Example of the Protocol: Generation of PNBs in EGFR-Positive Cancer Cells in Vitro

3.3.1 Materials

1. Primary culture of epidermal growth factor receptor (EGFR) positive cancer cells (for example, HN31).
2. Complete medium with a serum for cell culturing (for example, supplemented Dulbecco's Modified Eagle Medium (DMEM) with 10 % (v/v) a fetal bovine serum (FBS)) (*see* **Note 1**). Warm up the medium before use.
3. Sterile 1× phosphate-buffered saline (PBS).
4. Optically transparent cuvettes for cell culture (for example, μ-Slide VI (0.4), ibidi USA Inc, Madison, Wisconsin).
5. Nanoparticles: 20–200 nm gold spheres conjugated to anti-EGFR antibody.
6. CO_2 incubator.
7. Pulsed laser: wavelength 532 nm, pulse duration 0.07–10 ns (for example, 70 ps).
8. Lens with the focal distance 200–400 mm.

3.3.2 Preparation of Gold Nanoparticles and Incubation with Cells

1. Grow cells to 50–60 % of confluence. View cultures using an inverted microscope to check confluence and the absence of bacterial and fungal contaminants.
2. Shake a factory tube with nanoparticles for 10 s before taking an aliquot (*see* **Note 2**).
3. Sonicate the nanoparticle aliquot for 30 s in cold water.
4. Dilute the gold nanoparticles in the complete culture medium up to 2.4×10^{10} to 2.4×10^{11} GNPs/mL (*see* **Notes 1** and **3**).
5. Remove the medium from the culture cuvettes and wash the cell monolayer with PBS twice.
6. Fill up the cuvettes with the diluted nanoparticle suspension and incubate the cells during 24 h in the CO_2 incubator. View cultures using an inverted microscope to check confluence and the absence of bacterial and fungal contaminants and then wash the cells with PBS twice.
7. Fill up the cuvettes with a fresh PBS.

3.3.3 Laser Treatment

1. Measure the laser beam diameter and laser pulse energy to calculate and adjust the fluence of the single laser pulse in the sample plane (*see* **Note 4**).
2. Irradiate the individual cell or the number of cells (in a case of the broad laser beam) with a single laser pulse.
3. Detect the PNBs with the methods described above in the details.

3.3.4 Notes

1. Use the complete warmed medium *without* serum for incubation cells with the gold nanoparticles.
2. The nanoparticle aliquot should be no less than 30 μL.
3. Use the diluted nanoparticles suspension within 1 h. Shake and sonicate, if suspension been prepared more than 30 min before using.
4. For generation and detection of the PNBs in the individual cells, the excitation and detection schemes should be assembled on the inverted microscope to provide a positioning of the individual cells using the microscope. For the bulk treatment of cells by PNBs, the broad laser beam can be used for the PNB generation with the fluences which are above the threshold of the PNB generation. The details of the excitation and detection schemes are described in the main text.

References

1. Brinkmann R, Hüttmann G, Rögener J et al (2000) Origin of retinal pigment epithelium cell damage by pulsed laser irradiance in the nanosecond to microsecond time regimen. Lasers Surg Med 27:451–464
2. Leszczynski D, Pitsillides CM, Pastila RK et al (2001) Laser-beam-triggered microcavitation: a novel method for selective cell destruction. Radiat Res 156:399–407
3. Dou Y, Zhigilei LV, Winograd N et al (2001) Explosive boiling of water films adjacent to heated surfaces: a microscopic description. J Phys Chem A 105:2748–2755
4. Kotaidis V, Plech A (2005) Cavitation dynamics on the nanoscale. Appl Phys Lett 87: 213102
5. Farny CH, Wu T, Holt RG et al (2005) Nucleating cavitation from laser-illuminated nanoparticles. ARLO 6:138–143
6. Inasawa S, Sugiyama M, Noda S et al (2006) Spectroscopic study of laser-induced phase transition of gold nanoparticles on nanosecond time scales and longer. J Phys Chem B 110:3114–3119
7. Siems A, Webwr SAL, Boneberg J et al (2011) Thermodynamics of nanosecond nanobubble formation at laser-excited metal nanoparticles. New J Phys 13:043018
8. Lapotko D, Lukianova K, Shnip A (2005) Photothermal responses of individual cells. J Biomed Opt 10:014006
9. Lapotko D, Lukianova E, Oraevsky A (2006) Selective laser nano-thermolysis of human leukemia cells with microbubbles generated around clusters of gold nanoparticles. Lasers Surg Med 38:631–642
10. Lukianova-Hleb EY, Lapotko DO (2012) Experimental techniques for imaging and measuring transient vapor nanobubbles. Appl Phys Lett 101:264102
11. Baffou G, Polleux J, Rigneault H et al (2014) Super-heating and micro-bubble generation around plasmonic nanoparticles under cw illumination. J Phys Chem C 118:4890–4898
12. Anderson RR, Parrish JA (1983) Selective photothermolysis: precise microsurgery by selective absorption of pulsed radiation. Science 220:524–527

13. Hu M, Hartland GV (2002) Heat dissipation for Au particles in aqueous solution: relaxation time versus size. J Phys Chem B 106:7029–7033
14. Link S, El-Sayed MA (1999) Spectral properties and relaxation dynamics of surface plasmon electronic oscillations in gold and silver nanodots and nanorods. J Phys Chem B 103:8410–8426
15. Lukianova-Hleb E, Hu Y, Latterini L et al (2010) Plasmonic nanobubbles as transient vapor nanobubbles generated around plasmonic nanoparticles. ACS Nano 4:2109–2123
16. Lukianova-Hleb EY, Volkov AN, Wu X et al (2013) Transient enhancement and spectral narrowing of the photothermal effect of plasmonic nanoparticles under pulsed excitation. Adv Mater 25:772–776
17. François L, Mostafavi M, Belloni J et al (2001) Optical limitation induced by gold clusters: mechanism and efficiency. Phys Chem Chem Phys 3:4965–4971
18. Lapotko D, Lukianova E, Shnip A et al (2005) Photothermal microscopy and laser ablation of leukemia cells targeted with gold nanoparticles. Proc SPIE 5697:82–89
19. Hleb E, Lapotko D (2009) Influence of transient environmental photothermal effects on optical scattering by gold nanoparticles. Nano Lett 9:2160–2166
20. Lukianova-Hleb EY, Ren X, Sawant RR et al (2014) On-demand cancer cell-specific plasmonic nanobubble-mediated enhancement of intracellular drug release and radiation effects. Nat Med 20:778–784
21. Hleb EY, Lapotko DO (2008) Photothermal properties of gold nanoparticles under exposure to high optical energies. Nanotechnology 19:355702
22. Akchurin G, Khlebtsov B, Akchurin G et al (2008) Gold nanoshell photomodification under single nanosecond laser pulse accompanied by color-shifting and bubble formation phenomena. Nanotechnology 19:015701
23. Link S, El-Sayed MA (2003) Optical properties and ultrafast dynamics of metallic nanocrystals. Annu Rev Phys Chem 54:331–366
24. Hartland G (2004) Measurements of the material properties of metal nanoparticles by time-resolved spectroscopy. Phys Chem Chem Phys 6:5263–5274
25. Lukianova-Hleb EY, Volkov AN, Lapotko DO (2014) Laser pulse duration is critical for the generation of plasmonic nanobubbles. Langmuir 30:7425–7434
26. Vogel A, Linz N, Freidank S et al (2008) Femtosecond-laser-induced nanocavitation in water: implications for optical breakdown threshold and cell surgery. Phys Rev Lett 100:038102
27. Lukianova-Hleb EY, Oginsky EY, Samaniego AP et al (2011) Tunable plasmonic nanoprobes for theranostics of prostate cancer. Theranostics 1:3–17
28. Plech A, Kotaidis V, Lorenc M et al (2006) Femtosecond laser near-field ablation from gold nanoparticles. Nat Phys 2:44–47
29. Laser Institute of America. ANSI Z136.1–2007 (2007)
30. Braun GB, Pallaoro A, Wu G et al (2009) Laser-activated gene silencing via gold nanoshell-siRNA conjugates. ACS Nano 3:2007–2015
31. McLaughlan JR, Roy RA, Ju H et al (2010) Ultrasonic enhancement of photoacoustic emissions by nanoparticle-targeted cavitation. Opt Lett 35:2127–2129
32. Ibrahimkutty S, Kim J, Cammarata M et al (2011) Ultrafast structural dynamics of the photocleavage of protein hybrid nanoparticles. ACS Nano 5:3788–3794
33. Peeters S, Kitz M, Preisser S et al (2012) Mechanisms of nanoparticle-mediated photomechanical cell damage. Biomed Opt Express 3:435–446
34. Arita Y, Ploschner M, Antkowiak M et al (2013) Laser-induced breakdown of an optically trapped gold nanoparticle for single cell transfection. Opt Lett 38:3402–3405
35. Yuan F, Sankin G, Zhong P (2011) Dynamics of tandem bubble interaction in a microfluidic channel. J Acoust Soc Am 130:3339–3346
36. Zhao C, Liu Y, Zhao Y et al (2013) A reconfigurable plasmofluidic lens. Nat Commun 4:2305
37. Faraday M (1857) The Bakerian lecture: experimental relations of gold (and other metals) to light. Philos Trans R Soc Lond 147:145–181
38. Hu M, Hartland G (2004) Ultrafast dynamics of metal nanospheres and nanorods. In: Liz-Marzán L, Kamat P (eds) Nanoscale materials. Springer, New York, pp 97–118
39. Jain P, Lee KS, El-Sayed IH et al (2006) Calculated absorption and scattering properties of gold nanoparticles of different size, shape, and composition: applications in biological imaging and biomedicine. J Phys Chem B 110:7238–7248
40. Fang Z, Zhen YR, Neumann O (2013) Evolution of light-induced vapor generation at a

liquid-immersed metallic nanoparticle. Nano Lett 13:1736–1742

41. Link S, Burda C, Mohamed MB et al (1999) Laser photothermal melting and fragmentation of gold nanorods: energy and laser pulse-width dependence. J Phys Chem A 103: 1165–1170
42. Habenicht A, Olapinski M, Burmeister F et al (2005) Jumping nanodroplets. Science 309:2043–2045
43. Petrova H, Hu M, Hartland GV (2007) Photothermal properties of gold nanoparticles. Z Phys Chem 221:361–376
44. Kurita H, Takami A, Koda S (1998) Size reduction of gold particles in aqueous solution by pulsed laser irradiation. Appl Phys Lett 72:789–791
45. Werner D, Hashimoto S (2013) Controlling the pulsed-laser-induced size reduction of Au and Ag nanoparticles via changes in the external pressure, laser intensity, and excitation wavelength. Langmuir 29:1295–1302
46. Cavicchi RE, Meier DC, Presser C et al (2013) Single laser pulse effects on suspended-Au-nanoparticle size distributions and morphology. J Phys Chem 117:10866–10875
47. Lapotko D, Lukianova-Hleb E, Oraevsky A (2007) Clusterization of nanoparticles during their interaction with living cells. Nanomedicine 2:241–253
48. Chithrani BD, Ghazani AA, Chan WC (2006) Determining the size and shape dependence of gold nanoparticle uptake into mammalian cells. Nano Lett 6:662–668
49. Baffou G, Berto P, Bermúdez UE et al (2013) Photoinduced heating of nanoparticle arrays. ACS Nano 7:6478–6488
50. Volkov AN, Sevilla C, Zhigilei LV (2007) Numerical modeling of short pulse laser interaction with au nanoparticle surrounded by water. Appl Surf Sci 253:6394–6399
51. Yu YY, Chang SS, Lee CL et al (1997) Gold nanorods: electrochemical synthesis and optical properties. J Phys Chem B 101: 6661–6664
52. Dickerson EB, Dreaden EC, Huang X et al (2008) Gold nanorod assisted near-infrared plasmonic photothermal therapy (PPTT) of squamous cell carcinoma in mice. Cancer Lett 269:57–66
53. Garcia de Abajo FJ (2007) Colloquium: light scattering by particle and hole array. Rev Mod Phys 79:1267–1290
54. Kravets VG, Schedin F, Grigorenko AN (2008) Extremely narrow plasmonic resonances based on diffraction coupling of lacalized plasmons in arrays of metallic nanoparticles. Phys Rev Lett 101:087403
55. Lapotko DO (2009) Optical excitation and detection of vapor bubbles around plasmonic nanoparticles. Opt Express 17:2538–2556
56. Rayleigh L (1917) On the pressure developed in a liquid during the collapse of a spherical cavity. Philos Mag 34:94–98
57. Plesset MS (1949) The dynamic of cavitation bubbles. Trans ASME J Appl Mech 16:277–282
58. Askaryan GA, Prokhorov AM, Chanturiya GF (1963) The effects of a laser beam in a liquid. Soviet Phys JEPT 17:1463–1465
59. Barnes PA, Rieckhoff KE (1968) Laser-induced underwater sparks. Appl Phys Lett 13:282–284
60. Lauterborn W (1972) High-speed photography of laser-induced breakdown in liquids. Appl Phys Lett 21:27–29
61. Ohl CD, Philipp A, Lauterborn W (1995) Cavitation bubble collapse studied at 20 million frames per second. Ann Phys 4:26–34
62. Yavas O, Leiderer P, Park HK et al (1993) Optical reflectance and scattering studies of nucleation and growth of bubbles at a liquid-solid interface induced by pulsed laser heating. Phys Rev Lett 70:1830–1833
63. Vogel A, Lauterborn W (1988) Acoustic transient generation by laser-produced cavitation bubbles. J Acoust Soc Am 84:719–731
64. Marston PL (1979) Critical angle scattering by a bubble: physical-optics approximation and observations. J Opt Soc Am 69:1205–1211
65. Stroud JS, Marston PLJ (1993) Optical detection of transient oscillation associated with the underwater noise of rain. Acoust Soc Am 94:2788–2792
66. Asaki TJ, Thiessen DB, Marston PL (1995) Effect of an insoluble surfactant on capillary oscillations of bubbles in water: observation of a maximum in the damping. Phys Rev Lett 75:2686–2689
67. Fujimoto JG, Lin WZ, Ippen EP et al (1985) Time-resolved studies of Nd:YAG laser-induced breakdown. Plasma formation, acoustic wave generation, and cavitation. Invest Ophthalmol Vis Sci 26:1771–1777
68. Gaitan DF, Crum LA, Church CC et al (1992) Sonoluminescence and bubble dynamics for a single, stable, cavitation bubble. J Acoust Soc Am 91:3166–3183
69. Barber BP, Putterman SJ (1992) Light scattering measurements of the repetitive supersonic implosion of a sonoluminescing bubble. Phys Rev Lett 69:3839–3842

70. Jain KK (2010) Advanced in the field of nanooncology. BMC Med 8:83
71. O'Neill BE, Rapoport N (2011) Phase-shift, stimuli-responsive drug carriers for targeted delivery. Ther Deliv 2:1165–1187
72. Ashokkumar M (2011) The characterization of acoustic cavitation bubbles—an overview. Ultrason Sonochem 18:864–872
73. Boulais E, Lachaine R, Meunier M (2012) Plasma mediated off-resonance plasmonic enhanced ultrafast laser-induced nanocavitation. Nano Lett 12:4763–4769
74. Zharov V (2011) Ultrasharp nonlinear photothermal and photoacoustic resonances and holes beyond the spectral limit. Nat Photonics 5:110–116

Part III

Nanotechnology to Study Cancer

Chapter 12

Force Measurements for Cancer Cells

Vivek Rajasekharan, Varun K.A. Sreenivasan, and Brenda Farrell

Abstract

During cytoskeleton remodeling, cancer cells generate force at the plasma membrane that originates from chemical motors (e.g., actin). This force (pN) and its time course reflect the on and off-rates of the motors. We describe the design and calibration of a force-measuring device (i.e., optical tweezers) that is used to monitor this force and its time course at the edge of a cell, with particular emphasis on the temporal resolution of the instrument.

Key words Cell mobility, Membrane tube, Membrane force, Filopodium, Actin, Cytoskeleton, Motor kinetics, Optical tweezers, Time constant, Noise of signal

1 Introduction

1.1 Background

Most cancer-related mortalities occur when cancer cells migrate from the primary tumor site to form secondary tumors [1]. Transition to a mobile phenotype is triggered by gene mutations and growth factors (e.g., epidermal growth factor) that initiate cytoskeleton remodeling to form migratory structures (e.g., filopodia, invadopodia, and lamellapodia). These migratory structures enable cancer cells to breach the basement membrane and invade surrounding stroma both physically by generating force and chemically by secreting enzymes [2]; the presence of migratory structures is correlated with their metastatic potential [3, 4].

Cell mobility is commonly measured in vitro with the Boyden chamber assay [5] which counts the number of cells that move from one chamber to another through a porous membrane, and the scratch assay [6] which monitors the time it takes for cells to repopulate a dimple or scratch on a surface plate. These methods monitor the migration of hundreds of cells over long time frames (hours to days) and provide the average migration rate (e.g., $\mu m^2/h$, for scratch assay, number of cells/day for Boyden assay) of a population of cancer cells; they do not reveal the biophysical or molecular mechanisms of mobility. More modern methods that

Reema Zeineldin (ed.), *Cancer Nanotechnology: Methods and Protocols*, Methods in Molecular Biology, vol. 1530,
DOI 10.1007/978-1-4939-6646-2_12,

monitor the biophysical forces generated by cells reveal the characteristics of the motion. One example is traction force microscopy [7] which monitors the imprint on a matrix created by contractile stresses of the cell as it propels itself within the substrate, where this substrate is sometimes replaced by a bed of needles (spring constant ~ 32 nN/μm) that bend (>0.2 μm) in response to this force [8]. This adhesive traction force is ~10–300 nN when integrated over the area of a cell [8, 9]. Studies show that the magnitude of the contractile force correlates with the metastatic potential of cancer cells [9, 10]. This method has been scaled-up to monitor the average contractile force produced by a population of cells (10–40 cells per micropatterned plate) [11].

At the leading dynamic edges of a cell (e.g., filopodia, lamellipodia), pushing (protrusive) and pulling (retractive) forces are produced as the cytoskeleton undergoes remodeling. These forces are generated at an edge (as opposed to over the entire surface) and are in the pN range [12–17]. They result from work done on the membrane by chemical motors (e.g., actin, myosin, and tubulin) acting at or near the plasma membrane and are detectable with optical tweezers [12–17] and atomic force microscopy [18].

We describe two approaches that make use of optical tweezers [14–17, 19–21]. For the first, a dielectric bead is trapped by a focused laser beam and is only used to monitor force. In this case, the bead binds to the membrane at the edge of a cell (e.g., tip of a filopodia) and the position of the bead is monitored as the structure (e.g., filopodia) undergoes cytoskeleton remodeling [14, 15, 17]. For the second approach, a trapped bead is used both as a sensor to monitor force, and as a handle to exert force (Fig. 1a) to form a new filopodium-like structure [16, 19–21] sometimes coined a tether from a living cell. In this case, a trapped bead adheres to the cell membrane (Fig. 1b). To separate the plasma membrane from the cytoskeleton, the body of the cell is moved away from the bead (or the bead is moved away from the cell body) at a constant loading rate (pN/s) (Fig. 1c). A membrane tube forms once the membrane separates from the cytoskeleton. The extension of this tube to a fixed length happens by continued application of the load, then the tube relaxes towards a stationary force when this load is removed (Fig. 1d). When the tube is in this relaxed state we discern the magnitude of the stationary force, and detect the work done by chemical motors on the membrane (Fig. 1e). During this process (Fig. 1b–d), F-actin [20, 21] and sometimes β-tubulin [21] polymerize and fill the lumen of the tube. This method is adapted from techniques designed to form membrane tubes from vesicles and from cells including red blood cells [22], neurons [23], neutrophils [24] and outer hair cells [25]. It was initially used to estimate the nonlocal bending modulus for the membranes of vesicles [26] or the plasma membrane of red blood cells [22] and later used to

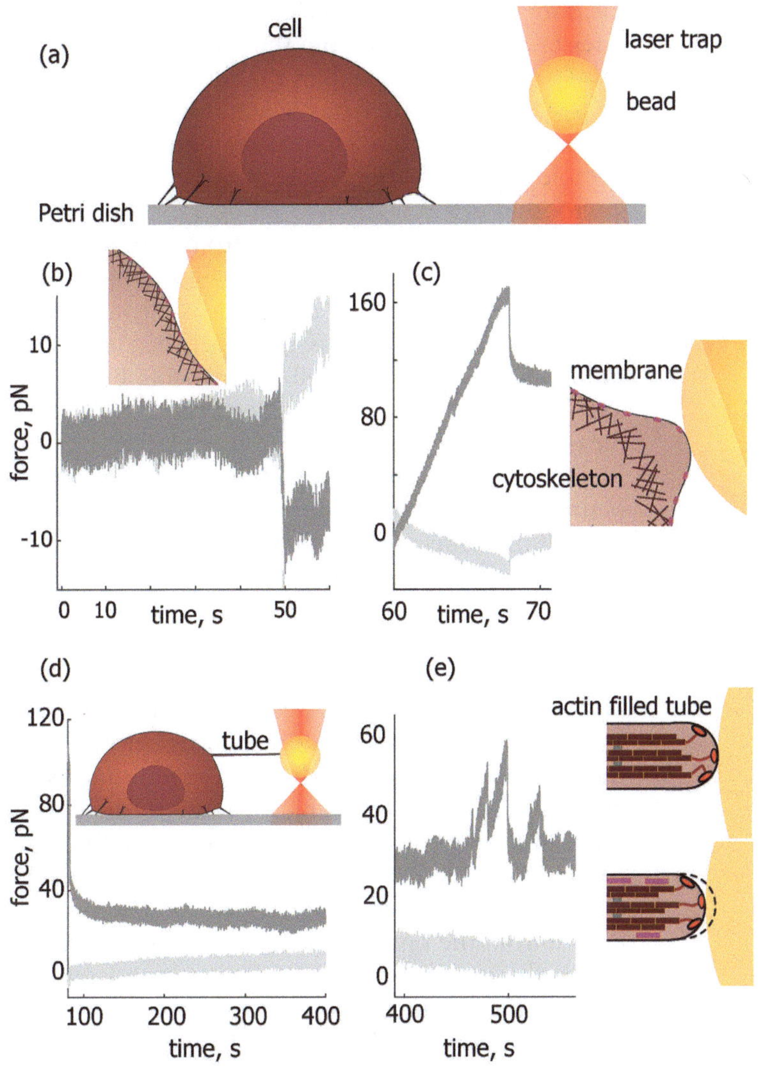

Fig. 1 Force measured during and after tube formation. (**a**) Initial positon of the two bodies: a cell firmly attached to a Petri dish and a trapped fluorescent bead. (**b**) The forces on the bead ($F(x)$ and $F(y)$) are recorded with the two bodies kept stationary and about 20 μm apart (time, *t*: 0–10 s). The cell is then brought towards the bead in the *X* direction (*see* Fig. 2) with the 3-D piezo stage at 0.5 μm/s (*t*: 10–50 s). At $t \sim 49$ s the bodies touch and the cell is pushed towards the bead and a negative force $F(x)$ is detected. The 3-D piezo stage is stopped (*t*: 50–60 s) to allow the bodies to adhere. Inset shows a deformed cell. (**c**) The cell is then pulled away from the bead in the *X* direction with the 3-D piezo stage at the same speed (*t*: 60–80 s) and a large positive force $F(x)$ is detected as the membrane separates from cytoskeleton. Inset shows separation and initiation of tube formation. (**d**) Once the pulling stops the tube relaxes and $F(x)$ decays to a stationary value. *Inset* shows the formed tube. (**e**) Sawtooths are observed to ride upon the stationary value. The inset shows filaments attached to membrane by linkers (*red*). Upon depolymerization the linkers attach to penultimate position on the filament and the monomers are lost to the cytoplasm. This results in a positive force $F(x)$ that adds to the stationary value. Experiment was conducted in PBS at 24 °C with a HN-31 cancer cell. The sampling frequency of both $F(x)$ (*dark gray*) and $F(y)$ (*light gray*) is 500 Hz except for (**c**) where it is 2 kHz

measure membrane-cytoskeleton adhesion [23] and the unbinding rates of the membrane from the cytoskeleton [27, 28].

In most of these studies the force was measured at slow rates (<100 Hz) or the tube was only stable for short times [27, 28]. By measuring the force at a faster sampling rate (1 kHz) at the edge of a stable structure we were able to detect nonstationary events (e.g., sawtooths) that ride upon a stationary value [16]. We reason that these nonstationary events arose from depolymerization and polymerization of F-actin that occurred at the tip of the structure, and estimated the on and off rates of this chemical motor within the cell. This provided the possibility that the kinetics of actin or other motor proteins within a cell are tractable by measuring the force and its time course at the membrane. Similar transients were measured when a trapped bead was placed at tips of filopodia of HeLa cells [17], and of membrane tubes formed from cultured neurons [19]. However, in these reports there was no description of the time course of the transients. One of these studies suggests that the transients are the result of actin filaments pulled rearward towards the cell cortex by myosin motors [19]. The other report does not provide an explanation for the transients, but suggests that retrograde flow of actin monomers drives retraction of filopodia and this pulling force requires membrane-actin linkages at the tip [17]. Our model also requires linkages between the filaments and the membrane at the tip, which act as transducers and convert the chemical energy to mechanical energy to drive membrane movement [16]. We suggest that the rise of the force during the sawtooth originates from depolymerization of actin at the barbed end (i.e., tip) by a type of stepping-end mechanism [29]. The linkers detach from the tip and re-attach at the penultimate position after which the monomers escape. This causes a pulling force, which adds to the stationary positive membrane force. Here, we show that we observe similar sawtooths at the edge of a cancer cell (Fig. 1e). In our previous report, the temporal response of the instrument was not measured [16]. In this work, we ensure that the time constant of our newer instrument is readily measurable, as one goal is to determine the kinetics of chemical motors like actin at the edge of a cancer cell from such transients (Fig. 1e) and the kinetics of the intrinsic membrane-cytoskeleton bonds (Fig. 1c). We do this by adding acousto-optic deflectors (AODs) to the optical path [25], as they enable rapid movement of the trapped fluorescent bead whose position is then tracked by monitoring an image of the bead with a fast quadrant photodiode. The instrument is based upon the design of Qian et al. [25] and the optical path is shown in Fig. 2.

1.2 Description of Instrument

A titanium (Ti)-sapphire laser serves as the trap (Fig. 2). It is pumped by a solid-state frequency-doubled neodymium-doped yttrium orthovanadate (Nd: YVO4) laser. A half-wave plate (not

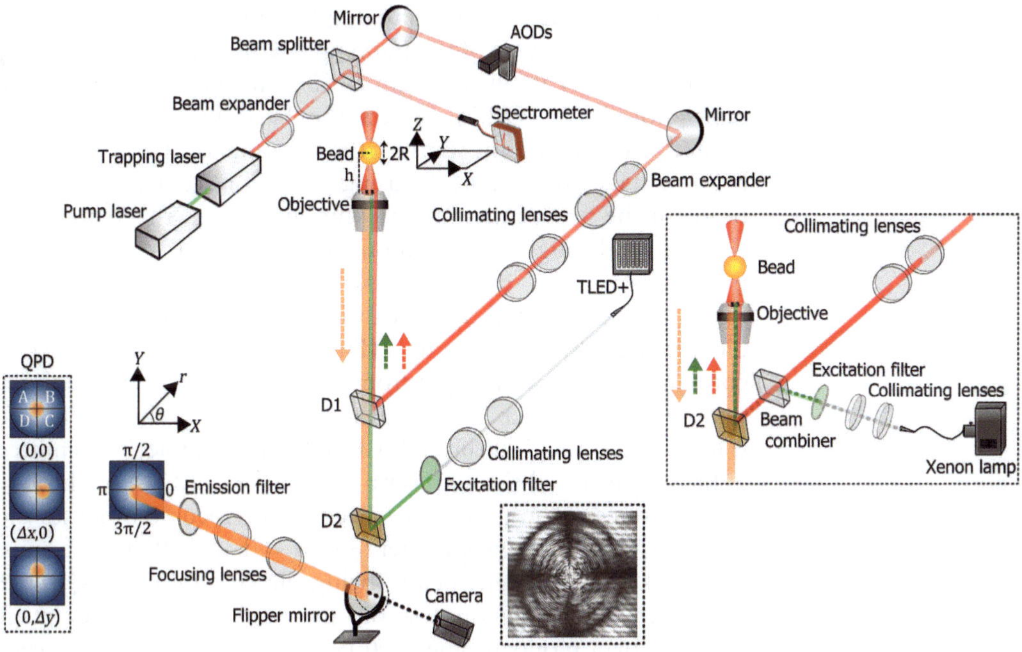

Fig. 2 Schematic diagram of the optical tweezers (not to scale). A laser beam (λ: 830 nm) that is focused by a high NA objective traps a fluorescent bead beyond its focal zone. The fluorescent bead is illuminated by a xenon (*right inset*) or TLED+ lamp where the change in position and intensity of the bead is measured with a quadrant photodiode (QPD) (*left inset*). The sample is moved in the transverse and focal directions with a 3-D piezo stage. A trapped bead is moved with the acousto-optic deflectors (AODs) and the fluorescence image of the bead is continuously projected onto the QPD. The trapping plane is at a constant height, *h* in the focal direction (*Z*) above the surface of a Petri dish shown in a cartesian (*X*, *Y*) plane. Center inset shows an image (projected by the camera onto the monitor) of a trapped bead in the center surrounded by fringes that reflect the distance from the trapping plane to the surface of the Petri dish

shown) rotates the plane of polarization of the trapping laser beam from vertical to horizontal. To set the wavelength of the trapping laser to 830 nm the beam is split, and the reflected beam is sent to a spectrometer. The transmitted beam is steered to fill the back aperture of an objective lens of high numerical aperture (NA) that is part of an inverted microscope.

Two acousto-optic deflectors (AODs) that are orthogonal (AODX and AODY) to each other control the laser power and position of the beam. Each AOD has two voltage inputs (V^a and V^f): V^f modifies the acoustic frequency to control beam position and V^a changes acoustic amplitude to control beam intensity. The laser beam is steered in the *XY* plane by changing the input frequency to the AODs. Two configurations were set-up depending upon the light source used to excite the bead (*see* **Note 1**). In the first configuration where a xenon lamp is used to excite the bead, the trapping laser beam is reflected by a dichroic, D2, that reflects at wavelengths > 723 nm (Fig. 2, right inset). In the second configuration where a transmitted light emitting diode (TLED+) lamp is used, the beam of the trapping laser is reflected by dichroic, D1, that reflects at a wavelength > 750 nm (Fig. 2). A fast quadrant photodiode (QPD) detects the bead fluorescence that is excited with either light source. It is mounted on a crossed-roller-bearing stage to facilitate focusing the fluorescent image of the bead. In the first configuration, white light from the xenon lamp is directed through an excitation filter (530 < T < 590 nm (T: transmission); the excitation peak of fluorescent bead is at 576 nm) and reflected by a dichroic beam combiner and then by dichroic D2 towards the sample (Fig. 2, right inset). In the second configuration, the white light from the TLED+ passes through the same excitation filter and is then reflected by dichroic D2 and transmitted through dichroic D1 towards the sample. The emitted light is transmitted through both dichroics (TLED+) or through one dichroic (xenon), this transmitted light is focused by lenses and then filtered by an emission filter (~600 < T < 700 nm; the emission peak is at 605 nm) before being directed onto the QPD. A computer monitor mounted on the wall projects the image acquired by a monochrome CMOS (complementary metal-oxide semiconductor) camera and tracks the position of the beam or bead during set-up.

A Petri dish that fits within an insert of a 3-D piezo stage is used to culture the cancer cells. This 3-D piezo stage facilitates movement of the sample along *X*, *Y* and *Z* directions and is mounted within the mechanical stage on the inverted microscope.

To operate the instrument we use hardware controlled by algorithms written in LabVIEW. The instrument is placed on an isolation table with feedback control that removes low frequency vibrations (starting below 1 Hz) in real time. Optical components are anchored firmly to the table and to each other to minimize the effects of any remaining acoustic sounds. The instrument is set-up in a dark room painted flat black and acoustically isolated from the control equipment found in the adjacent support rooms by insulation in the walls. The support equipment in the adjacent room includes two chillers (*see* **Note 2**) and the controls for Table, AODs, 3-D piezo stage, xenon or TLED+ lamps. This is safer as after optical alignment and set-up the experimentalist monitors and controls the modules with the computer in the adjacent well-lit room, and not in the dark room, which houses the lasers and other parts of the instrument.

1.3 Theoretical Framework to Measure the Temporal Response of the Trap

For displacements less than the radius of the bead (R) an optical trap acts like a Hookean spring [30], where the force, $\vec{F}(r,\theta)$ acting on the bead suspended above the surface of a dish at constant height (h) within the plane $0 \leq r \leq R$, $0 \leq \theta \leq 2\pi$ is

$$\vec{F}(r,\theta) = k_P[\hat{\imath}\,(r\,\mathrm{Cos}\,\theta) + \hat{\jmath}\,(r\,\mathrm{Sin}\,\theta)]$$
$$\vec{F}(x,y) = k_P[\hat{\imath}\,x + \hat{\jmath}\,y] \tag{1}$$

where r and θ describe the magnitude and direction of the force, k_P is the lateral stiffness at a power (P), (where the subscript indicates the power is held constant), within the plane and $\hat{\imath}$ and $\hat{\jmath}$ are unit vectors along the X and Y directions. Equation 1 states k_P is constant in the trapping plane, and there is no force acting on the bead when it is at the center ($r = 0$, $0 \leq \theta \leq 2\pi$). It also states there is only a component in the X direction if $0 < r \leq R$, $\theta \in \{0, \pi\}$ and only a component in the Y direction if $0 < r \leq R$, $\theta \in \{\frac{\pi}{2}, \frac{3\pi}{2}\}$. Specifically

$$F(x) = k_P x \tag{2a}$$

$$F(y) = k_P y \tag{2b}$$

where $-R \leq x \leq R$ and $-R \leq y \leq R$.

In the case when there is no force the measured resultant (r_m) reflects the noise of the recordings where the probability distribution function is described by the Rayleigh distribution [31]

$$P(r_m) = \frac{r_m}{\sigma^2} e^{-\frac{r_m^2}{2\sigma^2}} \tag{3}$$

where σ is the scale factor of the distribution with mean $\bar{r}_m$ and variance $\sigma_m{}^2$

$$\bar{r}_m = \sigma\sqrt{\frac{\pi}{2}}\ and\ \sigma_m^2 = \sigma^2\left(2 - \frac{\pi}{2}\right). \tag{4}$$

When a trapped dielectric bead is displaced from its lateral equilibrium position it experiences a restoring force proportional to the displacement, described in the X direction with

$$\beta\frac{dx}{dt} = -k_P x \tag{5}$$

where β is the Stokes damping constant (Nsm^{-1}) and t is the time. Note the inertial term [32] is not included, as it is negligible compared to the viscous term [33, p. 299]. Rearranging and integrating from the displaced position of the bead $x \equiv x_0$ at $t = 0$ back to the equilibrium position x_t at $t > 0$ Eq. 5 becomes

$$\int_{x_0}^{x_t} \frac{1}{x}\,dx = -\frac{k_P}{\beta}\int_0^t dt$$

$$x_t = x_0 e^{(-k_P/\beta)t} = x_0 e^{(-\tau_P)t} \tag{6}$$

where the reciprocal time constant (τ_P) for the bead trajectory is

$$\tau_P = \frac{k_P}{\beta}. \tag{7}$$

β is calculated with the Stoke's-Faxen law [34]

$$\beta = \frac{6\pi\eta R}{\left[1 - \frac{9}{16}\left(\frac{R}{h}\right) + \frac{1}{8}\left(\frac{R}{h}\right)^3 + \frac{45}{256}\left(\frac{R}{h}\right)^4 - \frac{1}{16}\left(\frac{R}{h}\right)^5\right]} \tag{8}$$

where the term in the denominator considers the additional effect on the hydrodynamic drag caused by proximity of the Petri dish to the bead and η is the viscosity of the solution.

We cannot readily measure P at the trapping plane; instead it is measured at the objective lens in the absence of a Petri dish i.e., $P_{\text{objective}}$. We assume that this power measured is directly proportional to power at the trapping plane and provide evidence that this is the case.

To calibrate the instrument we experimentally determine the:

1. Radius, R of the bead;
2. Viscosity, η of the solution at the temperature, T of the experiments;
3. Lateral displacement of the bead, x, y relative to the center of the plane;
4. Height, h of the trapped bead above the Petri dish;
5. Reciprocal time constant, τ_P of the trap at power P, and
6. Show that the τ_P and k_P are linear functions of P measured at the objective.

We then use Eq. 8 to calculate β, Eq. 7 to calculate k_P as a function of $P_{\text{objective}}$ and Eqs. 1 and 2 to determine the force, $\vec{F}(r,\theta)$, $F(x)$ and $F(y)$ for constant $P_{\text{objective}}$.

We first describe the reagents and equipment in Subheading 2. This is followed by a description of procedures that are either required to be executed each time an experiment is performed or only once (Subheadings 3.2 and 3.4, **step** 7 of Subheading 3.5, **step 3** of Subheading 3.6 and Subheadings 3.7 and 3.9). Briefly, we describe how to determine the drop in power upon movement of the beam with the AODs. We show it is insignificant within the linear range of the trap, avoiding the need for an extra feedback loop. Then we describe a method to determine whether the trap moves with the same linear slope in both directions (X, Y) in response to the AODs. We show this to be the case, which eliminates the requirement for calibration in both directions before each experiment. After which we describe the drag force method that we use to measure τ_B, and show it is linear with power. We then describe procedures to check reproducibility of the measurements, and to determine the typical noise within the signal. In the notes section, we suggest improvements. We conclude that the time constant of the instrument is sufficiently fast to enable monitoring the kinetics of chemical motors at the edge of a cancer cell.

2 Materials

2.1 Reagents

1. Buffered saline: 150 mM NaCl, 2 mM $CaCl_2$, 1 mM $MgCl_2$, 10 mM HEPES and 2.8 mM KOH, pH 7.2 and osmolality 300 mOsm/Kg.
2. Phosphate buffered saline (PBS): 1 mM KH_2PO_4, 154 mM NaCl, 5.2 mM Na_2HPO_4, pH 7.4 and osmolality 303 mOsm/Kg. Store buffered saline (above) and PBS at 4 °C. Filter them through 0.2 μm polyvinylidene fluoride (PVDF) filter before each experiment.
3. Petri dishes: 35 mm poly-D-lysine-coated glass bottom Petri dishes with 0.17 mm thick coverslips (MatTek Corp., Ashland, MA). The thickness of the coverslip is that recommended for use with the objective lens.
4. Beads: sulfate-coated fluorescent latex beads (FluoSpheres Sulfate Microspheres, F-8858, Life Technologies, Carlsbad, CA) with a nominal diameter of 4 μm. Beads are maximally excited at 576 nm and emit in the red region at ~605 nm.
5. Culture media for head and neck squamous cell carcinoma cell line, HN-31: Dulbecco's modified Eagle's medium with 10 % (v/v) fetal bovine serum, 250 U/ml penicillin—250 μg/ml streptomycin, 2 × concentration of vitamins found in minimal essential medium, 1 mM sodium pyruvate, 0.1 mM nonessential amino acids and 2 mM L-glutamine.

2.2 Equipment

1. Continuous wave Ti-sapphire laser with maximum power of 2 W tunable from 675 to 1100 nm (3900S Titanium:Sapphire CW Laser, Spectra-Physics, Santa Clara, CA, USA).
2. Solid-state frequency-doubled Nd: YVO_4 pump laser with maximum power of 6 W at 532 nm and controller (Millennia Prime, Spectra-Physics, Santa Clara, CA, USA).
3. Water-cooled chillers, one for each laser (1) Thermorack solid-state chiller, (Solid State Cooling Systems, Wappingers Falls, NY, USA) and a (2) 6360 T recirculator (Polyscience, Niles, IL USA) (*see* **Note 2**).
4. Polarizing beam splitter ($620 < T < 1000$ nm, CM1-PBS252, Thorlabs, Newton, NJ).

5. Objective with numerical aperture of 1.4 (Plan Apo VC 60×/1.40 Oil, Nikon Instruments Inc., Melville, NY, USA).
6. Inverted fluorescence microscope (Eclipse-Ti, Nikon Instruments Inc., Melville, NY, USA).
7. Spectrometer (USB2000+, Ocean Optics, Dunedin, FL).
8. Acousto-optic deflectors AODX and AODY and Radio Frequency, RF driver (72003 and R21.35-65-2ASVCO-2, Gooch & Housego, Melbourne, FL, USA). The amplitude signals from the RF driver are amplified with a custom-built audio class AB amplifier (NTE 1380, NTE Electronics, Inc., Bloomfield, NJ).
9. Quadrant photodiode (QPD, 2901, New Focus, Newport, NY USA) (*see* **Note 3**).
10. Crossed-roller-bearing stage (426 series, Newport Corporation, Irvine, CA) to mount the QPD.
11. Xenon (Lambda LS xenon arc lamp, 2.5 W output, Sutter Instrument Company, Novato, CA, USA) or TLED+ (LED transmitted light source, 75 W maximum output, Sutter Instrument Company, Novato, CA, USA) lamp.
12. Dichroic beam splitters, D1 (T < 750 nm) (Omega Optical, Inc., Brattleboro, VT) and D2 (605 nm < T < 723 nm) (Thorlabs, Newton, New Jersey).
13. Excitation filter (530 < T < 590 nm) (Thorlabs, Newton, New Jersey).
14. Emission filter (600 < T < 700 nm) (Thorlabs, Newton, New Jersey).
15. 3-D piezo stage and controller (p-545.xR7 PInano XYZ Piezo System, Physik Instrumente L.P., Auburn, MA, USA).
16. Monochrome CMOS (complementary metal-oxide semiconductor) camera (PL-B741, PixeLINK, Ottawa, ON, Canada), resolution 1.3 mega pixel.
17. STACIS iX LaserTable-Base and controller (Technical Manufacturing Corp., Peabody, MA).
18. Temperature data-logger with thermocouple (RDXL4SD, Omega Engineering, Stamford, CT).
19. Hand-held optical power meter (1916-R, Newport Corporation, Irvine, CA).
20. Glass slide with micrometer scale 10 μm.
21. Custom built photodetector with a Si photodiode (FDS1010, Thorlabs, Newton, New Jersey) with detection range: 400–1100 nm, and active area 10 mm × 10 mm.
22. Portable keyboard.

23. Wall-mounted monitor. Place the portable keyboard (above) and the wall-mounted monitor within the dark room to facilitate manipulations required during set up and calibration.
24. Virtual instrument written with LabVIEW (from v.12, National Instruments, Austin, TX) that controls a programmable gate array (FPGA; PCIc 7852R; 16-bit resolution; 40 MHz base clock; National Instruments, Austin, TX) and a data acquisition card (DAQ PCIe-6363; 16-bit resolution; National Instruments, Austin, TX) set at its lowest gain of ± 0.1 V. The FPGA enables synchronous (25 ns clock of the FPGA board) and continuous control of the two AODs and the 3-D piezo stage. Voltages from the FPGA to AODs control the position (± 10 V) and intensity (± 1 V) of the laser beam. Analog voltages (± 10 V) generated from the FPGA are also used to position the 3-D piezo stage. The resolution of the analog inputs of the FPGA card is 0.3 mV, which is of the order of the signal measured by the QPD (1–16 mV) and hence this FPGA is not suitable for collection of the sensor data. Instead, the voltage outputs from the QPD are monitored by the DAQ. A TTL pulse-train (200 kHz) generated with the FPGA synchronizes the data acquired with the DAQ, and the control signals produced by the FPGA.
25. MATLAB and toolboxes (from version R2011b, The Mathworks, Natick, MA) used for analysis.

3 Methods

3.1 Measuring P Along the Optical Path (See Note 4)

The power is measured with the hand-held optical power meter with AODX and AODY held at their center frequency (*see* Fig. 2).

1. Turn on pump laser that powers the trapping laser and let it warm up for 30 min.
2. Use the spectrometer to ensure the trapping laser is set to 830 nm. If the wavelength of the laser beam is not 830 nm, adjust the knob on the trapping laser while measuring the wavelength with the spectrometer.
3. Measure the power after the trapping laser (Fig. 2). Maximize the laser power with knobs located on the outside of the trapping laser box; this optimizes the alignment of mirrors within the housing. We operate the pump laser at 5 W, below the maximum of 6 W to prolong the life of the pump. The output power after the trapping laser is typically 1.4 W.
4. Measure the power after the half wave plate (not shown) positioned after the beam splitter (Fig. 2). Maximize the power at this position by aligning the mirrors up to the half wave plate. The power is typically 1.2 W after the half wave plate.

5. Measure the power after the AODs (Fig. 2). Maximize the power at this position by aligning the mirrors up to the AODs. The power drops to 0.55 W after the AODs, when the amplitude input to AODs is one half the maximum value at 0.5 V.
6. Measure $P_{\text{objective}}$: it should be maximal provided the beam is properly aligned. Reduce or increase the power at the pump to maintain $P_{\text{objective}}$ at a constant value for comparisons among (the same) experiments. This is 0.130 (± 0.001) W in our case.
7. When there is a need to vary $P_{\text{objective}}$, increase or decrease the power at the pump laser.

3.2 Measuring and Maintaining Constant P as the Beam is Moved with the AODs (See Note 5)

AODs are less efficient as they move from their center frequency [35, 36]. We now describe how to monitor P when the beam is moved by AODs. The laser beam is displaced by changing the voltage to the frequency inputs of the AODs. AODs control the intensity and position of the trapping laser beam at high rates (>100 kHz). Each AOD consists of a piezoelectric-based transducer across which a radio frequency voltage is applied. This generates a sound wave that is absorbed by the acousto-optic crystal. The sound wave produces a periodic mechanical stress in the crystal, varying its atomic density. This causes a change in refractive index that follows the period of the sound wave and produces a moving-phase grating which diffracts the laser beam into several orders. The first order is the most efficient when the amplitude input V^a is held at maximum value and the frequency input is held at f_{center}.

To steer the laser beam with an AOD, keep the amplitude input V^a constant at one half of the maximum value 0.5 V ($0 < V^a \leq 1$), and vary the frequency input by changing the voltage input V^f to the voltage-to-frequency converter. The f_{center} of the AOD, is 50 MHz (V_c^f: 6.2 V); as the frequency deviates from this center value diffraction efficiency decreases causing the power to drop. To determine this drop in power as a consequence of moving the beam with the AODs, we direct the beam on to a custom-built photodetector and record the output voltage and compare it with that recorded when the beam is in the center position. This ratio provides a measure of the drop in laser power.

1. Direct the laser beam into the custom-built photodetector placed after the AODs.
2. Vary the frequency input to AODX in steps (e.g., 0.395 MHz) through its maximal steering range with AODY fixed at one frequency. Record the output voltage from the photodetector at each step, and plot the voltage relative to voltage recorded at the center frequency as a function of the frequency of AODX (Fig. 3, left panel).
3. Repeat **steps 1–2** for the other 75 fixed frequencies of AODY (each increment 0.395 MHz).

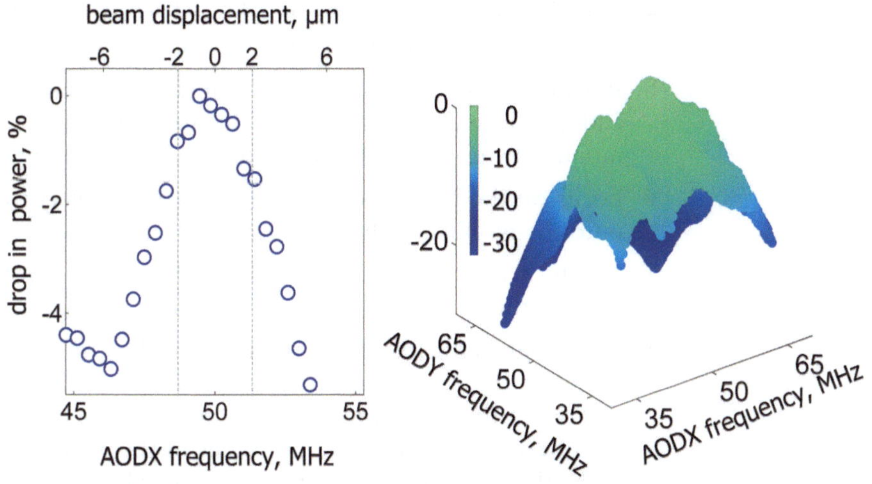

Fig. 3 The drop in laser power is small at ≤ 2 % within a 2×2 µm region of the trapping plane. *Left panel*: Drop in laser power with change in the acoustic frequency input to AODX with the input to AODY held constant at f_{center} (*open circles*). The *dotted vertical lines* represent the maximum range of the experiments. *Right panel:* A 3-D map of the power. Frequency input to AODX is steered between $\pm$ 15 MHz of f_{center} ($\Delta V^f = \pm$ 3.8 V) with AODY fixed at a frequency within the same range. Each data point was recorded upon changing the frequency by 0.395 MHz where the map was compiled from 76×76 measurements. The f_{center} of each AOD is 50 MHz and V^a was set at 0.5 V for both AODs in all shown experiments

A typical example of the drop in power is shown in Fig. 3, left panel. We observe a 4–5 % decrease in power as AODX is moved $\pm$ 5 MHz from f_{center} with AODY held at its center frequency. Each slice (like the left panel) is then concatenated to produce the 3-D map of the power. The right panel shows a 3-D view of the drop in laser power as the beam is moved through its maximal steering range of $\pm$ 15 MHz from f_{center}. Each data point is recorded upon changing the frequency by 0.395 MHz and the map is compiled from 76×76 measurements. Over this maximum steering range of the AODs the drop is considerable at up to 30 %. Fortunately, the experiments described require an AOD frequency range of within 1.5 MHz of f_{center} where the drop is less than 2 %. When significant steering ranges are required the amplitude input could be changed to compensate for the drop in power due to change in acoustic frequency (*see* **Note 6**). For strategies to increase power refer to Notes (*see* **Note 7**).

3.3 Preparation to Trap a Bead (See Note 4)

1. Aliquot 2 µl of the bead solution into 1 ml of water (18.0 MΩcm).
2. Centrifuge for 1 min at 10,000 × *g* and resuspend in 1 ml of buffered saline (*see* **Note 8**).
3. Place a Petri dish with 1 ml buffered saline into the insert of the 3-D piezo stage of the inverted microscope.

4. Pipette 2 μl of the resuspended bead-solution close to the coverslip edge of the Petri dish.
5. Ensure the laser is on and steered to focus at the trapping plane, and the bright field image of the beam projects onto the monitor by use of the CMOS camera (*see* Subheading 3.1).
6. Focus on the bottom of the Petri dish and project the image onto the monitor with CMOS camera.
7. Locate a bead that has not yet attached to the bottom by moving the dish laterally with the mechanical stage.
8. The image of the laser beam projected by the camera appears as a spot at the center surrounded by concentric fringes. While projecting the image onto the monitor with the camera, focus on a bead by adjusting the fine focus of the microscope, then move the bead into the center of the laser beam by use of the mechanical stage. The bead should enter the trap (*see* Fig. 2, center inset).

3.4 Determination of the Scale of the Trapping Plane (See Note 5)

We now establish whether the movement of the beam by each AOD is the same within the trapping plane and determine the V^f required to move the beam 1 μm.

1. Steer the laser beam by changing V^f in steps while tracking the displacement of the laser beam with the CMOS camera (Fig. 4).
2. Analyze the images captured with scripts written with the Image Processing Toolbox of MATLAB to determine the number of pixels the laser beam moves when V^f is changed by one (1) V. In the example shown, AODY is orthogonal to AODX as expected; however the beams move at an angle θ_D (−10.45°) to the trapping plane (Fig. 4, top panel). This results in primary and secondary components where the magnitude of the secondary component is about 20 % of the primary. We show that the beam moves linearly upon changing the voltage in AODX and AODY, and gets deflected by the same amount in X and Y for the same change in voltage (Fig. 4, center panel) to exhibit slopes (primary component) of 75.86 pixels/V (X) and 75.48 pixels/V (Y). We find that the slope of the secondary component is about 1/5th of the primary component with the magnitude 3 % less along Y relative to X. We associate this small difference with an error in fitting the data to this less steep slope.
3. To translate this deflection of the beam from pixels to μm, calibrate the CMOS camera with the slide micrometer by first setting the frame size of each image captured by the camera to ensure that the pixels are square and not distorted. This is achieved by capturing a region of interest of 1280 (X) pixels

× 1024 (Y) pixels for our camera. Then determine the number of pixels at each 10 μm increment in both the X and Y directions within each image. Plot the number of pixels as a function of distance and calculate the slope (pixels/μm). We make use of Image Processing Toolbox of MATLAB, and determine the slope in both directions to be 13.3 pixels/μm.

4. Alternatively, use a 3-D piezo stage (pre-calibrated with the slide micrometer) to move a bead firmly attached to the bottom of a Petri dish and track the center of the bead with the same camera (Fig. 4, bottom panel). Analyze the images as described in **step 2** and determine the conversion slopes. The slope for this relation is the same at 13.33 pixels/μm (X) and 13.32 pixels/μm (Y).
5. Determine the change in voltage V^f required to move the beam 1 μm by calculating the product of the two calibrations (V/pixels × pixels/μm) described in **steps 2** and **3** or **steps 2** and **4**. The change in voltage V^f required to move the beam 1 μm is the same for both AODs at 0.1757 V (X) and 0.1765 V (Y) within a 2 μm × 2 μm region of the trapping plane. We conclude that the beam can be steered with a resolution of ± 2 nm limited by the 16-bit resolution of the analog outputs of FPGA at ± 0.3 mV.

3.5 Description and Analysis of the Signal from the QPD: Determine the Lateral Displacement (x, y) Relative to the Center of the Plane

The position and intensity of the detected fluorescent light is translated to an electrical signal by the QPD. The emitted light is directed towards the center of the QPD such that the difference in intensity between the left and right quadrants and top and bottom quadrants is zero (Fig. 2, left inset). As the bead moves from this center position, there is a shift in intensity among the four quadrants. The X output is the difference in voltage between the left (B, C) and right (A, D) quadrants and the Y output is the difference in voltage between the top (A, B) and bottom (C, D) quadrants. The sum Σ is the total intensity in all four quadrants, and is used to normalize X and Y outputs to correct for intensity fluctuations especially due to photobleaching of the bead. The measured current, $I_M{}^Q$ in each quadrant $Q(Q \in \{A, B, C, D\})$ of the QPD is the sum of the current due to light emitted by the bead, $I_L{}^Q$ and a dark current, $I_D{}^Q$ present in the absence of the bead. This current is relayed through a first-stage amplifier of the QPD whose resistance (R1) is 200 kΩ. Specifically the measured output in volts for each quadrant $V_M{}^Q$ is

$$V_M^Q = I_M^Q \mathrm{R1} = (I_L^Q + I_D^Q)\mathrm{R1}, \quad Q \in \{A, B, C, D\}. \tag{9}$$

The signal is differenced and amplified by a second stage amplifier of the QPD with gain, G of 1, 3 or 10 (V/V) and the measured signal from the X and Y outputs are

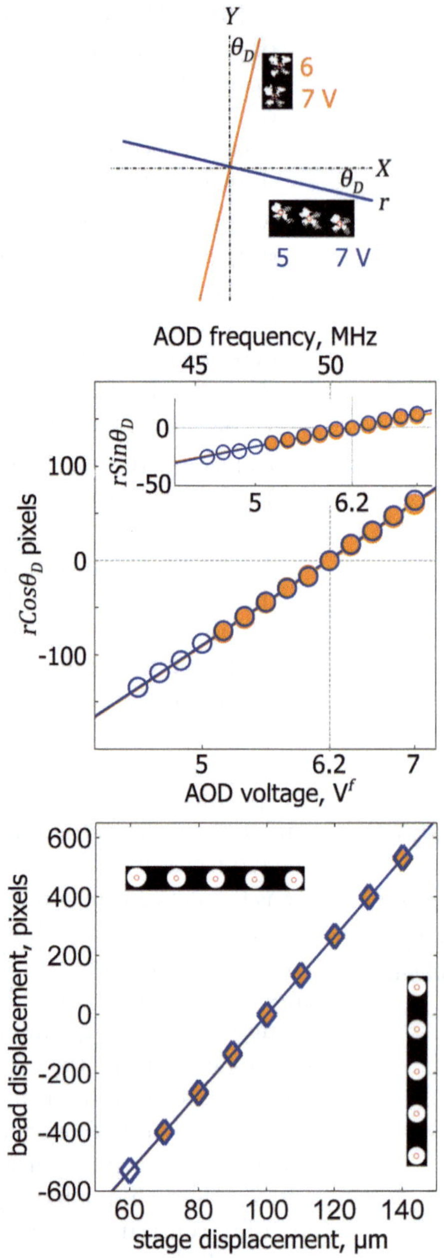

Fig. 4 The laser beam moves linearly with a change in V^f to the AODs and the magnitude of the displacement is the same in both directions. *Top panel*: Orientation of the steered beam within the cartesian plane of the trap (*see* Fig. 2). The insets show images of the beam recorded at described voltages for AODX (*bottom*) and AODY (*top*). The angle θ_D is $-10.45°$ relative to X (AODX steering) and Y (AODY steering) axes. *Center panel*: The primary component of the beam position detected with the CMOS camera upon changing the frequency to AODX (*open circles* with *blue* border) or AODY (*closed orange circles* with no border), where the center frequency is considered to be the origin. The solid lines

$$\Delta X_M = (\Delta X_L + \Delta X_D)G$$
$$= \left[\left(V_L^B + V_L^C - V_L^A - V_L^D\right) + \left(V_D^B + V_D^C - V_D^A - V_D^D\right)\right]G \tag{10a}$$

$$\Delta \Upsilon_M = (\Delta \Upsilon_L + \Delta \Upsilon_D)G$$
$$= [(V_L^A + V_L^B - V_L^C - V_L^D) + (V_D^A + V_D^B - V_D^C - V_D^D)]G. \tag{10b}$$

The output from the sum is

$$\sum\nolimits_{\text{M}} = \sum\nolimits_{\text{L}} + \sum\nolimits_{\text{D}}$$
$$= \left(V_L^A + V_L^B + V_L^C + V_L^D\right)$$
$$+ \left(V_D^A + V_D^B + V_D^C + V_D^D\right). \tag{10c}$$

The signal due to dark current is determined before each experiment by measuring ΔX_D, $\Delta \Upsilon_D$ and $\sum_{\text{D}}$ in the absence of a sample and in the dark. The signal due to the presence of the bead is found by writing Eq. 10 in terms of ΔX_L, $\Delta \Upsilon_L$ and $\sum_{\text{L}}$. To account for intensity fluctuations of the bead the signal is normalized by the sum (V/V)

$$\frac{\Delta X_L}{\sum_{\text{L}}} = \frac{\Delta X_M - (\Delta X_D G)}{\left(\sum_{\text{M}} - \sum_{\text{D}}\right)G}; \tag{11a}$$

$$\frac{\Delta \Upsilon_L}{\sum_{\text{L}}} = \frac{\Delta \Upsilon_M - (\Delta \Upsilon_D G)}{\left(\sum_{\text{M}} - \sum_{\text{D}}\right)G}. \tag{11b}$$

To convert this normalized voltage to nm a trapped bead is moved a known distance, Δx with AODX (by changing V^f) and the linear slope for X, m_{QPDX} (V/V/nm) is determined with

$$m_{QPDX} = \frac{\frac{\Delta X_L}{\Sigma_{\text{L}}}}{\Delta x} \tag{12a}$$

Fig. 4 (continued) are the robust linear least-squares fit to the primary component (r cos θ_D) with slopes 75.86 (0.62) pixels/V (*X*) and 75.48 (0.48) pixels/V (*Y*) (standard deviation in parenthesis). The inset shows the secondary component ($r\sin\theta_D$) with slopes 14.29 (0.63) pixels/V (*X*) and 13.09 (0.45) pixels/V (*Y*). *Bottom panel:* The 3-D piezo stage is used to move the Petri dish with fluorescent beads attached to the surface of the dish. The *insets* show position of the bead in pixels where the center-to-center distance between beads is 10 μm. Note the scale of the inset is not the same as shown on the abscissa. The solid lines are the robust linear least-squares fit to the data and exhibit slopes of 13.325 (0.014) pixels/μm (*X*) and 13.322 (0.030) pixels/μm (*Y*). The center (i.e., 100 μm) of the range of the 3-D piezo stage is taken as the origin. Each symbol (bottom and center panels) is the mean of three replicates where the standard deviation lies within the marker

In the same manner m_{QPDY} is

$$m_{QPDY} = \frac{\frac{\Delta Y_L}{\Sigma_L}}{\Delta y}. \tag{12b}$$

where Δy is the distance the trapped bead moves in nm in the Y direction when V^f to AODY is changed (data not shown) (*see* **Note 9**).

QPD scalar voltage signals (three channels) that monitor bead displacement and bead fluorescence are recorded at a sampling frequency of 200 kHz (each channel) and saved in TDMS format, a technical data management solution that is optimized for storing time series data and a propriety format of National Instruments. This format is fast and compact. For example, a TDMS file (6-digit precision i.e., μV) of 42 MB size, when converted to a text file (6-digit precision) requires 102 MB of storage. A properties file that contains the experimental conditions and metadata associated with the measurement is saved with every TDMS data file. The metadata includes dark current offsets of the QPD, voltages, and their durations at the frequency inputs of both AODs, voltages at the amplitude inputs of both AODs, and durations, positions, and velocities of the 3-D piezo stage.

To estimate the lateral displacement of a trapped bead, first determine the normalized signals i.e., left hand side of Eq. 11 which are described in **steps 1–6** and then convert them to a spatial measure described in **step 7** (*see* **Note 10**).

1. Move the QPD by adjusting the crossed-roller-bearing stage to align the focal spot of the light with the plane of the QPD and maximize the value of $\sum_L$.
2. Record the dark current before each experiment by measuring ΔX_D, ΔY_D and $\sum_D$ in the absence of a sample and in the dark. The typical voltage offset due to dark current exhibits a value of about 200 μV in the sum (range 80–600 μV).
3. Turn on the light source (xenon or TLED+ lamp) to excite the bead.
4. Position the bead at the center of the QPD with ΔX_L and ΔY_L at zero (Fig. 2, left inset).
5. Measure ΔX_M, ΔY_M, and Σ_M and relay to the DAQ at a sampling frequency of 200 kHz/channel (total bandwidth 600 kHz).
6. When the measurement is complete determine $\frac{\Delta X_L}{\Sigma_L}$ and $\frac{\Delta Y_L}{\Sigma_L}$ with Eq. 11. Typical values of ΔX_L and ΔY_L are $\leq$ 16 mV (*G*: 10) and Σ_L ~1–2.8 mV (*see* **Note 11**).
7. Displace a trapped bead (−5000 nm to 5000 nm, step size: 500 nm, period 80 ms) by changing the input V^f to AODX (making use of the calibrations shown in legend of Fig. 4 and

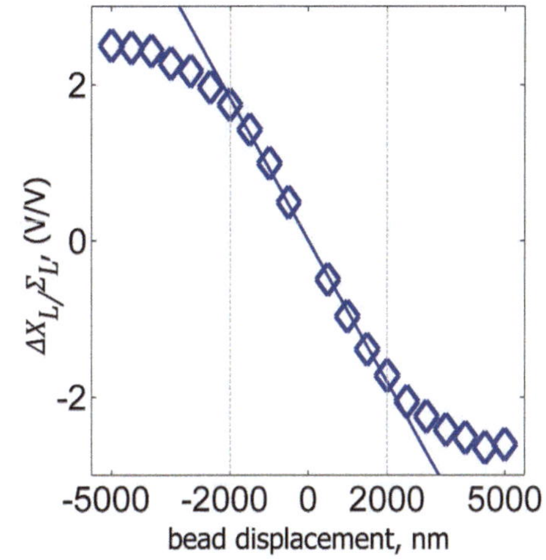

Fig. 5 Normalized voltage signal from the QPD varies linearly with displacement up to radius of the bead. An optically trapped fluorescent bead is displaced up to $\pm$ 5 μm by altering the input voltage of AODX while keeping the input to AODY at the center frequency and monitoring the intensity and position of the bead with the QPD. The symbols represent the primary component of the movement in the *X* direction after normalization (*see* Eq. 11a). The solid line is the best fit of data to the linear region ($\pm$ 2 μm) and exhibits a slope of 0.91 (V/V)/μm (*see* Eq. 12a). The experiments were conducted with a QPD-gain *G* of 3 V/V, resistance R1 of 200 kΩ (*see* Eqs. 9 and 10a), and a power of 130 mW at the objective

Subheading 3.4) with input to AODY kept constant. Figure 5 shows a representative example of the spatial position of the bead in the *X* direction (primary component) as a function of the normalized QPD voltage signal arising from the bead. The relationship is linear up to the radius of the bead, *R* (2000 nm) as expected by theory [30]. The slope of this relation (Eq. 12), m_{QPDX} or m_{QPDY}(V/V/nm) is used to convert the normalized QPD spatial voltage signal (numerator) into a distance measure i.e., nm for each direction.

3.6 Determination of Reciprocal Time Constant τ of the Trap Upon Varying P (See Note 12)

We use a variation of the drag force method called the step response method [37] to measure the reciprocal time constant.

1. Displace the trap rapidly with a square wave input ($\pm$ 350 nm, period 80 ms) to either AODX or AODY and measure the subsequent trajectory of the trapped bead with the QPD for one minute. Collect data at 200 kHz per channel and average 750 resulting waves. Figure 6 (left panel) shows a typical example of the bead trajectory during a step down. The bead trajectory is delayed relative to the step, due to the drag force exerted on the bead by the surrounding fluid (*see* **Note 13**).
2. Determine the reciprocal time constant of this exponential decay by fitting the data to Eq. 5 where the amplitude of the

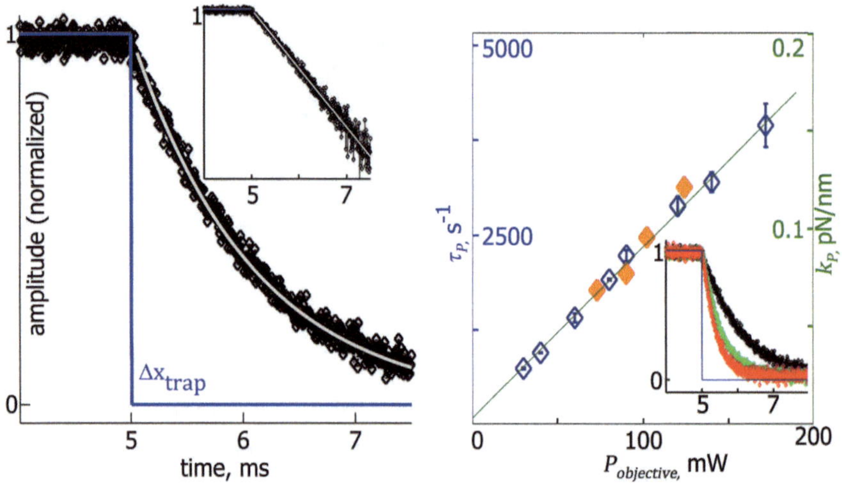

Fig. 6 The reciprocal time constant of the optical trap increases linearly with laser power. *Left panel*: The black open diamonds represent the trajectory of a trapped bead upon setting the bead in periodic motion ($\pm$ 350 nm, period 80 ms) by use of AODX (solid blue line, AODY constant). The solid *gray line* is the best fit of the decay to an exponential and the *inset* shows the fit on a log scale. The reciprocal time constant $\tau_{P \equiv P_{objective}}$ is calculated by fitting the data to Eq. 6 and is 920 s^{-1} at $P_{objective}$ of 40 mW. *Right panel:* τ_p varies linearly with power, where each open blue diamond represents the mean and standard deviation of four (4) to ten (10) measurements. The solid line is least squares fit of data to a linear function with slopes 22.66 s^{-1}mW^{-1} (*left* ordinate, *blue*) and 0.000878 pNnm^{-1}mW^{-1} (*right* ordinate, *green*). The filled diamonds (*orange*) are measurements in *Y* direction upon stimulation with AODY (AODX is kept constant). The inset shows the motion of the bead with powers 120 (fastest, *red*), 80 (*green*), and 40 (slowest, *black*) mW at the objective. Data was collected at 200 kHz for $\sim$ one (1) minute and 750 waves were averaged to retain a time resolution of 5 μs per point

square wave (x_o) is fixed at the size of the step, 350 nm and the subscript P of τ_P represents $P_{\text{objective}}$. For this example, we find $\tau_{P \equiv P_{\text{objective}}}$ to be 920 s^{-1} when $P_{\text{objective}}$ is 40 mW.

3. To show the reciprocal time constant increases linearly with $P_{\text{objective}}$, repeat **steps 1** and **2** for different $P_{\text{objective}}$ (*see* Subheading 3.1).

We show that

$$\tau_{P \equiv P_{\text{objective}}} = \tau(P_{\text{objective}}) = mP_{\text{objective}} \tag{13}$$

and determine a slope, m of 22.66 s^{-1}mW^{-1}. To determine k at each $P_{\text{objective}}$ we need to know β which depends upon R, η and h.

3.7 Determine the Radius, R of the Bead (See Note 5)

The R specified by the manufacturer is 2 μm and we describe a method to verify it.

1. Execute **steps 1–4** of Subheading 3.3 except ensure the beads adhere firmly to the coverslip.
2. Focus at the bottom (inside surface) of the dish while projecting the image of the beads onto the monitor by use of the CMOS camera.

3. Measure the diameter of the beads ($2R$) in pixels and use the linear slope determined in **step 3** or **4** of Subheading 3.4 to convert the pixels into μm. We verify R to be 2.13 ± 0.019 μm.

3.8 Determine the Viscosity, η of the Solution at the Temperature, T of Experiments (See Note 4)

The viscosity (η) depends upon the temperature (T) and the chemical composition of the saline. The main chemical component of our saline solutions is NaCl (150 mM). To determine T we place the thermocouple into the solution within the Petri dish. The average temperature of the solution is typically 24 °C, and we calculate η to be 0.920 mNsm^{-2}. It is calculated with an empirical expression (i.e., Eq. 11) found in Ozbek and others [38] which was formulated from a wide range of viscosity measurements (*see* **Note 14**).

3.9 Determination of the Height of the Trapped Bead h, from the Surface (See Note 15)

The size of the outermost fringe (Fig. 2, center inset) around the trapped bead (or laser spot) reflects the distance between the trapped bead and the Petri dish. This is used as a visual marker to ensure h is constant among measurements; h decreases as we move the Petri dish close to the bead and increases in the opposite direction. To measure the magnitude of h ($h = d + R$, where d is shortest distance between bead and Petri dish) we estimate the time the Petri dish takes to make impact with the bead when the dish is moved at a constant velocity towards the bead.

1. Trap a bead above the surface of the Petri dish (refer to Subheading 3.3).
2. Move the Petri dish with 3-D piezo stage to height, h by monitoring the size of the outermost fringe.
3. Set the trapped bead in motion with a square wave input to either AOD (refer to Subheading 3.6).
4. Move the Petri dish towards the bead at a speed, v_Z of 0.1 μms^{-1} with the 3-D piezo stage.
5. Determine the height of the bead from the time at the point of impact. Figure 7 demonstrates this measurement. The dish makes impact after time, t_Z of 74 s. Therefore, $d = 74\ (t_Z) \times 0.1\ (v_Z) = 7.4$ μm and $h = 7.4 + 2.1 = 9.5$ μm. The mean h determined for six independent measurements is 9.88 ± 0.04 μm.
6. Calculate β with Eq. 8. In this example, we calculate β to be 3.91×10^{-5} pNsnm^{-1} (*see* **Note 16**).
7. Calculate $k_{P \equiv P_{\text{objective}}}$ with Eq. 7 (*see* **Note 17**).
8. Determine the slope $m\beta$ from the linear plot of k_P as a function of $P_{\text{objective}}$

$$k_{P \equiv P_{\text{objective}}} = k(P_{\text{objective}}) = m\beta P_{\text{objective}}. \tag{14}$$

In this case $m\beta$ is 0.000878 pNnm^{-1}mW^{-1} (Fig. 6, right panel).

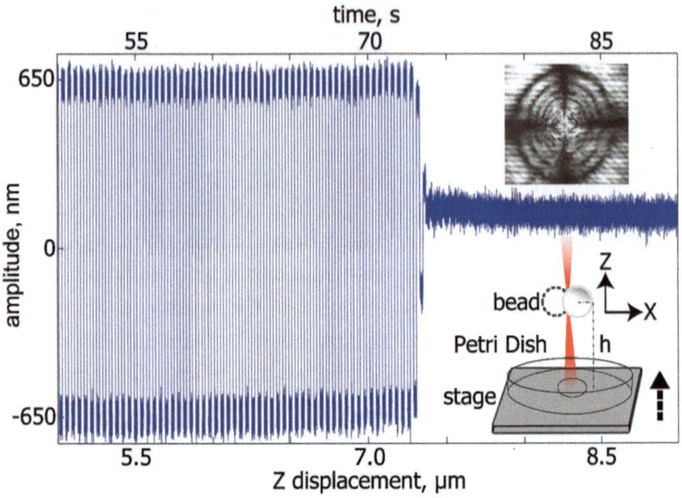

Fig. 7 Measuring the height, *h* of the bead above the surface of the Petri dish. The *left plot* shows the trajectory of a trapped bead upon setting the bead in periodic motion (± 650 nm, period 80 ms) by use of AODX (*solid* (*blue*) *line*) with AODY constant. This motion is arrested when the surface of the Petri dish impacts the bead. This is carried out by moving the dish in the focal (*Z*) direction towards the bead with the 3-D piezo stage at a rate of 0.1 μms^{-1} (indicated by the *arrow*). The *bottom right inset* shows the geometry of the experiment

Our data show that τ_P and k_P are linear with $P_{\text{objective}}$ with slopes m and $m\beta$ that are reflective of our instrument. This linear relationship allows us to compare our measured τ_P and k_P with values determined with other instruments provided they also exhibit a linear function with power. We make these comparisons by adjusting β for R where h is taken to be ~10 μm because R is often reported, but h is not. There is one report where the reciprocal time constant was measured by rapidly perturbing the trapped bead with AODs [37]; Simmons and colleagues showed τ_P and k_P were linear with power. The measured τ_P for a k_P of 0.11 pNnm^{-1} is ~12,000 s^{-1} for a bead with R of 0.5 μm. For a R of 2 μm used in our experiments the reciprocal time constant would be four times lower at 3000 s^{-1}, which is comparable to our measured value of 2840 s^{-1} (Fig. 6, right panel) and corroborates the measurements.

Other reports perform power spectrum analysis [34, 39–41] to determine the angular corner frequency, f_c. We compare our data with these measurements as f_c relates to τ_P by

$$f_c = \frac{\tau_P}{2\pi}. \tag{15}$$

We calculate τ_P from the measured f_c and scale to adjust for variation in bead size. We determine τ_P to be 450, 584, 1601, and 1908 s^{-1} for a range of k_P at 0.0183 [39], 0.021 [40], 0.06 [41] and 0.08 [34] pNnm^{-1} which are comparable to our measured values of τ_P at 472, 542, 1548, and 2065 s^{-1} for the same k_P (Fig. 6, right panel). This corroboration of measurements from different laboratories and instruments suggests that it is reasonable to assume that $P_{\text{objective}}$ is proportional to the power at the trapping plane (see Subheading 1.3).

This data show that events occurring at rates slower than the corner frequency of 469 s^{-1} (calculated with Eq. 13 for $\tau_{P\equiv0.130\ W}$: 2946 s^{-1}) can be detected with high fidelity. This corner frequency is of the order of the rate for actin polymerization in cells [42], tubulin polymerization [43], and the fast kinetic steps of kinesins [44] and unconventional myosins [45, 46]. It is faster than the reported rate (~100 s^{-1}) we observed for actin polymerization, and confirms the measurements were not limited by the temporal response of the instrument [16].

3.10 Reliability and Consistency of Measurements (See Note 4)

Before each experiment, calibrate the position sensor and determine the stiffness and reciprocal time constant to compare consistency among experiments. In our case we conduct experiments at the same $P_{\text{objective}}$ of 0.130 W (*see* Subheading 3.1).

1. Trap a bead above the surface of the Petri dish (refer to Subheading 3.3).
2. Send square wave inputs of amplitudes ± 500 and ± 800 nm with a period of 80 ms to one of the AODs to displace the optical trap (refer to Subheading 3.6). Then record the deviation in the voltage signal of the trapped bead between the baseline and peak positions with the QPD as it follows the square wave generated by AOD. Figure 8 (top panel) shows a plot of this sensor response relative to the amplitude of the input square waves in nm. The bead displacement varies linearly with the resulting normalized voltage signal to exhibit a slope m_{QPDX} of 0.00028 V/V/nm. The slopes measured on different days are consistent and exhibit a normal distribution with mean $\overline{m}_{QPDX}$ of 0.00027 (± 0.00002) V/V/nm (Fig. 8, center panel).
3. Check whether $k_{P\equiv P_{\text{objective}}}$ is consistent among experiments by first measuring $\tau_{P\equiv P_{\text{objective}}}$, and then calculating $k_{P\equiv P_{\text{objective}}}$ (refer to Subheadings 3.6–3.9). We determine $\tau_{P\equiv P_{\text{objective}}}$ as described in **steps 1** and **2** of Subheading 3.6, except in this case we move the beam with square waves of four different amplitudes (*see* square waves described in **step 2** above). The reciprocal time constant in response to each square wave input is measured, and the average value of the four measures is then used to calculate $k_{P\equiv P_{\text{objective}}}$. Figure 8 (bottom panel) shows the normal distribution of $k_{P\equiv0.130\ W}$ with a mean and standard deviation of 0.116 (± 0.011 pNnm^{-1}) (*see* **Note 18**).

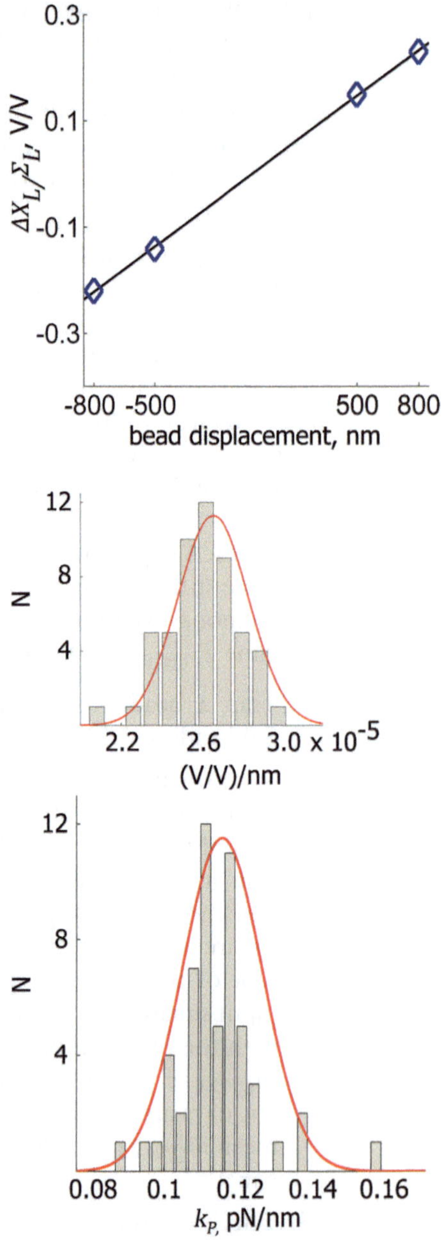

Fig. 8 Position sensor is calibrated and k_P is measured before each experiment. A trapped bead is displaced by initiating periodic movement of the bead with AODX (square waves: amplitudes of $\pm$ 500 nm and $\pm$ 800 nm and period 80 ms) with AODY constant. The trajectory of the trapped bead is recorded with the QPD and is further analyzed. *Top panel*: The diamonds (*blue*) show the normalized voltage signal in V/V recorded for the displacements of the trapped bead between the baseline and peak positions. The *solid line* is a least squares fit to the data and exhibits a slope of 0.00028 V/V/nm. *Center panel:* Histogram for 54 independent measurements of m_{QPDX} (V/V/nm). The solid line (*red*) is a fit of the data to a normal distribution with mean and standard deviation 0.00027 $\pm$ 0.00002 V/V/nm. *Bottom panel*: Histogram for 56 independent

3.11 Quantifying the Displacement of a Trapped Bead in the Absence of a Force: Estimating the Signal to Noise Ratio, SNR

The projection of the fluorescent bead on the QPD can be described by the position vector (r, θ). In the absence of a force the bead occupies each quadrant for an equivalent amount of time. This position vector (r_m, θ) of the bead is transformed to the X and Υ components by the electronics of the QPD and further transformed to displacements (nm) x and y with Eq. 12. Each component, exhibits a probability distribution that is Gaussian. These signals do not reflect the true noise, it is described by the magnitude of the scale factor determined upon fitting r_m to a Rayleigh distribution (Eq. 3). We also determine whether the detector exhibits bias by examining the distribution of θ. To do this we analyze 10 s of data (Fig. 9, top panel) before each experiment (Fig. 1), which were collected at 200 kHz/channel, and further averaged to sampling rates between 2000 and 100 Hz with scripts written in MATLAB.

1. Determine the displacement in nm i.e. x and y (*see* Subheading 3.5) from the first 10 s of data. Figure 9, top panel shows typical example at a sampling frequency of 2 kHz.
2. Calculate r_m (with Eq. 3) and θ from x and y and fit to Rayleigh and uniform probability distributions, respectively. We find θ exhibits values between 0° and 360° with equal probability (center panel, left) to fit a uniform distribution function with a mean of 0.0028 per degree (center panel, right). r_m exhibits a Rayleigh distribution with σ, $\overline{r}_m$, and ${\sigma_m}^2$ of 18.6 nm, 23.3 nm and 145 nm^2 (*see* Eqs. 3 and 4). We calculate a mean value for σ to be 21.9 nm ($15 \leq \sigma \leq 30$, at sampling frequency of 2 kHz) for 11 recordings. At 2 kHz we can reliably resolve displacements of ~45 nm (signal to noise displacement ratio is 2:1), while at 100 Hz the resolution is ~12 nm.

σ decreases with the logarithm of the sampling frequency to exhibit an intercept of 0.8 nm at zero sampling frequency (Fig. 9, lower right panel). This is of the order of the resolution of the DAQ card at 0.4–0.9 nm (It is calculated with Eq. 11a and 12a with $\overline{m}_{QPDX}$ of 0.00027 V/V/nm, $\sum_L$ of 1–2.8 mV, G of 10, and ΔX_M of 3 μV, assuming no dark current). The xenon lamp was used as the excitation source for these measurements (*see* Fig. 2, right inset) (*see* **Note 19**).

3.12 Summary of Methods

A flow chart summarizing the methodology is shown in Fig. 10. Improvements are described in notes and include: (1) strategies to improve temporal resolution (*see* **Note 20**) and spatial resolution

Fig. 8 (continued) measurements of k_P (pN/nm). *Solid line* (*red*) is a fit of the data to a normal distribution with mean and standard deviation 0.116 ± 0.011 pN/nm. The experiments were conducted with G at 10 V/V (Eq. 10a) and resistance of R1 at 200 kΩ (Eq. 9), and power at the objective of 130 mW

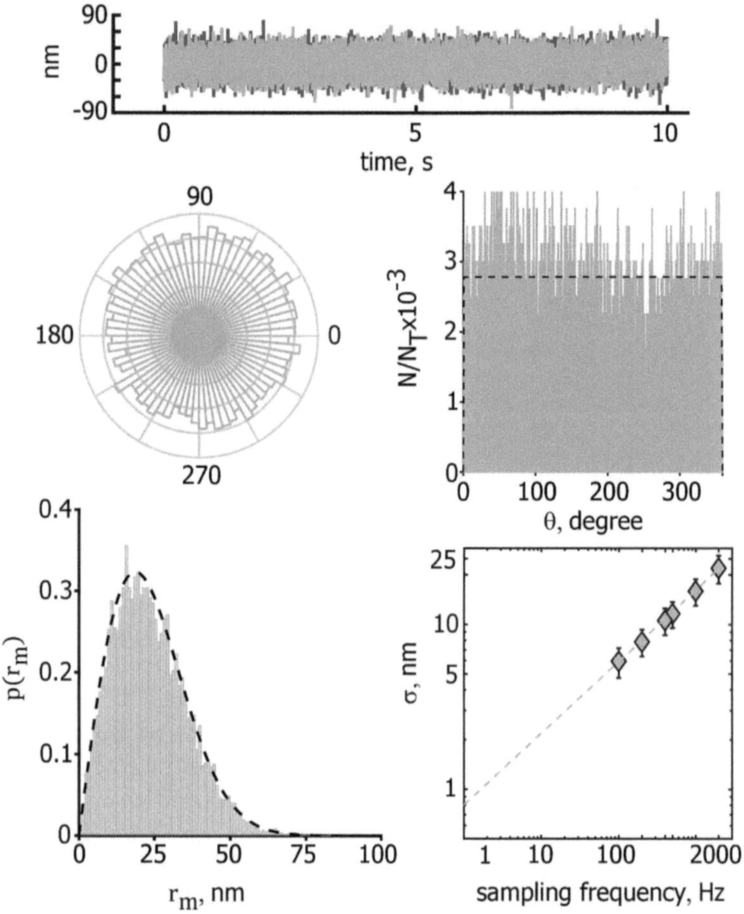

Fig. 9 In the absence of a force, r_m exhibits a Rayleigh distribution and θ is described by a uniform distribution. *Top panel:* Measured displacement (*x: dark gray, y: light gray*) of a trapped bead before onset of an experiment. Sampling frequency is 2 kHz. *Center panel left:* A histogram of θ calculated from the data (2 seconds of data) where the four concentric circles represent 50, 100, 150, and 200 counts per division. *Center panel right:* θ is fit to a uniform distribution (*dashed line*) with mean 0.0028 per degree. The width of each bin is 0.3125° where N_T is total count at 4000. *Bottom panel left:* r_m is described with a Rayleigh distribution with σ of 18.6 nm, $\bar{r}_m$ of 23.3 nm and σ_m^2 of 145 nm^2. *Bottom panel right:* σ scales with the log of the sampling frequency. Each data point represents the mean and standard deviation of 11 independent measurements calculated upon averaging the data sampled at 200 kHz, 100-2000 times, and determined upon fitting to Rayleigh distribution. The dashed line is the fit of the data to a power function with exponent of 0.435 nmHz$^{-0.435}$ and σ of 0.8 nm at zero sampling frequency

(*see* **Note 21**); (2) how to monitor the real-time position of the 3-D piezo stage (response time) (*see* **Note 22**) and improved data management strategies (*see* **Note 23**).

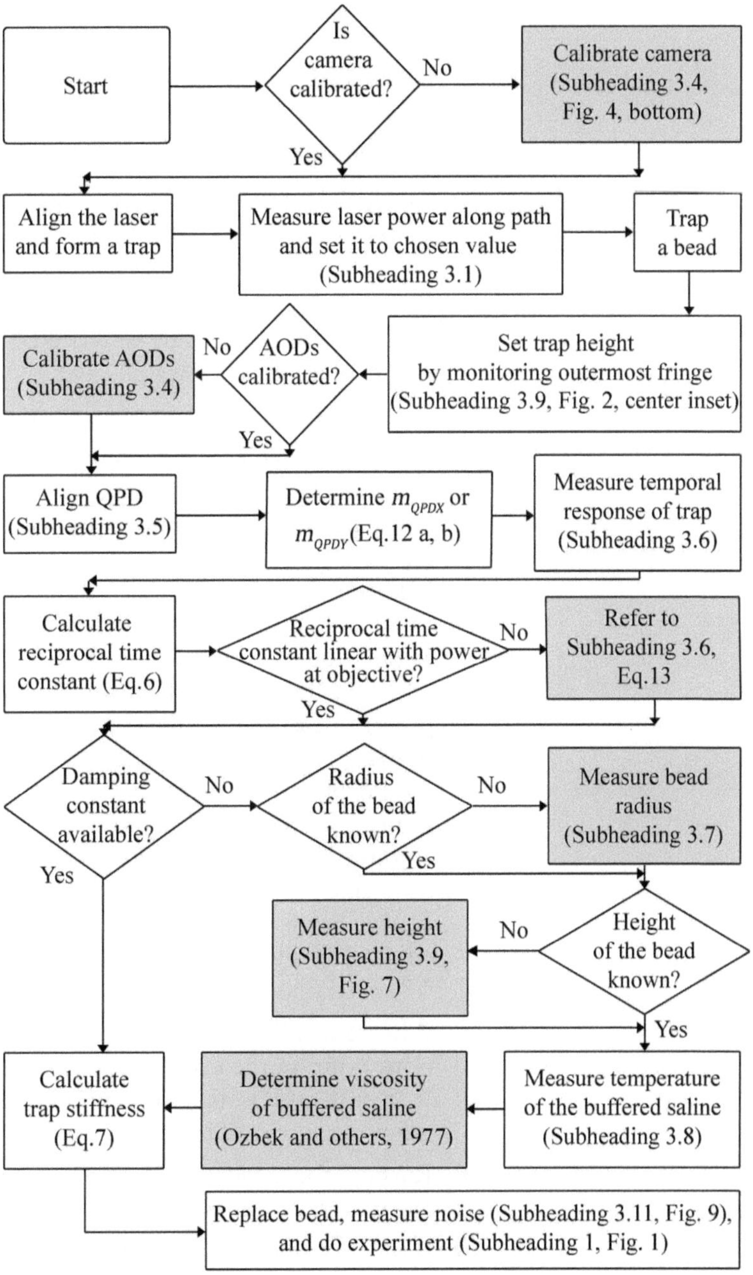

Fig. 10 Flow chart summarizing key steps of experimental methods. The shaded areas identify procedures that only require to be performed once

4 Notes

1. Initially a xenon lamp was used. As the xenon lamp ages, the attachment point of the arc on the cathode wobbles, causing fluctuations in the brightness of the arc. This process is coined

arc wander and results in extra frequency components within the signal. Given that the bulbs are expensive to replace we exchanged the xenon lamp for a TLED+ lamp.

2. The chillers use distilled water purchased from retail stores, as recommended by Spectra Physics engineers.
3. The QPD is powered by a nine (9) V battery (cf. power supply) to reduce electrical line noise. If it is possible, all electrical equipment should be battery-powered to reduce electrical noise.
4. This procedure needs to be repeated before each set of experiments (e.g., once a day).
5. This procedure needs to be performed only once.
6. This can be achieved by reference to a look-up table. The data shown in Fig. 3 was recorded with V^a set at its center value. To construct a look-up table many more measurements at different V^a would be needed (e.g., incrementing by 0.005 V between 0 and 1 V is an additional 200 values). For each value of V^a, vary the frequency inputs to AODX and AODY as described in **steps 2** and **3** over the desired steering range and then determine the drop in laser power relative to the power measured at the center frequency. Plot the loss of power as a function of V^a at each frequency; in this case there are 76 plots each with 201 points for each AOD. Store the values in a look-up table. When the beam is moved a significant amount by each AOD refer to the look-up table to discern by how much V^a needs to be changed to keep the power constant as the beam is moved a significant distance. This requires writing an algorithm to execute the feed-back loop to adjust V^a based upon the reference data within the look-up table.
7. When a feedback loop is not necessary to maintain a constant power during the experiments, V^a can be increased to one (1) V at both AODs and the pump laser could be set to its maximum value of 6 W to obtain maximum power at the objective.
8. Rinsing the beads is necessary to remove additives and to facilitate their adhesion to surfaces.
9. If the movement of the beam by both AODs is not the same, it would be necessary to determine m_{QPDX} and m_{QPDY} separately before each experiment.
10. **Steps 1–6** need to be repeated before each set of experiments (e.g., once a day). **Step** 7 needs to be performed to check the linearity for distances beyond R only once, after which only the slope is calculated for distances $< R$ each time (*see* **step 2** of Subheading 3.10).
11. This is at least 300 times more than the nominal resolution of the DAQ at 3 μV. In addition, we verified this resolution to be

of this order (i.e., 2–5 μV) by measuring the analog inputs at the DAQ terminals when they are not connected to the instrument. This magnitude is below the integrated bandwidth (up to 100 kHz) noise of the QPD calculated with 2 μV rms/(Hz)$^{1/2}$.

12. **Steps 1** and **2** need to be repeated before each set of experiments (e.g., once a day). **Step 3** needs to be performed only once.
13. The AODs are moved with an input square pulse from the FPGA of frequency 12.5 Hz (period: 80 ms). Data acquisition starts when the DAQ card receives the first pulse from the FPGA.
14. A temperature control unit can be implemented to make measurements at physiological temperature i.e., 37 °C.
15. **Steps 1–6** and **8** are performed only once provided all experiments are conducted with the trapped bead at the same height. The stiffness needs to be calculated for each set of experiments from the value for the reciprocal time constant determined for that set.
16. This β is larger than that calculated when the proximity of the Petri dish to the bead is not considered i.e., 3.47×10^{-5} pNsnm^{-1}.
17. There is a 13 % increase in the stiffness when h is considered, which demonstrates that this parameter needs to be kept constant and preferably measured when $h \to 2R$.
18. Deviation in $k_{P \equiv 0.130\ W}$ could be due to: (1) errors in the measurement of $P_{\text{objective}}$; (2) deviations in h or R among experiments; and (3) variation of power at the trapping plane due to differences in the optical properties of coverslips.
19. The xenon lamp was later replaced with a TLED+ lamp. The first prototype tested (loaner from Sutter Instruments) exhibited a bias in θ with σ 5–10 nm greater than that observed with the xenon lamp. The scale factor returned to ~22 nm, and the detector became unbiased when this old controller for the TLED+ was replaced with a new one.
20. A higher dynamic range ($f_c > 500$ s^{-1}) could be achieved by increasing the reciprocal time-constant of the instrument through reduction of the bead radius (Eqs. 7 and 8). However, this improved temporal fidelity will result in reduced spatial range and decreased bead brightness at the sensor. A second strategy to extend the dynamic range is to increase power at the objective. When the pump laser is set to 6 W we find $P_{\text{objective}}$ is 0.243 W and τ_P is 5500 s^{-1}, k_P is 0.215 pNnm^{-1} and f_c is greater at 875 s^{-1}. Other strategies to increase power include: increasing V^a of AODs from 0.5 to 1 V, or by bypassing the

AODs in the laser path once calibration is complete. AODs result in a 50 % drop in laser power; though they are used to measure the reciprocal time constant, they are unused during experimental manipulations with cells. However, an increase in the trapping power will increase the likelihood that cells will exhibit phototoxic effects, although this should be less pronounced at 830 nm which is the wavelength of our trapping laser [47, 48].

21. The spatial resolution can be improved by reducing the sampling rate, but this comes at a loss of temporal precision. One strategy to improve spatial resolution is to increase the QPD output voltage i.e., Σ. This can be achieved by enhancing the input signal intensity by use of brighter fluorescent beads or by increasing the power of the excitation illumination (i.e., TLED+ or xenon lamps). There is a limit to this power as it will increase the photo-bleaching rate of beads, which will impact the duration of experiments. A better strategy is to use sensors that exhibit greater optical-sensitivity. For example, Single Photon Avalanche Diode (SPAD) devices are optical detectors that comprise an array of avalanche photodiodes [49]. They offer single photon sensitivities at visible wavelengths and the capability of parallel read-outs from individual pixels at > 10 MHz. The bead can be monitored with improved sensitivity and time resolution when a SPAD array is used in conjunction with a sensitive FPGA as this will enable fast on-board signal processing and live tracking of a bead. This would enable active feedback control of the V^f input to the AODs, and facilitate implementation of the instrument in force-clamp mode. In this case, the data card would require to exhibit higher resolution than we currently use. Finally, there have been major advancements in signal processing techniques that remove noise from measurements [50, 51] while retaining the temporal fidelity of the signal. They include denoising algorithms that utilize wavelets [50] and empirical mode decomposition which make use of the intrinsic functions of the signal [51]. We have tested these techniques, and started to incorporate them into the analysis and will report this in a later communication.

22. The durations, positions, and velocities of movements of 3-D piezo stage are currently saved as metadata in the TDMS properties file (*see* Subheading 3.5). This is normally sufficient to match the QPD data with the stage position, as the stage control (FPGA) and QPD acquisition (DAQ) systems are synchronized to within 5 μs with a TTL pulse-train (200 kHz). However, as the temporal response of the stage is in the order of ms (mean: 10 ms), not μs, it is sometimes necessary to monitor the real-time position of the 3-D piezo stage. This

can be performed with the existing FPGA card. The DAQ card is not a satisfactory option, because round-robin scanning mode of the analog-to-digital converter exhibits significant signal cross-talk, when the input voltages differ by more than an order of magnitude. The position signal from 3-D piezo stage is in the order of a few volts, whereas the voltage of the QPD channels is in the order of millivolts. Secondly, the net DAQ bandwidth of 600 kHz is shared between the input terminals and would reduce from 200 to 100 kHz per channel if the DAQ is used to record the 3-D piezo stage location.

23. The TDMS file format is a proprietary file type developed by National Instruments. TDMS files are not readily imported into other workspaces. Currently, we use a custom developed LabVIEW VI to convert TDMS data to text files to facilitate analysis within MATLAB and other software packages. A better option is to translate the TDMS file to the Hierarchical Data Format version 5 (HDF5) (www.hdf5.org) which is becoming the standard for technical data. This format can be imported, and manipulated by many free wares and proprietary software packages, including MATLAB.

Acknowledgements

Research supported by NIH grants S10 RR027549-01, R21CA152779, and RO1DC00354 and by the Alliance for Nanohealth 1W81XWH-10-2-0125. We thank Dr. W. E. Brownell who contributed to the design of the instrument, and Dr T. Yuan who also contributed to the design helped assemble and collected the data shown in Fig. 3. We thank Dr. J. N. Myers for providing the HN-31 cancer cell line, and are grateful for discussions with Dr. F. A. Pereira.

References

1. Monteiro J, Fodde R (2010) Cancer stemness and metastasis: therapeutic consequences and perspectives. Eur J Cancer 46(7):1198–1203. doi:10.1016/j.ejca.2010.02.030, S0959-8049(10)00157-7 [pii]
2. Wolf K, Wu YI, Liu Y, Geiger J, Tam E, Overall C, Stack MS, Friedl P (2007) Multi-step pericellular proteolysis controls the transition from individual to collective cancer cell invasion. Nat Cell Biol 9(8):893–904. doi:10.1038/ncb1616, ncb1616 [pii]
3. Baugher PJ, Krishnamoorthy L, Price JE, Dharmawardhane SF (2005) Rac1 and Rac3 isoform activation is involved in the invasive and metastatic phenotype of human breast cancer cells. Breast Cancer Res BCR 7: R965–74. doi: 10.1186/bcr1329
4. Vignjevic D, Schoumacher M, Gavert N, Janssen KP, Jih G, Lae M, Louvard D, Ben-Ze'ev A, Robine S (2007) Fascin, a novel target of beta-catenin-TCF signaling, is expressed at the invasive front of human colon cancer. Cancer Res 67(14):6844–6853. doi:10.1158/0008-5472.CAN-07-0929
5. Boyden S (1962) The chemotactic effect of mixtures of antibody and antigen on polymorphonuclear leucocytes. J Exp Med 115:453–466
6. Liang CC, Park AY, Guan JL (2007) In vitro scratch assay: a convenient and inexpensive

method for analysis of cell migration in vitro. Nat Protoc 2(2):329–333. doi:10.1038/nprot.2007.30, nprot.2007.30 [pii]

7. Dembo M, Wang YL (1999) Stresses at the cell-to-substrate interface during locomotion of fibroblasts. Biophys J 76(4):2307–2316. doi:10.1016/S0006-3495(99)77386-8, S0006-3495(99)77386-8 [pii]
8. Tan JL, Tien J, Pirone DM, Gray DS, Bhadriraju K, Chen CS (2003) Cells lying on a bed of microneedles: an approach to isolate mechanical force. Proc Natl Acad Sci U S A 100 (4):1484–1489. doi:10.1073/pnas.0235407100, 0235407100 [pii]
9. Kraning-Rush CM, Califano JP, Reinhart-King CA (2012) Cellular traction stresses increase with increasing metastatic potential. PLoS One 7(2):e32572. doi:10.1371/journal.pone.0032572, PONE-D-12-00385 [pii]
10. Indra I, Undyala V, Kandow C, Thirumurthi U, Dembo M, Beningo KA (2013) An in vitro correlation of mechanical forces and metastatic capacity. Phys Biol 8(1):015015. doi:10.1088/1478-3975/8/1/015015, S1478-3975(11)69851-2 [pii]
11. Tseng Q, Wang I, Duchemin-Pelletier E, Azioune A, Carpi N, Gao J, Filhol O, Piel M, Thery M, Balland M (2011) A new micropatterning method of soft substrates reveals that different tumorigenic signals can promote or reduce cell contraction levels. Lab Chip 11 (13):2231–2240. doi:10.1039/c0lc00641f
12. Amin L, Ercolini E, Shahapure R, Bisson G, Torre V (2011) The elementary events underlying force generation in neuronal lamellipodia. Sci Rep 1:153. doi:10.1038/srep00153
13. Amin L, Ercolini E, Shahapure R, Migliorini E, Torre V (2012) The role of membrane stiffness and actin turnover on the force exerted by DRG lamellipodia. Biophys J 102 (11):2451–2460. doi:10.1016/j.bpj.2012.04.036, S0006-3495(12)00510-3 [pii]
14. Cojoc D, Difato F, Ferrari E, Shahapure RB, Laishram J, Righi M, Di Fabrizio EM, Torre V (2007) Properties of the force exerted by filopodia and lamellipodia and the involvement of cytoskeletal components. PLoS One 2(10):e1072. doi:10.1371/journal.pone.0001072
15. Sayyad WA, Amin L, Fabris P, Ercolini E, Torre V (2015) The role of myosin-II in force generation of DRG filopodia and lamellipodia. Sci Rep 5:7842. doi:10.1038/srep07842, srep07842 [pii]
16. Farrell B, Qian F, Kolomeisky A, Anvari B, Brownell WE (2013) Measuring forces at the leading edge: a force assay for cell motility. Integr Biol (Camb) 5(1):204–214. doi:10.1039/c2ib20097j
17. Bornschlogl T, Romero S, Vestergaard CL, Joanny JF, Van Nhieu GT, Bassereau P (2013) Filopodial retraction force is generated by cortical actin dynamics and controlled by reversible tethering at the tip. Proc Natl Acad Sci U S A 110(47):18928–18933. doi:10.1073/pnas.1316572110, 1316572110 [pii]
18. Manoussaki D, Shin WD, Waterman CM, Chadwick RS (2015) Cytosolic pressure provides a propulsive force comparable to actin polymerization during lamellipod protrusion. Sci Rep 5:12314. doi:10.1038/srep12314, srep12314 [pii]
19. Datar A, Bornschlogl T, Bassereau P, Prost J, Pullarkat PA (2015) Dynamics of membrane tethers reveal novel aspects of cytoskeleton-membrane interactions in axons. Biophys J 108(3):489–497. doi:10.1016/j.bpj.2014.11.3480, S0006-3495(14)04744-4 [pii]
20. Pontes B, Viana NB, Salgado LT, Farina M, Moura Neto V, Nussenzveig HM (2011) Cell cytoskeleton and tether extraction. Biophys J 101(1):43–52. doi:10.1016/j.bpj.2011.05.044, S0006-3495(11)00614-X [pii]
21. Pontes B, Ayala Y, Fonseca AC, Romao LF, Amaral RF, Salgado LT, Lima FR, Farina M, Viana NB, Moura-Neto V, Nussenzveig HM (2013) Membrane elastic properties and cell function. PLoS One 8(7):e67708. doi:10.1371/journal.pone.0067708, PONE-D-13-05775 [pii]
22. Hochmuth RM, Mohandas N, Blackshear PL Jr (1973) Measurement of the elastic modulus for red cell membrane using a fluid mechanical technique. Biophys J 13(8):747–762. doi:10.1016/S0006-3495(73)86021-7, S0006-3495(73)86021-7 [pii]
23. Dai J, Sheetz MP (1995) Mechanical properties of neuronal growth cone membranes studied by tether formation with laser optical tweezers. Biophys J 68(3):988–996. doi:10.1016/S0006-3495(95)80274-2, S0006-3495(95)80274-2 [pii]
24. Shao JY, Hochmuth RM (1996) Micropipette suction for measuring piconewton forces of adhesion and tether formation from neutrophil membranes. Biophys J 71(5):2892–2901. doi:10.1016/S0006-3495(96)79486-9, S0006-3495(96)79486-9 [pii]
25. Qian F, Ermilov S, Murdock D, Brownell WE, Anvari B (2004) Combining optical tweezers and patch clamp for studies of cell membrane electromechanics. Rev Sci Instrum 75 (9):2937–2942. doi:10.1063/1.1781382
26. Bo L, Waugh RE (1989) Determination of bilayer membrane bending stiffness by tether formation from giant, thin-walled vesicles.

Biophys J 55(3):509–517. doi:10.1016/S0006-3495(89)82844-9, S0006-3495(89)82844-9 [pii]

27. Evans E, Heinrich V, Leung A, Kinoshita K (2005) Nano- to microscale dynamics of P-selectin detachment from leukocyte interfaces. I. Membrane separation from the cytoskeleton. Biophys J 88(3):2288–2298. doi:10.1529/biophysj.104.051698, S0006-3495(05)73288-4 [pii]
28. Heinrich V, Leung A, Evans E (2005) Nano- to microscale dynamics of P-selectin detachment from leukocyte interfaces. II. Tether flow terminated by P-selectin dissociation from PSGL-1. Biophys J 88(3):2299–2308. doi:10.1529/biophysj.104.051706, S0006-3495(05)73289-6 [pii]
29. Dickinson RB (2009) Models for actin polymerization motors. J Math Biol 58(1–2):81–103. doi:10.1007/s00285-008-0200-4
30. Ashkin A (1992) Forces of a single-beam gradient laser trap on a dielectric sphere in the ray optics regime. Biophys J 61(2):569–582. doi:10.1016/S0006-3495(92)81860-X, S0006-3495(92)81860-X [pii]
31. Gudbjartsson H, Patz S (1995) The Rician distribution of noisy MRI data. Magn Reson Med 34(6):910–914
32. Lemons DS (1997) Paul Langevin's 1908 paper "On the theory of brownian motion" ["Sur la théorie du mouvement brownien," C. R. Acad. Sci. (Paris) 146, 530–533 (1908)]. American Journal of Physics 65(11):1079. doi:10.1119/1.18725
33. Klafter J, Lim SC, Metzler R (2012) Fractional dynamics : recent advances. World Scientific, Singapore; Hackensack, NJ
34. Neuman KC, Block SM (2004) Optical trapping. Rev Sci Instrum 75(9):2787–2809. doi:10.1063/1.1785844
35. Warner AW (1972) Acousto-optic light deflectors using optical activity in paratellurite. J Appl Phys 43(11):4489. doi:10.1063/1.1660950
36. Chang IC, Hecht DL (1975) Doubling acousto-optic deflector resolution utilizing second-order birefringent diffraction. Appl Phys Lett 27(10):517–517. doi:10.1063/1.88290
37. Simmons RM, Finer JT, Chu S, Ja S (1996) Quantitative measurements of force and displacement using an optical trap. Biophys J 70(4):1813–1822. doi:10.1016/s0006-3495(96)79746-1
38. Ozbek H, Fair JA, Phillips SL (1977) Viscosity of aqueous sodium chloride solutions from 0 to 150 °C. (No. LBL-5931). Ernest Orlando Lawrence Berkeley National Laboratory, Berkeley, CA (US)
39. Le Gall A, Perronet K, Dulin D, Villing A, Bouyer P, Visscher K, Westbrook N (2010) Simultaneous calibration of optical tweezers spring constant and position detector response. Opt Express 18(25):26469–26474, doi: 208584 [pii]
40. Berg-Sørensen K, Flyvbjerg H (2004) Power spectrum analysis for optical tweezers. Rev Sci Instruments 75(3):594. doi:10.1063/1.1645654
41. Sarshar M, Wong WT, Anvari B (2014) Comparative study of methods to calibrate the stiffness of a single-beam gradient-force optical tweezers over various laser trapping powers. J Biomed Opt 19(11):115001. doi:10.1117/1.JBO.19.11.115001, 1934601 [pii]
42. Higashida C, Miyoshi T, Fujita A, Oceguera-Yanez F, Monypenny J, Andou Y, Narumiya S, Watanabe N (2004) Actin polymerization-driven molecular movement of mDia1 in living cells. Science 303(5666):2007–2010. doi:10.1126/science.1093923, 303/5666/2007 [pii]
43. Caplow M (1994) The free energy for hydrolysis of a microtubule-bound nucleotide triphosphate is near zero: all of the free energy for hydrolysis is stored in the microtubule lattice. J Cell Biol 127(3):779–788. doi:10.1083/jcb.127.3.779
44. Cross RA (2004) The kinetic mechanism of kinesin. Trends Biochem Sci 29(6):301–309. doi:10.1016/j.tibs.2004.04.010, S0968-0004(04)00103-3 [pii]
45. Greenberg MJ, Ostap EM (2013) Regulation and control of myosin-I by the motor and light chain binding domains. Trends Cell Biol 23(2):81–89. doi:10.1016/j.tcb.2012.10.008
46. Rief M, Rock RS, Mehta AD, Mooseker MS, Cheney RE, Spudich JA (2000) Myosin-V stepping kinetics: a molecular model for processivity. Proc Natl Acad Sci U S A 97(17):9482–9486, doi: 97/17/9482 [pii]
47. Liang H, Vu KT, Krishnan P, Trang TC, Shin D, Kimel S, Berns MW (1996) Wavelength dependence of cell cloning efficiency after optical trapping. Biophys J 70(3):1529–1533. doi:10.1016/S0006-3495(96)79716-3, S0006-3495(96)79716-3 [pii]
48. Leitz G, Fallman E, Tuck S, Axner O (2002) Stress response in caenorhabditis elegans caused by optical tweezers: wavelength, power, and time dependence. Biophys J 82(4):2224–2231. doi:10.1016/S0006-3495(02)75568-9, S0006-3495(02)75568-9 [pii]

49. Li DD, Ameer-Beg S, Arlt J, Tyndall D, Walker R, Matthews DR, Visitkul V, Richardson J, Henderson RK (2012) Time-domain fluorescence lifetime imaging techniques suitable for solid-state imaging sensor arrays. Sensors (Basel) 12 (5):5650–5669. doi:10.3390/s120505650
50. Donoho DL (1995) De-noising by soft-thresholding. IEEE Transactions on Information Theory 41(3):613–627
51. Huang N, Shen Z, Long, SR, Wu M, Shih H, Zheng Q, Yen N, Tung C, Liu H (1998) The empirical mode decomposition and the Hilbert spectrum for nonlinear and nonstationary time series analysis. Proceedings of the Royal Society A: Mathematical, Physical and Engineering Sciences 454 (1971):995, 903–995, 903. doi:10.1098/rspa.1998.0193

Chapter 13

Fractal Analysis of Cancer Cell Surface

Igor Sokolov and Maxim E. Dokukin

Abstract

Fractal analysis of the cell surface is a rather sensitive method which has been recently introduced to characterize cell progression toward cancer. The surface of fixed and freeze-dried cells is imaged with atomic force microscopy (AFM) modality in ambient conditions. Here we describe the method to perform the fractal analysis specifically developed for the AFM images. Technical details, potential difficulties, points of special attention are described.

Key words Fractal analysis, Cancer progression, Physics of cancer

1 Introduction

Fractal geometry is one of the intriguing mathematical constructs. If a surface is fractal, its geometry repeats itself periodically at different scales [1]. These complex disorderly patterns are typically formed under far-from-equilibrium conditions [2], or emerge from chaos [1].

Examples of fractal shape range from the large-scale structure of the universe [3] to forms of continental coastlines [4], trees [5], grain structures of many metals, ceramics and minerals [6], clouds [7], and even some artistic creations [8]. Some biological tissues [9] show fractal patterns. Recently a fractal structure of chromatin has been used to show how the cell's nucleus holds molecules that manage nuclear DNA in the right location [10].

The idea of a possible connection between cancer and fractals (self-affinity) has been suggested in a number of works [11–13]. It was proposed that disbalance of various biochemical reactions, which is typically associated with cancer, could result in chaotic formation of various geometrical characteristics of cancer, and consequently, appearance of fractal geometry because chaos typically results in the appearance of fractals. It was indeed demonstrated that tumor vasculature and antiangiogenesis demonstrated explicit fractal behavior [12, 14]. Cancer-specific fractal behavior of tumors

Reema Zeineldin (ed.), *Cancer Nanotechnology: Methods and Protocols*, Methods in Molecular Biology, vol. 1530, DOI 10.1007/978-1-4939-6646-2_13, © Springer Science+Business Media New York 2017

at the macroscale has been recently found when analyzing the tumor perimeters [9, 15]. Fractal geometry was also found in the structure of tumor antiangiogenesis [12, 14]. Similar analysis at the micro- and submicron scales was done in both neoplastic and normal cells. Various morphometric analyses have been applied to analyze individual cells [16, 17] and cell nuclei [18]. One-dimensional perimeter of cross sections of cells or cell nuclei was analyzed in those works. However, the fractal analysis at the micro- and submicron scales did not show the transition to fractal when cells become cancerous. Both cancer and normal cells demonstrated good fractal behavior, although with different fractal dimension [17, 18]. Moreover, those works were descriptive in nature; they were based on the analysis of the previously well-known morphometric features of the cell boundary (pseudopodia) and did not provide any noticeable improvement in identification of cancer cells [19].

Recently it has been shown that the analysis of fractal dimension of cell surface imaged with atomic force microscopy (AFM*atomic force microscopy*) showed a strong segregation between normal, immortal (precancerous), and malignant human cervical epithelial cells [20, 21]. However, fractal dimension can be calculated for any surface, not necessarily fractal (fractal dimension can formally be assigned to any surface). The study of the emergence of fractal geometry in itself on the cell surface has been reported just recently [22, 23]. It was shown that there was a strong correlation between multi-fractality (a parameter introduced to characterize the deviation from fractal) and the stage of progression to cancer. Multi-fractality is reaching zero, which corresponds to a simple or ideal fractal, at the stage when immortal cells turn into cancerous. Moreover, cancer cells deviate from ideal fractal with the increase of the number of divisions of cancer cells, which is typically associated with the cancer progression.

Here we describe the method to perform the fractal analysis which was used in the AFM works cited above. This method was specifically developed for the AFM images. Non-resonant AFM modes (as well as HarmoniX) allow recording maps of topography (surface image), rigidity, adhesion, dissipation energy, maximal (peak) force, and sometime phase (shift of the oscillating cantilever due to the interaction with cell surface). For the purposes of fractal analysis, it was found that the adhesion map channel gives the best results [20].

Technical details, potential difficulties, points of special attention are described. Application of this method is demonstrated for human cervical epithelial cells at different stages of progression to cervical cancer, from normal to immortal (premalignant), to malignant.

There are different methods of processing images to analyze their fractal behavior. Fractal analysis is typically done by calculating self-correlation function. A power law dependence of the self-correlation function on the geometrical scale is a definitive behavior of fractal. The fractal behavior can also be tested by utilizing Fourier analysis [24]. Because the Fourier analysis of two-dimensional images is typically present at any AFM software, we found the latter method to be particularly suitable to do the fractal analysis of AFM images. Here we describe the method and technical steps needed to do the analysis.

2 Materials

2.1 Cell Preparation

1. Freeze-dryer (*see* **Note 1**).
2. Phosphate-buffered saline (PBS): 0.01 M phosphate buffered saline, 0.138 M NaCl, 0.0027 M KCl, pH 7.4. Store at or below 4 °C.
3. Karnovsky's Fixative—Paraformaldehyde-Glutaraldehyde Solution (Karnovsky's fixative) (SPI-Chem, Structure Probe, Inc., West Chester, PA, USA): Mix 16 % 20 ml of paraformaldehyde solution, 8 ml of 50 % glutaraldehyde EM grade solution, 25 ml of 0.2 M sodium phosphate buffer, and 25 ml of distilled water (*see* **Note 2**). Store at or below 4 °C for up to 6 months.

2.2 Atomic Force Microscopy and Image Processing

1. 3100/Dimension Icon (Bruker/Veeco, Inc., Santa Barbara, CA) atomic force microscopes equipped with Nanoscope V controller.
2. HarmoniX, PeakForceQMN (Bruker/Veeco, Inc., Santa Barbara, CA) imaging modes (*see* **Note 3**).
3. The Ringing imaging mode (NanoScience Solutions, Arlington, VA, USA) (*see* **Note 4**).
4. Standard AFM cantilever holders for operation in air (Bruker/Veeco, Inc., Santa Barbara, CA).
5. Bruker ScanAssyst cantilevers for imaging in air (Bruker/Veeco, Inc., Santa Barbara, CA) (*see* **Note 5**).
6. HarmoniX standard cantilevers for imaging in air (Bruker/Veeco, Inc., Santa Barbara, CA) (*see* **Note 5**).
7. Standard tip-check sample TIP001 (Aurora NanoDevices, Canada).
8. NanoScope Analysis software (Bruker/Veeco, Inc., Santa Barbara, CA).
9. Scanning Probe Image Processor (SPIP) software (Image Metrology A/S, Hørsholm, Denmark).
10. Origin 9.0 or higher software (OriginLab Corp., Northampton, MA, USA).

3 Methods

For the purpose of fractal analysis, individual cells should be used (*see* **Note 6**). Cells can be either cultured and attached to a culture dish, or extracted from a tissue, or scratched from a tissue surface, or collected from body fluids (*see* **Note 7**).

3.1 Cell Preparation for AFM Study

1. Wash cells cultured in tissue culture dishes two times with PBS (*see* **Note 8**). Drain all excessive liquid and add 4 ml of Karnovsky's fixative solution. Keep for 12 h at 4 °C. Remove Karnovsky's fixative solution and wash with PBS.
2. Drain all excessive liquid and add 4 ml of PBS. Keep for 2 h at room temperature.
3. Repeat **step 2**.
4. Drain all excessive liquid and add 5 ml of deionized (DI) water. Keep for 12 h at 4 °C.
5. Wash cells with 5 ml of DI water twice before freeze drying (*see* **Note 9**). Keep cells in 5 ml of DI water at 4 °C before freeze-drying.
6. Place cells in DI water in the freezer with temperature −40 °C or below to freeze cells (*see* **Note 10**). After a sample is frozen transfer it in to the freeze-dryer and keep it there until sample is completely dried (*see* **Note 11**).
7. After freeze-drying, keep cells in a desiccator (*see* **Note 12**). After removing from desiccator cells should be imaged under AFM directly in culture dishes (*see* **Note 13**).

3.2 AFM Imaging of Cell Surface

1. Calibrate the deflection sensitivity and the spring constant of the AFM cantilever (*see* **Note 14**).
2. Estimate the radius of the AFM probe: Collect the image of the standard TIP001 tip-check sample. Use NanoScope Analysis or SPIP software to reconstruct shape/radius of the AFM probe (*see* **Notes 15–17**).
3. Locate the AFM probe over the surface of a cell using an optical microscope which is typically built in or attached to virtually all AFMs.
4. Choose appropriate load force (also called "peak force" or maximum force) which should be kept constant through all imaging. The key criteria for the choice of the right force are (a) independence of the fractal dimension of small variations of the load force, and (b) stability of the image after multiple scanning of the same area (*see* **Notes 18** and **19**).
5. Choose an appropriate imaging speed: The most accurate way to estimate the maximum possible speed which gives still no

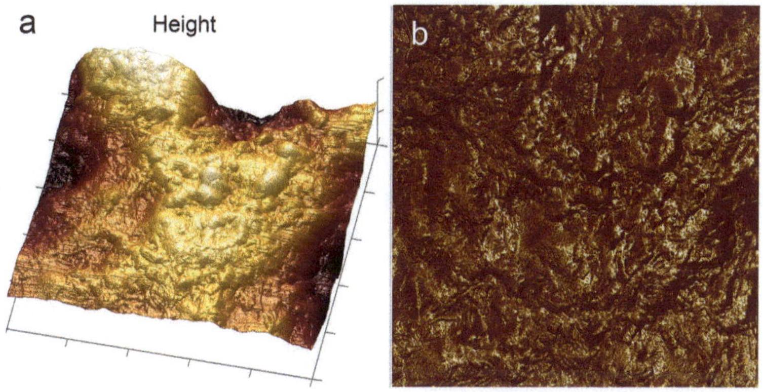

Fig. 1 A 10 × 10 μm^2 example of an AFM scan of the surface of a human cervical epithelial cancer cell. (**a**) Height image (the vertical scale is 2 μm) and (**b**) adhesion map (the vertical scale is 25 nN) are shown. The images/maps were recorded with 512 × 512 pixels with 0.4 Hz scan speed

artifacts is to calculate the fractal dimension as a function of scanning speed. It is advisable to work with the speeds which are at least 10 % lower than the value at which one can see a clearly visible change of the fractal parameter (*see* **Note 20**). To increase the imaging speed, the bidirectional scanning mode can be used (*see* **Note 21**).

6. Collect the images at the scan size of 10 × 10 μm (at the resolution of 512 × 512 pixels) (*see* **Note 22**). An example of human cervical epithelial cancer cell imaged with HarmoniX mode is shown in Fig. 1.

3.3 Fractal Analysis

1. Choose which type of map/image to analyze. It is recommended to work with adhesion images since the map of adhesion allows to detect the surface feature on the cell surface down to 1 nm [22]. This is substantially higher than features resolved on the height images of cells. Moreover, the analysis of the height images show that both normal and cancer cells are perfect fractals. Whereas the analysis of maps of adhesion demonstrate a substantial deviation from fractal behavior for different cell phenotypes (Fig. 2) (*see* **Note 23**).
2. Split each 10 × 10 μm^2 cell map into four 5 × 5 μm^2 zoomed images. This can be done with a built in AFM NanoScope Analysis software or within SPIP directly. The zoomed images only without or with small number artifacts should be processed (*see* **Notes 24** and **25**).
3. Use each zoomed image, which is obtained as described in **step 2**, to calculate Fourier magnitude using the following equation:

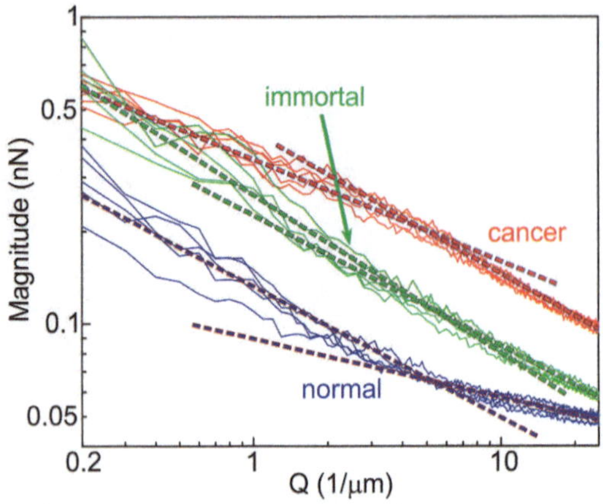

Fig. 2 Examples of representative magnitude dependences $\langle F(Q)\rangle$ for normal, pre-malignant, and malignant cells. (Taken with permission from [22])

$$F(u,v) = \sum_{x=0}^{N_x-1} \sum_{y=0}^{N_y-1} z(x,y)\exp\left[-i2\pi\left(ux/N_x + vy/N_y\right)\right]/N_xN_y, \tag{1}$$

where $z(x, y)$ is the value of the image at a point/pixel (x,y), N_x, N_y are the number of pixels in the x, y directions and u and v are Fourier coordinates. Such calculation can be done through the Fourier transformation using SPIP software (*see* **Note 26**).

4. Calculate the average of the Fourier magnitude $\langle F(Q)\rangle$ spectra (or self-correlation function) in polar coordinates as follows:

$$\langle F(Q)\rangle = \frac{1}{\pi}\int_0^{\pi} F(Q\cos\varphi, Q\sin\varphi)d\varphi. \tag{2}$$

Here the averaged Fourier magnitude $\langle F(Q)\rangle$ is a function of reciprocal space Q (inverse lateral size of the geometrical features on the AFM image—L). The linear behavior of $\langle F(Q)\rangle$ in the log–log scale (or $\langle F(Q)\rangle \tilde{} Q^b$) is a defining feature of fractals. By analyzing $\langle F(Q)\rangle$ one can define if the surface of interest is fractal or not. Figure 3 shows the results of processing of a map of adhesion through the Fourier transform of SPIP software. Initially the Fourier transform is done at a range of polar angles. To average the magnitude, we averaged the spectra along radial lines as an average cross section for the polar angles from 0 to 180 for the top half-plane as shown in Fig. 3a. The averaged (one-dimensional) Fourier spectrum, the Fourier magnitude, as a function of reciprocal space Q is shown in Fig. 3b.

5. Fit the obtained spectra with the allometric law function $\langle F(Q)\rangle = aQ^b$ using Origin 9.0 software to determine an

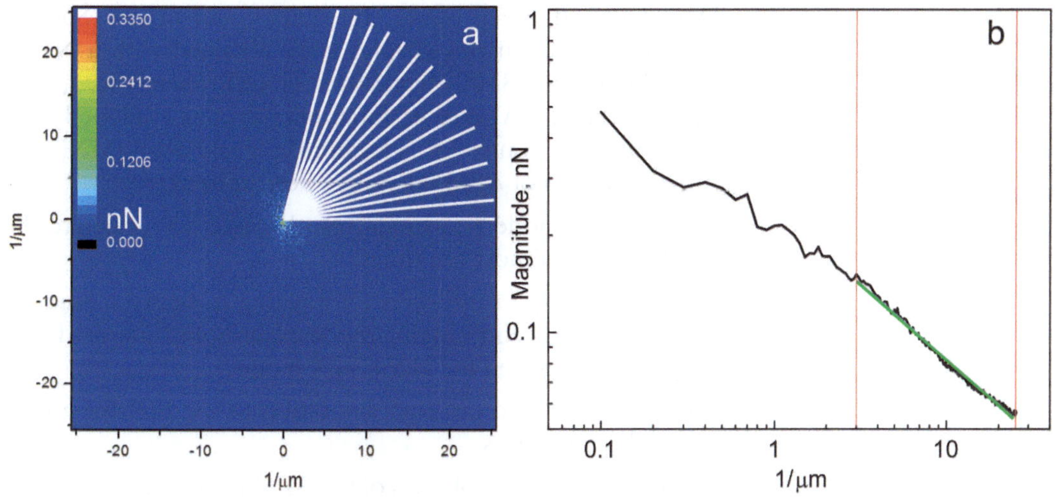

Fig. 3 (**a**) A typical Fourier magnitude spectrum map and (**b**) the results of the averaging of the Fourier magnitude $\langle F(Q) \rangle$ over the polar angle

important parameter of fractals, the fractal dimensionality, by doing a linear fitting in log–log scale using $\log(F) = \log(a) + b\log(Q)$ in the reciprocal range of interest. The slope b of the fitting curve defines the fractal dimension α as follows $\alpha = 2 - b$ (*see* **Note 27**).

6. Calculate the multi-fractality parameter: find the fractal dimension for two reciprocal intervals, and subtract one fractal dimension from the other. For the example of human cervical epithelial cells, those intervals were 0.1–5 and 5–25 μm^{-1}. The specific point to split the entire interval of reciprocal parameter Q can be found for other cell types by plotting $\langle F(Q) \rangle$ in log–log scale (Fig. 3b). The split point should be seen as a break position between two straight lines (*see* **Note 28**).

4 Notes

1. Labconco Lyph-Lock 12 freeze dryer was used.
2. Karnovsky's Fixative—Paraformaldehyde-Glutaraldehyde Solution Ready to mix-and-use kit contains: 16 % Formaldehyde 2 × 10 ml ampoules; 50 % Glutaraldehyde 1 × 10 ml ampoules and Sodium Phosphate Buffer, 0.2 M 1 × 50 ml vial. Final mixture is 78 ml with 5 % Glutaraldehyde, 4 % Paraformaldehyde in 0.064 M Buffer. This mixture is extremely hypertonic, with an osmolarity of more than 2000 mOsm.
3. Any AFM which can operate in a special HarmoniX or one of the non-resonant modes can be used. The latter include ScanAssyst, PeakForceQMN (by Bruker), HybriD (by NT-MDT),

Digital Pulsed Force Mode (by Witec), and others. Specific examples shown in this chapter were obtained with a Nanoscope Dimension 3100/Dimension Icon (Bruker/Veeco, Inc., Santa Barbara, CA) atomic force microscopes equipped with Nanoscope V controller. HarmoniX, PeakForceQMN, and Ringing modes of AFM operation were utilized.

4. The Ringing mode attachment can be used to accelerate the AFM imaging almost ten times.
5. Bruker ScanAssyst cantilevers for imaging in air were used for PeakForceQMN and Ringing modes; HarmoniX standard cantilevers were utilized for HarmoniX mode.
6. Though there is no principal limitation to use the tissue with exposed cell surfaces.
7. To increase lateral resolution of the AFM images, and to mimic the processing of cells in the screening liquid cytology tests, cells should be fixed and dried before the imaging with AFM. To avoid drying artifacts, freeze-drying should be used. Cells collected in suspension should be freeze-dried on glass slide or plastic culture dish.
8. For specific examples shown in this chapter cells were cultured in 60 mm tissue culture dishes. The cells were analyzed when the cells reach <50 % confluency.
9. The cell samples thus prepared can be preserved for several weeks with DI water at 4 °C before freeze drying.
10. Cell should be frozen rapidly to avoid ice crystals formation. Though freezer with temperature of −40 °C can be used it is preferable to use temperature of −80 °C.
11. Fractal parameters can depend on cell drying time [20]. To check the influence of a different drying time on the results of fractal analysis, one cancer cell line and one normal cell strain were investigated. Culture dishes with fixed cells were filled with a similar amount of water, fast frozen, and kept in a freeze-drier for 2, 4 and 12 h (the minimal time (2 h) was chosen by visible absence of any traces of water or ice in culture dishes. After that, the cells were immediately imaged using AFM. There was no statistically significant difference observed in the fractal dimension parameter for samples dried different times.
12. The dried samples can be preserved at least for several weeks in a desiccator.
13. There is concern that samples can be rehydrated after freeze-drying if ambient humidity is high. The cells should be imaged under AFM directly in culture dishes after not more than 30 min after removing from desiccator. Although humidity can be controlled during the AFM scanning, the role of

humidity can be evaluated. As has been shown and tested by Dokukin and coworkers [20], the fractal geometry recovered from the AFM images is rather stable up to a relative humidity of 60 %. The imaging here should be done below that level and samples should be kept in ambient conditions for not more than 4 h.

14. The deflection sensitivity has to be calibrated when measuring a deflection of the AFM cantilever on a rigid surface, for example, a clean silicon wafer or glass slide. The spring constant of the AFM cantilever can be found using the thermal tuning, an option which exist in virtually all new AFMs. The HarmoniX mode requires an additional calibration of the torsional spring constant.

15. To avoid possible error coming from probe contamination/damage, the probe radius should be checked before and after each experiment.

16. The calibration of the AFM probe allows for precise control of the acquisition of data which is used for fractal analysis. Although we demonstrate that the precise knowledge of the data acquisition parameters is not critical for the fractal analysis, it is still important to be within some allowable range. Therefore, the above steps are important to verify if the data acquisition (scanning parameters, such as the load force and probe radius) are within the allowable range.

17. Fractal parameters may depend on the AFM probe radius. Although possible, it is practically inconvenient to try to keep the radius AFM apex the same for all imaging. Variation of the radius of curvature of commercially available sharp AFM probes is typically within 5–20 nm. If we assume no specific chemical interactions between the AFM probe and the cell surface (it can be seen/verified by the lack of specific force signatures [25], which is not typically observed when scanning cells), the adhesion force could be simulated as a contact of two spherical surfaces [26]. Using this approximation, it is possible to recover the change of the adhesion at each particular pixel for different probe radii. Figure 4 shows the predicted dependence of the fractal dimension and multi-fractality parameter on the value of $R_t/10$ nm, where R_t is the radius of the AFM probe. One can see that both parameters of the modeled images are virtually constant for a wide range of the probe radii. Specifically, both parameters change within 1 % when an initial probe diameter of 10 nm changes within the range of 4–18 nm. Another point to take into consideration for the probe radius is possible probe contaminations. As one can judge from the weak dependence of the probe radius, small

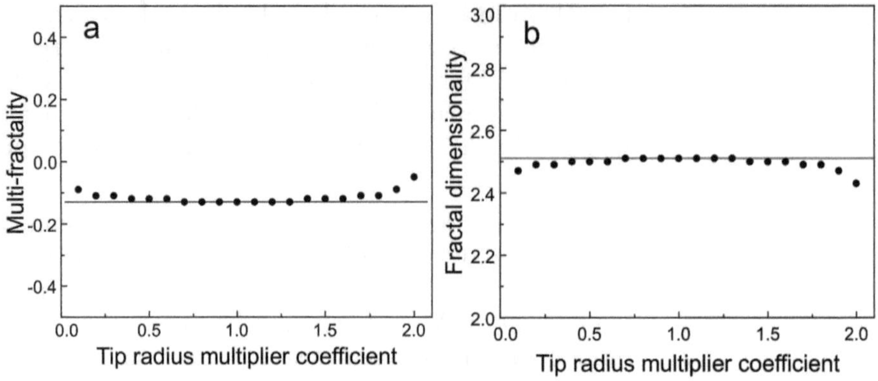

Fig. 4 Dependence of the fractal dimension (a) and multi-fractality (b) on the coefficient R_t/10 nm, where R_t is the AFM probe radius (Adapted with permission from [22])

contaminations on the AFM probe that do not change the probe radius substantially are not dangerous for robust measurements of fractal properties. In previously reported measurements [20–22], no statistically detectable change of fractal parameters was observed when imaging at least 30 cells. Contaminated probes typically can be cleaned with water plasma cleaners and reused. All large contaminations are easily detectable by a sudden change of the image during scanning.

18. Although the particular characteristic of the fractal geometry, the fractal dimension is almost independent of the load force, it is a good idea to keep this force constant through all imaging. That way one can see possible artifacts related to abnormal change of the sample or quality of the AFM probe. As to the specific value of the load force, it depends on the chosen scanning mode. For example, this force was equal to ~40 nN when doing HarmoniX mode imaging [20]. PeakForce QNM and Ringing mode allowed working with much smaller forces (less than 1 nN; though the used load force of 5 nN is preferable for the cell scanning).

19. The load force is to be chosen by the AFM operator. Therefore, independence of our results from this parameter is important to verify. It is quite natural to expect weak dependence on the fractal parameters on the load force because the values of adhesion should not depend on it. In reality, the adhesion may depend on it because of viscous retardation of the probe-surface contact upon the probe withdrawal. Therefore, it is advisable to test the limits of the load forces suitable for the fractal study for each particular sample type. One can study the dependence of multi-fractality as the function of the load force as follows: The same area of the sample surface is scanned with different forces of increasing values (it is important to return back to the minimum force to verify repeatability to avoid the

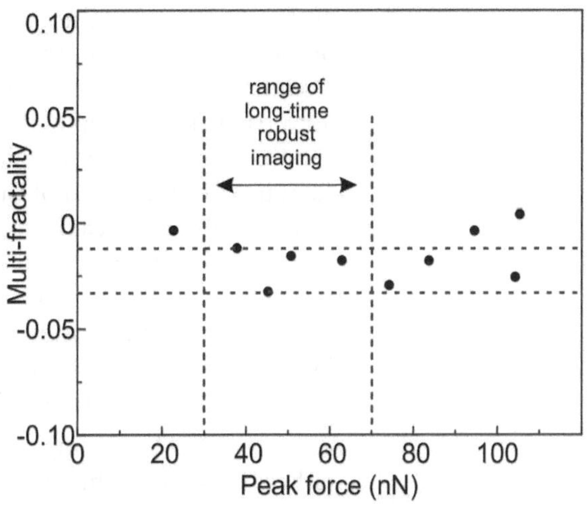

Fig. 5 The multi-fractality of adhesion maps of a cancer cell calculated on the same surface imaged with different load forces (Taken with permission from [22])

artifacts due to potential damaging of the sample by the action of the AFM probe). Then the images are tested with one of the fractal parameters. For example, while working in HarmoniX mode and using standard HarmoniX AFM cantilevers, one can get reliable imaging starting from the scan force of ~20 nN and until the force reaches ~105 nN. The dependence of the multi-fractality on the scan force is shown in Fig. 5. One can see that the multi-fractality is practically independent of the scanning force. The standard deviation of calculated multi-fractality is just 0.01. To avoid the danger of sample destruction by the AFM probe, it is advisable not to use too high forces. On the other hand, the use of two small force may result in unstable scanning (this is particularly true when scanning in HarmoniX mode). As an example, a range of 30–70 nN was found to be the best for a robust imaging for the time needed to get several scans of the cell surface.

20. The speed of data acquisition is typically chosen as a compromise between the speed and quality (excessively fast scanning will create artifacts that should be avoided). Obviously the faster speed is preferable to complete imaging faster. As to the specific numbers, when working with human epithelial cells, the maximum scanning speed without artifacts was 0.5 Hz (2 s per line) when working in HarmoniX mode, 0.1 Hz for the PeakForce QNM mode, and 0.5–1 Hz for the Ringing mode. Although the HarmoniX and Ringing modes are both faster, the Ringing mode seems to demonstrate higher long-term imaging stability. As it was mentioned above the HarmoniX

mode requires an additional (torsional) calibration of the AFM cantilever. In addition, the feedback of controlling HarmoniX scanning is not as robust as the one of the non-resonant modes. For a particular example of human cervical epithelial cells, the scanning may require retuning the scanning parameters when changing from one area of the sample to another (for example, another cell). The PeakForce QNM mode very rarely required retuning the scan parameters when moving to another part of the sample. The Ringing mode (which is essentially an advanced data processing add-on for nonresonant modes (like PeakForce QNM) uses the feedback of the parent nonresonant mode, and therefore, inherits its stability.

21. A standard AFM scanning records only one part of each scan line (either the left to right or right to left). This is done to avoid an internal creep of the AFM scanner. Although it is technically possible to record both forward and backward lines, and therefore, scan twice faster (the so-called bidirectional recording), it is not recommended for the majority of scanners because it creates substantial artifacts. One can, however, check if the artifacts are substantial, for example, by comparing the value of the fractal dimension calculated for the same area recorded with and without bidirectional scanning. If the difference is within a tolerable level, it is advisable to use bidirectional scanning to accelerate the image recording.
22. This is a typical size of cell images studied so far. The key criteria for choosing the right scan size and the digital (pixel) resolution are (a) the size should cover the largest possible area of the cell without artifacts, and (b) the lateral size of each pixel has to be 20 nm or smaller (while smaller numbers are preferable for the analysis, they increase the time of acquisition).
23. It was shown that the AFM height images are not sensitive enough to segregate between cancer and normal cells [21].
24. It is allowed to taking into account some small artifacts sometimes found on the cell surface (such artifacts are typically obvious features on many cell surface images). Technically it can be done, for an example of calculating of fractal dimension, by taking the mean value of four values obtained for the zoomed images. If the amount of artifacts is too high, up to 1×1 μm zoomed images could still be processed because the fractal dimension doesn't depend on the area. The images used for surface analysis should not be processed by any other way than mentioned above. Many software have a default initial preprocessing (like flattening and plane fit) to make images easy to see. These default preprocessing has to be switched off.

25. Dependent on the growth conditions, some cells can grow well-developed filopodia. Figure 6 demonstrates an example of such features imaged on the cell surface with HarmoniX mode. A filopodium can substantially alter fractal parameters.

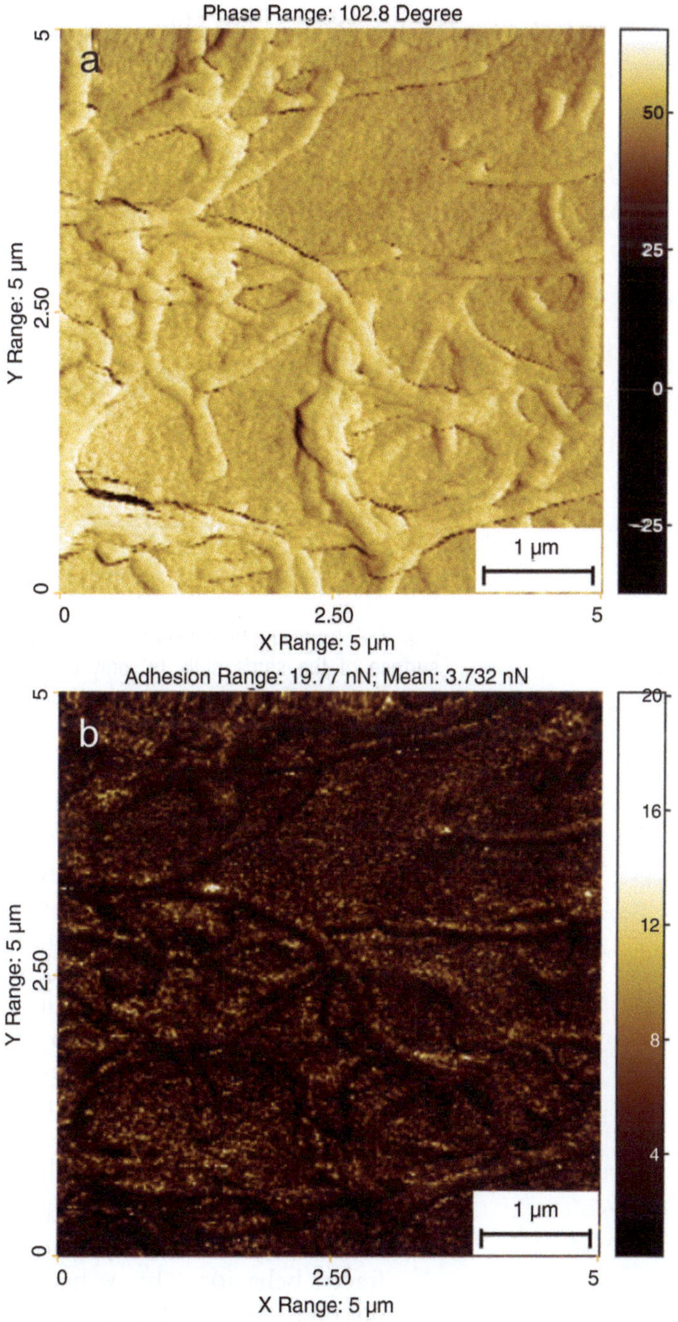

Fig. 6 (**a**) Phase and (**b**) adhesion maps of normal cell surface with filopodia (large fibers seen on the surface)

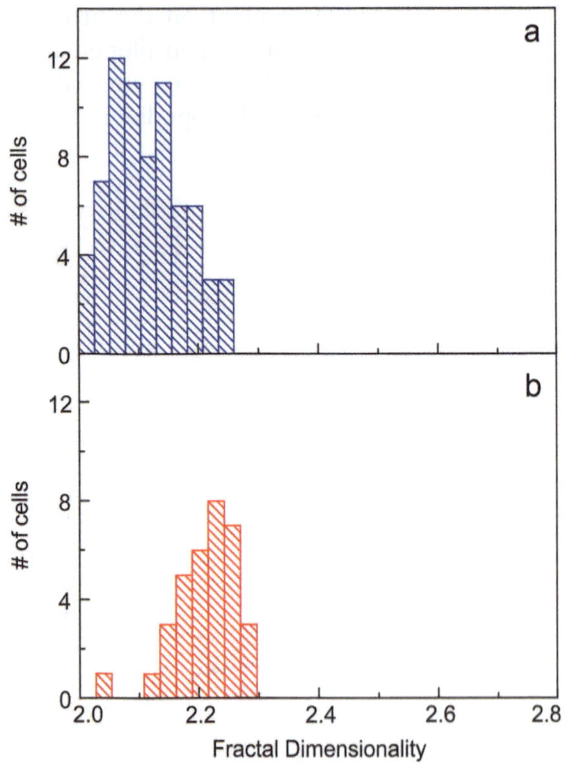

Fig. 7 A representative example of fractal dimensionality calculated on the surface of the same cells (**a**) only over the area without filopodia, and (**b**) averaged over the entire surface (including filopodia)

Figure 7 demonstrates that the change of fractal dimension of the adhesion maps depends on filopodia. We compare fractal dimension for a partially covered and clear membrane. Figure 7 shows the fractal dimension calculated on the surface of the same cells averaged over the entire surface (including filopodia) and only over the area without filopodia. One can see that the presence of filopodia can result in a shift of fractal dimensionality to a higher value. We found that it was possible to avoid the issue by zooming to the area without filopodia fibers (it was possible to find such areas between 1×1 to 5×5 μm^2). The fractal dimensionality is well defined and rather homogeneous on such areas within each cell.

26. Here it becomes clear why the Fourier analysis is more suitable to find the self-correlation function needed to define fractal behavior. This is because the coordinates (x, y) are discrete, and therefore, the calculation of the self-correlation function would require extrapolation which is quite a complicated procedure (in particular, when the noise has to be

taken into account). The Fourier coordinates (u,v) are continuous, and consequently, one doesn't have the problem for extrapolation.

27. Such a definition of the fractal dimension gives $\alpha = 2$ for flat and $\alpha = 3$ for infinitely rough surfaces, which correspond to a common definition of dimensionality of space. Strictly speaking, it is impossible to obtain the exact fractal behavior from the maps observed for any realistic surface. According to the classical definition of fractal, the power dependence of the magnitude which defines the fractal should be observed in the entire geometrical (infinite) scale of Q. However, this is impractical because of natural limitations [27] due to the finite size of data and finite digitalization/pixelization of any image. It implies that the fractal geometry cannot be even considered for the size of geometrical features L $(=Q^{-1})$ that are either greater than the size of the recorded image or smaller than the size of each pixel. It is worth noting that, one could technically consider infinite scales by extrapolating Eq. 2 to arbitrary scales. It should be clear that such extrapolation would be an artifact of the use of the Fourier method. For example, if the image of 5×5 μm^2 is recorded with 256×256 pixels, the fractal behavior can be analyzed for L ranging between ~5 μm and 20 nm (~5 μm/256). Thus, the fractal geometry described in this work is defined within these limits.

28. The analysis of $\langle F(Q) \rangle \tilde{} Q^b$ shows that the fractal behavior can be nontrivial. Specifically, it may show different values of b and different scales. Such behavior is called multi-fractal [27, 28]. This is shown in Fig. 2 in which the function $\langle F(Q) \rangle$ is plotted in log–log scale. A straight line in the log–log scale of Fig. 2 indicates the power law dependence, i.e., fractal. One can see from Fig. 2 that the magnitude can be approximated as a straight line in the log–log scale on the whole range of scales Q (reciprocal of the range $L = 5$ μm–20 nm) for only some immortal and malignant cells. For other pre-malignant, most of the malignant, and all normal cells, the magnitude $A(Q)$ plotted in log–log scale can be well-approximated as a broken straight line with the break point at $Q \sim 5$ μm^{-1} ($L \sim 200$ nm). This multi-fractal geometry can be described with two fractal dimensions. A parameter of "multi-fractality" was introduced in [22] to describe the deviation of the observed geometry from a simple fractal. It is equal to the difference between two fractal dimensions below and above a break point. In the other words, the multi-fractality is defined as the change of the fractal dimension when defined above and below $Q = 5$ μm^{-1}. The multi-fractality is zero for the ideal (simple) fractal.

Acknowledgments

We gratefully acknowledge partial funding for this work by NSF CMMI-1435655. Veeco Award "HarmoniX Innovation" is thankfully acknowledged by I.S.

References

1. McCauley JL (1993) Chaos, dynamics, and fractals: an algorithmic approach to deterministic chaos, vol 2, Cambridge nonlinear science series. Cambridge University Press, Cambridge
2. Meakin P (1998) Fractals, scaling, and growth far from equilibrium, vol 5, Cambridge nonlinear science series. Cambridge University Press, Cambridge, UK
3. Wu KKS, Lahav O, Rees MJ (1999) The large-scale smoothness of the Universe. Nature 397 (6716):225–230
4. Burrough PA (1981) Fractal dimensions of landscapes and other environmental data. Nature 294(5838):240–242
5. Morse DR, Lawton JH, Dodson MM, Williamson MH (1985) Fractal dimension of vegetation and the distribution of arthropod body lengths. Nature 314(6013):731–733
6. Chopard B, Herrmann HJ, Vicsek T (1991) Structure and growth mechanism of mineral dendrites. Nature 353(6343):409–412
7. Lovejoy S (1982) Area-perimeter relation for rain and cloud areas. Science 216 (4542):185–187. doi:10.1126/science.216.4542.185, 216/4542/185 [pii]
8. Jones-Smith K, Mathur H (2006) Fractal analysis: revisiting Pollock's drip paintings. Nature 444(7119):E9–E10, discussion E10–11. doi:10.1038/nature05398, nature05398 [pii]
9. Losa GA (2005) Fractals in biology and medicine, vol 4, Mathematics and biosciences in interaction. Birkhäuser, Basel
10. Lieberman-Aiden E, van Berkum NL, Williams L, Imakaev M, Ragoczy T, Telling A, Amit I, Lajoie BR, Sabo PJ, Dorschner MO, Sandstrom R, Bernstein B, Bender MA, Groudine M, Gnirke A, Stamatoyannopoulos J, Mirny LA, Lander ES, Dekker J (2009) Comprehensive mapping of long-range interactions reveals folding principles of the human genome. Science 326(5950):289–293. doi:10.1126/science.1181369, 326/5950/289 [pii]
11. Sedivy R, Mader RM (1997) Fractals, chaos, and cancer: do they coincide? Cancer Invest 15 (6):601–607
12. Baish JW, Jain RK (2000) Fractals and cancer. Cancer Res 60(14):3683–3688
13. Pansera F (1994) Fractals and cancer. Med Hypotheses 42(6):400
14. Less JR, Skalak TC, Sevick EM, Jain RK (1991) Microvascular architecture in a mammary carcinoma: branching patterns and vessel dimensions. Cancer Res 51(1):265–273
15. Mashiah A, Wolach O, Sandbank J, Uziel O, Raanani P, Lahav M (2008) Lymphoma and leukemia cells possess fractal dimensions that correlate with their biological features. Acta Haematol 119(3):142–150. doi:10.1159/000125551, 000125551 [pii]
16. Mango LJ, Valente PT (1998) Neural-network-assisted analysis and microscopic rescreening in presumed negative cervical cytologic smears. A comparison. Acta Cytol 42 (1):227–232
17. Meerding WJ, Doornewaard H, van Ballegooijen M, Bos A, van der Graaf Y, van den Tweel JG, van der Schouw YT, Habbema JD (2001) Cost analysis of PAPNET-assisted vs. conventional Pap smear evaluation in primary screening of cervical smears. Acta Cytol 45(1):28–35
18. Pierard GE, Ezzine-Sebai N, Fazaa B, Nikkels-Tassoudji N, Pierard-Franchimont C (1995) Karyometry of malignant melanoma cells present in skin strippings. Skin Res Technol 1:177–179
19. Doornewaard H, van der Schouw YT, van der Graaf Y, Bos AB, van den Tweel JG (1999) Observer variation in cytologic grading for cervical dysplasia of Papanicolaou smears with the PAPNET testing system. Cancer 87 (4):178–183
20. Dokukin ME, Guz NV, Gaikwad RM, Woodworth CD, Sokolov I (2011) Cell surface as a fractal: normal and cancerous cervical cells demonstrate different fractal behavior of surface adhesion maps at the nanoscale. Phys Rev Lett 107(2):028101
21. Guz NV, Dokukin ME, Woodworth CD, Cardin A, Sokolov I (2015) Towards early detection of cervical cancer: fractal dimension of AFM images of human cervical epithelial cells at different stages of progression to cancer. Nanomedicine 11(7):1667–1675. doi:10.1016/j.nano.2015.04.012

22. Dokukin ME, Guz NV, Woodworth CD, Sokolov I (2015) Emerging of fractal geometry on surface of human cervical epithelial cells during progression towards cancer. New J Phys 17:033019
23. Sokolov I (2015) Fractals: a possible new path to diagnose and cure cancer? Future Oncol 11 (22):3049–3051. doi:10.2217/fon.15.211
24. Falconer KJ (1990) Fractal geometry: mathematical foundations and applications. Wiley, Chichester
25. Fisher TE, Marszalek PE, Fernandez JM (2000) Stretching single molecules into novel conformations using the atomic force microscope. Nat Struct Biol 7(9):719–724. doi:10.1038/78936
26. Israelachvili JN (1985) Intermolecular and surface forces: with applications to colloidal and biological systems. Academic, London
27. Kant R (1996) Statistics of approximately self-affine fractals: random corrugated surface and time series. Phys Rev E 53(6):5749–5763
28. Barabasi AL, Vicsek T (1991) Multifractality of self-affine fractals. Phys Rev A 44 (4):2730–2733

Chapter 14

Quantitative Evaluation of the Enhanced Permeability and Retention (EPR) Effect

Luisa M. Russell, Charlene M. Dawidczyk, and Peter C. Searson

Abstract

Quantitative evaluation of nanoparticle delivery to a tumor site can be invaluable for cross-platform comparison, a consideration not currently taken into account by many in the field of cancer nanomedicine (Dawidczyk et al., Front Chem 2:69, 2014). Standardization of measured parameters and experimental design will facilitate nanoparticle design and understanding in the field. Here, we present a broadly applicable in vivo protocol for preclinical trials of nanomedicines, including pharmacokinetic modeling and recommendations for parameters to be reported for nanoparticle evaluation. The proposed protocol is simple and not prohibitively mouse-heavy, using procedures that are not overly complicated or difficult to learn, yet is a powerful way to analyze the effectiveness of new cancer nanomedicines against standard or more developed ones.

Key words Tumor uptake, Nanoparticles, Enhanced permeability and retention (EPR) effect, Drug delivery systems, Pharmacokinetics

1 Introduction

In order to compare nanoparticle-based drug delivery systems, it is critical to maintain consistency across experimental evaluations. Unfortunately, it is commonplace to design experiments around qualitative clinical efficacy instead of around quantitative metrics. In the following chapter, we put forth a generic protocol for cross-platform evaluation of pharmacokinetics and tumor accumulation of nanoparticle delivery systems [2]. These parameters are important in determining in vivo behavior as well as providing a quantitative standard by which nanoparticle delivery systems for cancer treatment can be compared.

Though many groups use in vivo techniques for nanoparticle evaluation of nanomedicines, few include quantitative pharmacokinetic analysis. The intersection of pharmacokinetics and common metrics of preclinical trials, such as survival, can yield important insight into possible efficacy in human models. The second key

Reema Zeineldin (ed.), *Cancer Nanotechnology: Methods and Protocols*, Methods in Molecular Biology, vol. 1530,
DOI 10.1007/978-1-4939-6646-2_14,

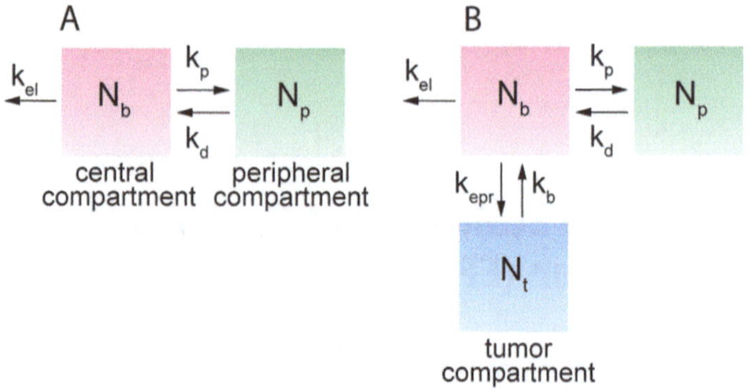

Fig. 1 Schematic illustrating the role of rate constants related to both a two (**a**) and three (**b**) compartment pharmacokinetic model, where transport between the compartments is defined by the rate constants k_p, k_d, k_{epr}, and k_b and elimination by other pathways is defined by the rate constant k_{el}

component of the protocol we put forth is inclusion of a three-compartment pharmacokinetic model to fit the data collected in the proposed experiments. The three compartments in this model are: (1) vasculature, (2) healthy tissue, and (3) the tumor itself. Inclusion of the tumor as the third compartment allows quantitative analysis of tumor accumulation kinetics for any nanoparticle delivery system. The nanomedicine is initially injected into the vascular compartment and transport between the compartments is defined by the rate constants k_p, k_d, k_{epr}, and k_b (where k_p and k_d are the rate constants for entry and exit into normal tissues, and k_{epr} and k_b are the rates of entry and exit from a solid tumor mass, respectively), while elimination by other pathways is defined by the rate constant k_{el} (Fig. 1). Identification of these rate constants provides insight into mechanisms of action, including potential for negative side effects, as well as tumor accumulation.

Adoption of this protocol and associated modeling will allow for the eventual development of cross-platform design rules by which the field of cancer nanomedicine can continue to innovate and grow. Defining design rules for new nanoparticle delivery systems is difficult because standardized protocols do not exist. To adequately compare new nanoparticles, it becomes imperative to have identical testing methods. For example, tumor accumulation of gold nanoparticles cannot be compared with accumulation in liposomes if one study is performed in subcutaneous colorectal adenocarcinoma and the other in orthotopic breast adenocarcinoma. Unfortunately, current practice for nanoparticle evaluation not only varies tumor type but time point, success metric (i.e., tumor accumulation vs. mouse survival), among others. With the adoption of protocols like this one as standards, cross-platform comparison of nanoparticle types will be possible.

The protocol proposed below is intended as a limited set of additional experiments to allow direct comparison and benchmarking of different drug delivery systems. It is because of this that relatively few time points are proposed. The results from this protocol are intended to be reported as a standard characterization metric, not as a study unto itself.

To that end, an in vivo mouse protocol is described in which nanoparticles are administered to mice bearing LS 174T subcutaneous xenografts. LS 174T is a human colorectal adenocarcinoma cell line. This cell line is chosen for the standardized experiment not only because of its relatively fast growth time and ease of culture, but also because tumors produced by inoculation of these cells display highly leaky vasculature without any notable negative impact on the mice such as formation of metastatic tumors or cachexia. The particular mouse type is chosen for its ability to grow subcutaneous tumors as well as their even temperament and lack of fur, making them ideal candidates for possible fluorescent imaging. Time points for measurement are chosen based on the peak tumor accumulation ranges of many nanoparticle delivery systems administered to tumor-bearing mice [1, 2].

In brief, nude mice subcutaneously xenografted with LS 147T cells are injected with a standardized number of nanoparticles, then sacrificed at each time point for quantitative analysis of both blood concentration and quantitative tumor uptake. A modeling method is then be described to which the quantitative data may be applied for kinetic analysis of tumor uptake ability (*see* **Note 1**).

2 Materials

1. LS 174T cells from American Type Cell Culture (ATCC).
2. Cell culture medium: Eagle's Minimum Essential Medium (EMEM) with 10 % fetal bovine serum (FBS) and 1 % penicillin–streptomycin (P/S).
3. Athymic nude mice from Charles River.
4. Mouse plasma from Innovative Research.
5. A cordless motorized pestle.
6. Liposomal doxorubicin from LipoCure through Avanti.
7. BDS Hypersil C18 column.

3 Methods

1. Inoculate subcutaneous LS 174T xenografts into athymic nu/nu mice and allow to grow to 5–7 mm in diameter. It is suggested to use 7 mice for each of 3 time points, a total of 21 mice.
2. Inject on the order of 10^{13} nanoparticles (25 mg/m^2 of liposomal doxorubicin) via tail-vein injection.
3. At 6, 24, and 48 h post injection, sedate mice using isoflurane gas until heartbeat slows but does not stop.
4. Extract blood via cardiac puncture. Centrifuge immediately to extract plasma. Confirm mouse death.
5. Excise mouse tumor. Homogenize tumor with 300 μL of mouse plasma using a motorized pestle for 20 min.
6. Quantitatively measure the number of nanoparticles in the blood and the tumor at each time point. For the specific case of liposomal doxorubicin (*see* **Note 2**).
7. Centrifuge blood plasma and homogenized tumor at 7500 × *g* for 20 min, reserve supernatant.
8. Add 10 μL of Triton X-100 and 1 μL of daunorubicin (as a standard) to glass vials with rubber lids. Next, add the samples (100 μL of blood plasma and all of plasma from tumor samples) to each vial. Finally, add 600 μL of acetonitrile to each sample.
9. Mix vials vigorously on a rocker for 30 min.
10. Centrifuge for 10 min at 7500 × *g*. Transfer each supernatant to a vial and dry in a water bath set to 37 °C under argon flow.
11. Resuspend samples in 100 μL of 30 % (v/v) methanol in deionized water, transfer to HPLC vials.
12. Run a calibration curve and then blood and tumor samples on the HPLC using 1 mL/min of 70 % (v/v) methanol in deionized water with 0.1 % formic acid through a reverse phase Hypersil BDS C18 column (200 × 4.6 mm, 5 μm bead size) until both the doxorubicin and daunorubicin are eluted, about 35 min.
13. Using a calibration curve, correlate the area under each doxorubicin peak back to the percent injected dose (%ID) for the tumors and blood at each time point, Fig. 2.
14. Plot %ID vs. time for both blood and tumor.
15. Repeat this section for tumor-free mice, analyzing blood as a control.

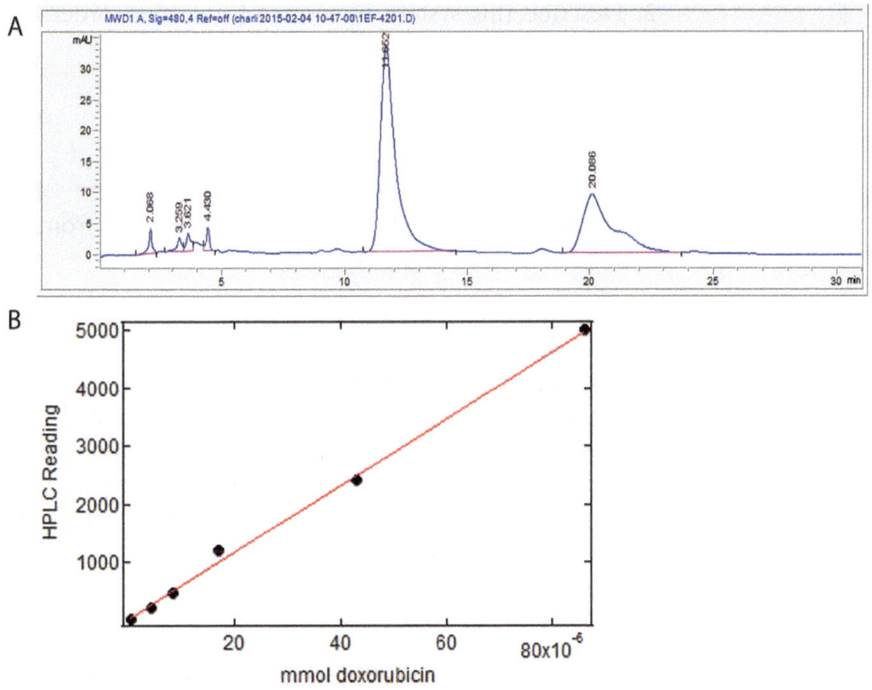

Fig. 2 Example HPLC graphs. (**a**) Example HPLC curve using the method described, where the sample in question is taken from the blood at 6 h post-injection. The first few peaks to elute are a solvent front, with the first major peak to elute being the doxorubicin in the sample, and the second major peak being the daunorubicin added as a standard. Note that both peaks are well-defined, with flat base-lines and low noise, and are fully resolved. (**b**) Calibration curve fit to a linear regression to show robustness of this quantification method, correlating HPLC area under the peak to mmol of doxorubicin in the sample

4 Modeling

1. A two-compartment model can be used to describe pharmacokinetics from tumor-free mice. Mass balance equations for the vascular and peripheral compartments are shown in Eqs. 1 and 2, respectively:

$$V_{\mathrm{b}}\frac{\mathrm{d}c_{\mathrm{b}}}{\mathrm{d}t} = V_{\mathrm{p}}k_{\mathrm{d}}c_{\mathrm{p}} - V_{\mathrm{b}}k_{\mathrm{p}}c_{\mathrm{b}} - V_{\mathrm{b}}k_{\mathrm{el}}c_{\mathrm{b}} \quad (1)$$

$$V_{\mathrm{p}}\frac{\mathrm{d}c_{\mathrm{p}}}{\mathrm{d}t} = V_{\mathrm{b}}k_{\mathrm{p}}c_{\mathrm{b}} - V_{\mathrm{p}}k_{\mathrm{d}}c_{\mathrm{p}} \quad (2)$$

where V is volume, c is concentration, and k is the kinetic rate parameter corresponding to transfer of mass between compartments.

2. Describe this system in terms of a second order differential equation:

$$\frac{d^2 c_b}{dt^2} + A\frac{dc_b}{dt} + Bc_b = 0 \quad (3)$$

where A and B are fitting parameters derived from the blood concentration curve over time.

3. The solution to this is of the form shown in Eq. 4, where the y-intercepts for the distribution and elimination phases are described by A and B, respectively. Similarly, α and β describe the half lives of, respectively, distribution and elimination phases. Fit the experimental blood concentration data collected over time in Excel to a piecewise fit of two exponential curves. These curves will yield values for A, B, α, and β, using the equation described below:

$$C_b(t) = Ae^{-\alpha t} + Be^{-\beta t} \quad (4)$$

4. Use the initial condition that at $t = 0$ the full concentration of doxorubicin is injected into the vasculature to solve for the rate constants, where dose is usually calculated in terms of mg:

$$A + B = \text{Dose} \quad (5)$$

$$k_d = \frac{A\beta + B\alpha}{A + B} \quad (6)$$

$$\alpha\beta = k_{el}k_d \quad (7)$$

$$\alpha + \beta = k_d + k_{el} + k_p \quad (8)$$

5. Next, fit data from the tumor-bearing mice to a three-compartment model where the compartments represent the vasculature, the peripheral tissue, and the tumor.
6. Mass balance equations for each compartment (Eqs. 9–11), assuming first order kinetics,

$$V_b\frac{dc_b}{dt} = V_p k_d c_p - V_b k_p c_b + V_t k_b c_t - V_b k_{epr} c_b - V_b k_{el} c_b \quad (9)$$

$$V_p\frac{dc_p}{dt} = V_b k_p c_b - V_p k_d c_p \quad (10)$$

$$V_t\frac{dc_t}{dt} = V_b k_{epr} c_b - V_t k_b c_t \quad (11)$$

where we assume k's remain constant across the tumor-bearing and tumor-free mice.

Solve for the kinetic rate constants k_{epr} and k_b, assuming k_{el}, k_p, and k_d remain constant. Using a numerical iterative fitting process written in MatLab in which deviation of points from the predicted fit is minimized, values for k_{epr} and k_b can be identified from a best fit derived from a three-compartment pharmacokinetic model. For a MatLab code to solve for these rate constants given amounts of drug in the blood and tumor over time, refer to Wong et al. [3]. In the case specific to the protocol above, this code is modified to include the ability to fit to data by the size of the error bars.

Briefly, code is written to both produce a best fit to the data for blood concentration and tumor accumulation based on this three-compartment pharmacokinetic model and to produce figures to display these fits against the original data. To accomplish this, first the time points that the mice were analyzed at are defined as a variable. The first step in derivation of the rate parameters, as mentioned above, is to determine the rate parameters corresponding to the case without the tumor (k_p, k_d, and k_{el}). We can then apply these values to the fit with the tumor, modifying the fit using the rate parameters that apply to a tumor model (k_{epr} and k_b). In the no tumor case, we define concentrations over time in mg/L, convert to amount by multiplying by the volume (in this case, 0.00053 L of mouse blood plasma), and also define the corresponding error bars in the same way. We then define A1, A2, alpha, and beta from fits of two exponential curves to the data in Excel. The rate constants k_p, k_d, and k_{el} are then solved for as described above, with the fit being graphed alongside it according to the form of Eq. 4. The same set of parameters is defined for the tumor-bearing mice, and both are graphed together as shown in Fig. 1.

To fit to the tumor accumulation data, an iterative fitting process is written in MatLab. Briefly, amounts of doxorubicin in the tumor over time are entered as a variable, with another variable corresponding to their error bars. Ranges are then set for modification of k_{el}, k_{epr}, and k_b with start, end, and step widths. A for-loop is then written to minimize the distance of the fit from the points, taking into account the size of the error bars at each point. The tumor accumulation and corresponding fit are then graphed as in Fig. 2, in amount (mg) versus time (h), and the code is finished by displaying the values it calculated for k_b, k_{epr}, k_{el}, and the minimum total error.

5 Notes

1. This protocol was developed by the authors to allow comparison and benchmarking of nanoparticle delivery systems in preclinical trials. Though several aspects of the protocol above can and should be modified based on the requirements of each nanoparticle type, the overall methodology should remain consistent to enable comparison of tumor accumulation of nanoparticles developed for cancer imaging/therapy. Above all, to enable comparison, the same mouse model should be used, with measurements of the same metrics at the same time points. This protocol is designed for comparison of nanoparticle delivery systems for treatment of solid tumors, where tumor accumulation is mediated by the enhanced permeability and retention effect. For comparison of nanoparticle delivery systems in other tumor types, similar protocols could be developed.
2. Tumor accumulation of liposomes remote-loaded with doxorubicin can be quantified via HPLC analysis. However, this method of quantitative analysis might not be most suited to inorganic nanoparticle delivery systems, for which other methods (including ICP-MS) are more suitable.

References

1. Dawidczyk CM, Russell LM, Searson PC (2014) Nanomedicines for cancer therapy: state-of-the-art and limitations to pre-clinical studies that hinder future developments. Front Chem 2:69
2. Dawidczyk CM, Russell LM, Searson PC (2015) Recommendations for benchmarking preclinical studies of nanomedicines. Cancer Res 75 (19):4016–4020
3. Wong AD, Ye M, Ulmschneider MB, Searson PC (2015) Quantitative analysis of the enhanced permeation and retention (EPR) effect. PLoS One 10(5)

Part IV

Nanotechnology for Prevention and Detection/Imaging of Cancer

Chapter 15

Nanotechnology-Based Cancer Vaccine

Aws Alshamsan

Abstract

Nanotechnology offers invaluable tools to tailor cancer vaccines in order to generate robust antitumor immune response. Among the types of vehicles for cancer vaccines, nanoparticles (NPs) are easier to produce with better scalability. Several nanostructures have been discussed in literature as potential delivery systems for cancer antigens. Here, we focus on polymeric NPs fabricated from poly(D,L-lactic-*co*-glycolic) acid (PLGA). We describe how to prepare and characterize such NPs loaded with ovalbumin (OVA) antigen and immune adjuvant monophosphoryl lipid A (MPLA). We further describe methods to test the immune efficacy of such NPs in vitro and in vivo.

Key words Cancer vaccine, Nanoparticle (NPs), Poly(D,L-lactic-*co*-glycolic) acid (PLGA), Immunotherapy, Dendritic cell (DC)

1 Introduction

Immunotherapy has emerged as a new therapeutic modality of cancer with promises of higher specificity and longevity outcomes. It is based either on supplementing effector immune components (passive immunotherapy), e.g., monoclonal antibody (mAb), or generating robust immune response (active immunotherapy) by cancer vaccine. The latter carries a potential of eliciting multifaceted antitumor immune response accompanied with immunological memory [1]. Cancer vaccine types include: (1) cell-based vaccines such as ex vivo manipulated tumor cells, activated peripheral-blood or bone-marrow derived monocytes, dendritic cells (DCs), or lymphocytes, (2) subunit antigen such as synthetic peptide, purified peptide, or tumor cell lysate, (3) viral and plasmid vectors expressing desired antigens, and (4) nanotechnology-based cancer vaccine, which involves fabricated nanosystems that deliver cancer-specific antigens to target antigen-presenting cells (APCs) especially DCs [2]. Several nanotechnology-based delivery systems have been introduced in the literature as potential carriers for cancer antigens [3, 4]. Among them, polymeric nanoparticles (NPs) offer greater

Reema Zeineldin (ed.), *Cancer Nanotechnology: Methods and Protocols*, Methods in Molecular Biology, vol. 1530,
DOI 10.1007/978-1-4939-6646-2_15, © Springer Science+Business Media New York 2017

versatility with respect to manipulating physical and chemical properties in order to accommodate a wide range of antigens and immune adjuvants and to enhance DC targeting, as well as higher scalability potential [5]. Here, we describe how to prepare NPs made of poly(D,L-lactic-*co*-glycolic) acid (PLGA) loaded with chicken ovalbumin (OVA) protein and monophosphoryl lipid A (MPLA). PLGA NPs gained special interest as a vaccine delivery system due to its biocompatibility, biodegradability, ability to encapsulate a wide range of antigens and immune adjuvants, and most importantly the ability of cross-presentation and reactivation of tumor-suppressed DCs [6–8]. This chapter will focus on how to prepare PLGA NPs by emulsification solvent-evaporation technique and how to characterize such NPs for their size, surface charge, and surface morphology. We also describe in detail how to generate and maintain a primary culture of bone-marrow derived dendritic cells (BMDC) from hematopoietic stem cells that were isolated from mouse bone marrow. Moreover, we describe how to isolate $CD4^+$ and $CD8^+$ T cells from mouse spleen and how to test the immunologic efficacy of OVA/MPLA-loaded PLGA NPs in vitro and in vivo using B16-OVA melanoma bearing mice.

2 Materials

All glassware, small animal surgery kits, and general laboratory equipment must be sterile, autoclaved, or disinfected. Opening of sterile material must be under aseptic environment (*see* **Note 1**).

2.1 Nanoparticle Preparation

1. Ester-terminated poly(D,L-lactide-*co*-glycolide) also called poly (D,L-lactic-*co*-glycolic) acid (PLGA), lactic-to-glycolic ratio 50:50, inherent viscosity 0.15–0.25, molecular weight 7000–15,000 Da (*see* **Note 2**).
2. Grade V albumin from chicken egg white (also known as ovalbumin or OVA protein).
3. MPLA from *Salmonella enterica* or any other gram-negative bacteria.
4. Pierce™ Microplate BCA Protein Assay Kit (Thermo Fisher Scientific).
5. Phosphate buffer saline 1× solution: in 800 mL sterile double-distilled water, dissolve 8 g NaCl, 0.2 g KCl, 1.44 g Na_2HPO_4, 0.24 g KH_2PO_4. Adjust the pH to 7.4 with HCl, then complete to 1 L with sterile double-distilled water. Filter-sterile under aseptic environment. Cover and seal with PARAFILM® and store at room temperature (*see* **Note 3**).

6. 9 % (w/v) polyvinyl alcohol (PVA, sometimes referred to as PVOH) solution in PBS: add 9 g PVA powder to 1 L stirring PBS. Heat the mixture gradually to 90 °C. After completely dissolving the polymer, cool the solution and store at room temperature. PVA molecular weight 31,000–50,000 Da (*see* **Note 4**).
7. HPLC grade chloroform and methanol.

2.2 Bone-Marrow Derived Dendritic Cells (BMDC) Culture

1. C57BL/6 mice, age: 4–6 weeks (The Jackson Laboratory) (*see* **Note 5**).
2. Dissection board (*see* **Note 6**), small animal surgery kit, sterile Corning® non-treated culture dishes ($D \times H$ 35 mm × 10 mm) (*see* **Note 7**), Corning® Soda Lime Silica glass Petri Dish with Cover ($D \times H$ 60 mm × 15 mm), sterile individually-wrapped Corning® cell strainer (size 70 μm).
3. Complete RPMI-1640 culture medium: sterile liquid RPMI-1640 supplemented with 100 IU/mL penicillin, 100 μg/mL streptomycin, 80 μg/mL gentamicin, 2 mM L-glutamine, and 10 % HyClone™ heat-inactivated Fetal Bovine Serum (*see* **Note 8**).
4. Recombinant Granulocyte-Macrophage Colony-Stimulating Factor (GM-CSF) from mouse: dissolve 100 μg GM-CSF in 500 mL complete culture medium. Then, dilute 1 mL of the prepared solution in 10 mL complete culture medium to reach final concentration of GM-CSF 20 ng/mL. Store the 10 mL aliquots in −20 °C for further use.
5. 70 % (v/v) ethanol: pour 70 mL of 95 % (v/v) ethanol in a measuring cylinder then add double-distilled water to 95 mL.

2.3 $CD4^+$ and $CD8^+$ Lymphocyte Isolation and Activation and Tumor-Cell Innoculation

1. OT-I mice (containing $CD8^+$ T cells) and OT-II (containing $CD4^+$ T cells) mice, age: 4–6 weeks (*see* **Note 5**).
2. EasySep™ mouse $CD4^+$ T cell and $CD8^+$ T cell isolation kits (StemCell™ Technologies) (*see* **Note 9**).
3. Tetrazolium-based cell proliferation reagent for microculture tetrazolium assays (*see* **Note 10**).
4. FACS buffer: PBS with 5 % (v/v) FBS and 0.09 % (w/v) sodium azide.
5. Monoclonal antibodies: anti-mouse CD16/CD32, fluorescence-conjugated CD3, CD4, CD8, CD90, CD11a, CD44, CD62L, and CD69.
6. Enzyme-linked immunosorbent assay (ELISA) kits of tumor-necrosis factor (TNF)-α, interleukin (IL)-12, interferon (IFN)-γ, IL-2, IL-6 and vascular endothelial growth factor (VEGF).
7. 96-well filter plates for IFN-γ Enzyme-Linked ImmunoSpot (ELISPOT) assay.

8. H2-K^b restricted OVA epitope: $OVA_{257\text{-}264}$ (SIINFEKL) and H-2^b restricted irrelevant epitope. These commercially available peptides are used in this particular mouse model because they can be presented by the H-2^b haplotype of Class-I major histocompatibility complex (MHC-I).
9. C57BL/6 mice, age: 4–6 weeks (The Jackson Laboratory).
10. B16-OVA cell lines: this cell line can be generated by transfection of B16.F1 or B16.F10 cells with OVA cDNA.
11. Geneticin® reagent (G-418) (*see* **Note 11**).

3 Methods

3.1 Preparation and Characterization of Pathogen Mimicking PLGA Nanoparticles

1. Dissolve 25 mg OVA protein in 50 μL PBS in an autoclaved glass vial (aqueous phase). Dissolve 100 mg PLGA in 300 μL chloroform and mix with in an autoclaved glass vial (organic phase). Dissolve 200 μg MPLA in 100 μL of 1:4 methanol: chloroform mixture in an autoclaved glass vial and add to the organic phase containing PLGA (*see* **Note 12**).
2. Pour the aqueous phase on the organic phase and emulsify using probe sonication for 15 s at level 2 out of 10 or 20 out of 100.
3. Pour the primary water-in-oil (w/o) emulsion on 2 mL of PVA solution (9 % w/v in PBS) and emulsify by probe sonication for 45 s at level 4 out of 10 or 40 out of 100 (*see* **Note 13**).
4. Add the secondary (w/o/w) emulsion dropwise into stirring 8 mL PVA solution (2 % w/v in PBS). Leave in stirring for 3 h then centrifuge at 40,000 × *g* for 10 min at 4 °C.
5. Wash the collected nanoparticles twice with cold deionized water using the same centrifugation conditions. Free-dry and store at −20 °C (Fig. 1).
6. To determine the loaded amount of OVA protein, disperse 5 mg of PLGA NPs in 3 mL solution of 0.1 M NaOH containing 5 % (w/v) sodium dodecyl sulfate (SDS). Keep the suspension in high-speed orbital shaking overnight. Then, centrifuge at 15,000 × *g* for 10 min and collect supernatant. Determine OVA protein concentration by micro BCA protein assay. Calculate encapsulation efficiency (EE%) as $\frac{\text{Amount of OVA in PLGA particles}}{\text{Total amount of OVA used}} \times 100$. Calculate OVA loading in PLGA NPs as $\frac{\text{Amount of OVA in mg}}{\text{Amount of PLGA in mg}}$ and expressed as (w/w). The latter is used to calculate the dose of PLGA NPs needed for in vitro and in vivo treatment.
7. To measure particle size and surface net charge, employ dynamic light scattering (DLS) and zeta potential measurement,

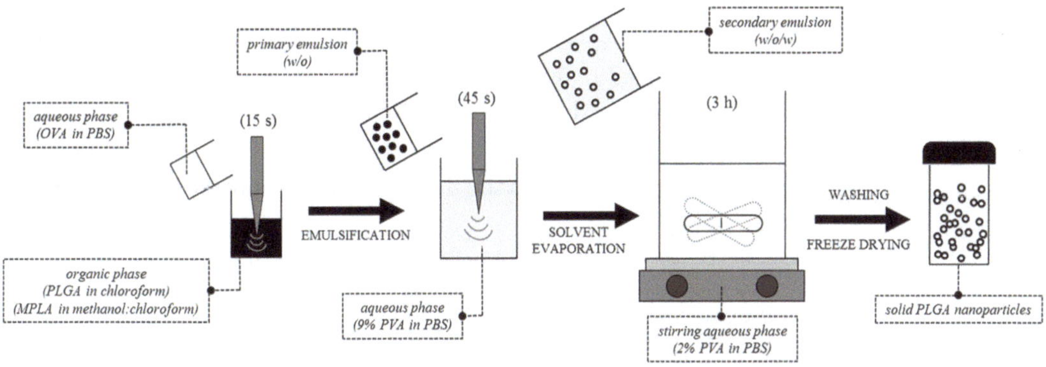

Fig. 1 Preparation of OVA/MPLA-loaded PLGA NPs by emulsification solvent-evaporation technique. Schematic depiction represents sequential processes of NP-vaccine preparation by emulsification solvent-evaporation technique. It is worth noting that changing the parameters of the process such as sonication time, stirring time, organic solvent, etc. may significantly affect NP characteristics

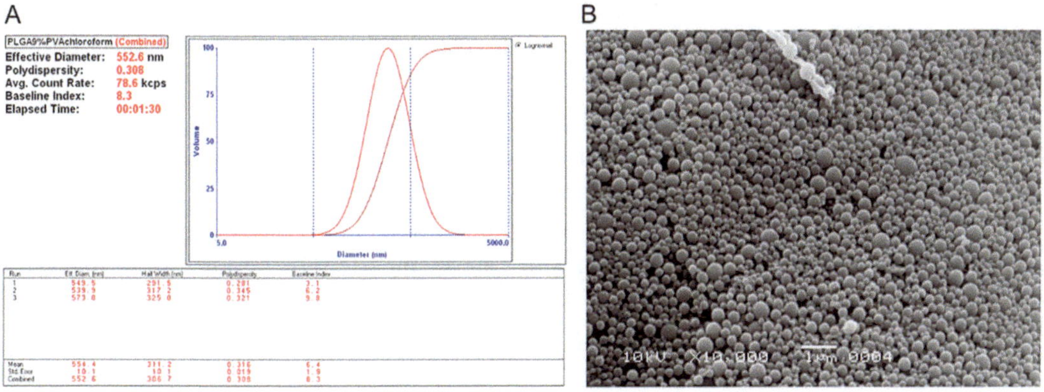

Fig. 2 Characterization of PLGA NPs. (**a**) Dynamic Light Scattering shows average effective diameter (hydrodynamic diameter) of 552.6 nm (*see* **Note 15**). (**b**) Scanning Electron Microscope image shows uniform spherical structures with smooth surface (*see* **Note 16**)

respectively, using suitable particle size/zeta potential analyzer such as Zetasizer Nano ZS or Brookhaven 90Plus Particle Size Analyzer (*see* **Note 14**). Study particle morphology by scanning electron microscopy (SEM) (Fig. 2).

3.2 Generation of Bone-Marrow Derived Dendritic Cells (BMDC)

1. Pin a mouse to dissection board (*see* **Note 6**), pour 70 % ethanol, and cut skin across thigh to ankle. Expose the bone by removing the entire muscle layer. To free the femur bone, cut just above the joints and pick the femur gently with tweezers.
2. Soak the isolated femur in 70 % ethanol for 2 min for disinfection, then soak in sterile PBS for 30 s to wash.

3. Carefully cut both ends of the femur bone with scissors. Flush the bone marrow with 1 mL sterile PBS using a 1 cc BD ™ U-100 insulin syringe with a 26 G (0.45 mm diameter) needle into a 50 mL sterile tube. Repeat the process for at least three times (*see* **Note 17**).
4. Add sterile PBS to the flushed marrow to make the final volume 30 mL.
5. Filter the cell suspension through 70 μm cell strainer (mesh) into a new sterile 50 mL tube. Centrifuge the filtrate at 300 × *g* for 5 min. Remove the supernatant and suspend the pellet in 10 mL of sterile PBS, then perform cell count with hemocytometer. From each femur, 1–1.5 × 10^7 cells should be obtained.
6. Centrifuge as mentioned above and suspend the pellet in complete RPMI-1640 culture medium.
7. Seed 2 × 10^6 cells in 10 mL complete culture medium containing 20 ng/mL GM-CSF per 100 mm petri dish (*see* **Note 7**).
8. At day 3, add to the plate another 10 mL of complete culture medium containing 20 ng/mL GM-CSF.
9. At day 6, withdraw 10 mL from the petri dish and replace with fresh complete culture medium containing 20 ng/mL GM-CSF (*see* **Note 18**).
10. At day 7, harvest semi-adherent cells by pipetting up and down gently using 5 mL sterile pipette. DC population in harvested cells will be around 70 % based on CD11c expression [9, 10].
11. Pulse the BMDC on day 6 with OVA-MPLA NPs, OVA NPs, and soluble OVA. Calculate PLGA NPs dose based on 1 μg/mL OVA concentration per dish. Negative controls include groups pulsed with PBS, soluble MPLA, and empty NPs.
12. After overnight incubation, harvest, irradiate, wash, and transfer BMDC groups to 96-well plates at 2 × 10^4 BMDC per well in at least three replicates per group.

3.3 In Vitro T Cell Activation

1. Pour 5 mL of culture medium in small petri dish and keep in ice.
2. Euthanize then soak OT-I mouse (containing $CD8^+$ T cells) and OT-II (containing $CD4^+$ T cells) mouse in 70 % ethanol.
3. To harvest spleen, make a small snip in the mouse abdomen using sterile scissors and remove the skin to expose the peritoneal cavity. The spleen is the lengthened slightly curve-shaped organ located in the left superior abdominal quadrant. Cut through the muscle layer and remove the intact spleen using tweezers.

4. Put the spleen in the dish and cut it to two pieces. Put each piece between two rough surfaces of frosted microscope slides and smash it to disrupt the splenocytes. Use a dropper to wash the smashed cells into the dish and discard any connective tissue.
5. Suspend isolated splenocytes three times in the dish using 5 mL syringe with 18 G needle. Repeat the process with 22 G and 26 G needles, sequentially (*see* **Note 19**). Transfer the cell suspension into 15 mL sterile centrifuge tube. Wash the dish with 5 mL culture medium and add it to the 15 mL tube.
6. Isolate $CD8^+$ T cells and $CD4^+$ T cells with EasySep™ mouse $CD4^+$ T cell and $CD8^+$ T cell isolation kits (StemCell™ Technologies) (*see* **Note 9**).
7. Coculture isolated T cells with BMDC groups at 2×10^5 T cells per well. This protocol will produce BMDC:T cell ratio of 1:10. You can optimize the ratio to the desired response but coculture each ratio on a separate plate.
8. After 72 h, perform microculture tetrazolium assay (*see* **Note 10**). Quantify the produced color by spectrophotometry at the appropriate wavelength. This depends on the tetrazolium reagent you are using. The color intensity is proportionally related to T cell proliferation.
9. In another set of experiment, measure the protein levels of IL-2 and IFN-γ in coculture supernatants over time range (0–96 h) by ELISA.
10. After 96 h, collect 1×10^6 cells from each well, wash twice with sterile PBS at $300 \times g$ for 5 min, and suspend the pellet in FACS buffer.
11. To each sample, add 0.25 μg anti-mouse CD16/CD32 mAb in order to block FcγRIII/FcγRII receptors to prevent nonspecific binding. Incubate for 30 min at 37 °C in 5 % CO_2.
12. Wash and suspend the pellet in FACS buffer and appropriately stain relevant T cell surface markers, i.e., CD3, CD4, CD8, CD90 with fluorescence-conjugated mAb (*see* **Note 20**). Also appropriately stain previously mentioned groups with activation markers CD11a, CD44, CD62L, and CD69.
13. After 30 min incubation at 37 °C, wash and suspend the pellet in FACS buffer and perform flow cytometry immediately or keep at 4 °C for no longer than 6 h after final washing. If flow cytometry will be performed at a later time point, fix the cells by the addition of formaldehyde or paraformaldehyde to final concentration 2–4 %.

3.4 Vaccination of Tumor-Bearing Mice

1. In 25 cm^2 tissue culture treated plastic flask, seed B16-OVA cells (*see* **Note 21**) in complete RPMI-1640 culture medium

supplemented with 500 μg/mL Geneticin® reagent (G-418) (*see* **Note 11**).

2. At 90 % confluence, subculture according to American Type Culture Collection (ATCC) recommendation.
3. After three passages, isolate 90 % confluent culture and suspend 1×10^5 cells in 100 μL normal saline (0.9 % NaCl) or PBS.
4. Inoculate suspended B16-OVA cells subcutaneously (s.c.) in the upper right flank of C57BL/6 male mice (4–6 weeks of age) (*see* **Note 5**).
5. Observe the inoculation site daily and measure tumor size throughout the experiment with Vernier caliper (also known as Vernier scale). Record the longest diameter and the diameter perpendicular to the longest length of the tumor mass in order to calculate tumor area and volume at the end of the experiment [11].
6. After 3 days, randomly assign five mice to each treatment group. Immunize each group s.c. in the lower right flank with corresponding treatment OVA-MPLA NPs, OVA NPs, or empty NPs. Calculate PLGA NPs dose based on 20 μg OVA per dose. Give booster immunization dose at day 7 and at day 10. Use a group of untreated tumor-bearing mice as control.
7. On day 21, euthanize all mice and shave around tumor mass then take a photo of each group for comparison.
8. Harvest spleens and draining lymph nodes of each group and prepare single-cell suspensions as mentioned earlier.
9. Harvest and record the tumor weight of each mouse. Calculate the percentage of mice in each group that have tumor less than 0.3 g.
10. Similar to preparing splenocytes single-cell suspension, smash isolated tumors between two rough surfaces of frosted microscope slides and prepare single-cell suspensions.
11. Filter the cell suspension through 70 μm cell strainer into a new sterile 50 mL tube. Centrifuge the filtrate at $300 \times g$ for 5 min.
12. Measure the protein levels of TNF-α, IL-12, IFN-γ, IL-2, IL-6, and VEGF by ELISA and normalize the results to the total protein weight available in each sample by micro BCA protein assay.
13. Wash the precipitated cells twice with sterile PBS and suspend 1×10^6 cells in FACS buffer.
14. Properly stain cells for CD3, CD4, and CD8 surface marker to detect percentage of tumor-infiltrating lymphocytes by flow cytometry (*see* **Note 20**).

15. Prepare single-cell suspension from isolated spleens and lymph nodes as mentioned above. From each group, isolate $CD8^+$ T cells, wash twice with PBS at $300 \times g$ for 5 min and suspend 1×10^7 cells/mL in complete culture RPMI-1640 medium (*see* **Note 9**).
16. Coat 96 well filter plate with 100 μL/well IFN-γ-specific capture antibody at 4 °C overnight prior to T cell isolation.
17. Decant coating solution and wash the plate twice with sterile PBS (200 μL/well) then add culture medium (200 μL/well) for 1 h at room temperature to block the plate.
18. Decant medium and place 1×10^6 isolated $CD8^+$ T cells (almost equal to 100 μL per well). Consider 5–8 replicates per group to reduce standard error.
19. Stimulate cells with 20 μM $CD8^+$ recall positive epitope $OVA_{257-264}$ (SIINFEKL), H-2^b restricted irrelevant epitope, or free medium as negative control. Incubate plates at 37 °C for 18 h in 5 % CO_2.
20. After 18 h, wash the plate three times with 0.05 % Tween 20 in sterile PBS (washing solution).
21. Add 100 μL anti-mouse IFN-γ detection antibody diluted according to manufacturer's instruction. Incubate at room temperature for 2 h.
22. Wash four times with washing solution.
23. Add streptavidin-HRP reagent and keep at room temperature for 45 min.
24. Wash three times with washing solution then twice with PBS.
25. To each well, add 100 μL freshly prepared AEC Chromogen/Substrate solution.
26. Stop the reaction after 30 min by washing three times with distilled water.

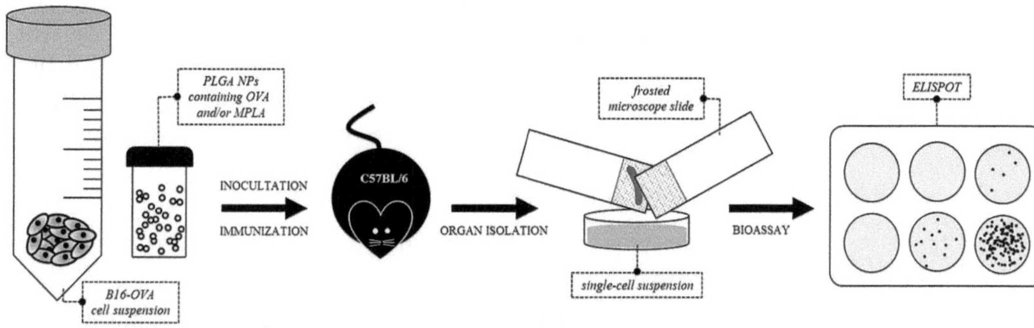

Fig. 3 Testing nanoparticle-based vaccine strategy on tumor-bearing mouse model. Schematic depiction represents sequential processes of inducing antitumor immune response. Site of tumor inoculation and rout of vaccination may significantly affect the immune response outcome

27. Dry the plate and read the developed spots using proper ELISPOT reader (Fig. 3) (*see* **Note 22**).

4 Notes

1. Individually wrap surgical tools before autoclaving. Open the tools inside laminar-flow biosafety cabinet to ensure aseptic environment. Disinfect the mouse before dissection by 70 % ethanol.
2. PLGA is provided as ester-terminated or acid-terminated forms. It also comes in several molecular weights and monomer ratios. They are NOT interchangeable because their half-life, drug release kinetics, and drug encapsulation efficiency are different. Prepare an aliquot of PLGA crystals in a small vial and apply gentle stream of nitrogen gas in the aliquot vial for 15 s to prevent oxidation. Cover the vial, seal it with PARAFILM®, put in Ziploc® bag with desiccant silica gel crystals, and store at −20 °C. Also store the original PLGA stock at −20 °C.
3. A 10× PBS stock can be prepared in 1 L by multiplying all salts amounts by a factor of 10. Alternatively, premixed PBS powder and solution are commercially available. However, checking and adjusting pH of the final solution is always needed.
4. PVA viscosity varies according to the molecular weight. This change in viscosity will significantly affect the size and encapsulation efficiency of PLGA NPs. Dissolving PVA may take up to several hours. Swollen polymer tends to stick to the stirring bar. Remove any sticking pieces for rapid dissolution.
5. Make sure you are certified to handle laboratory animals in your institution. Always wear gloves when handling laboratory animals. C57BL/6 mice (the black ones) tend to bite the handler fingers and they are generally more aggressive than BALB/c mice (the white ones). Mice used in this protocol must be of the same gender. Male mice were reported to be inferior to female mice in immunologic functions [12]. They are also more aggressive than female mice and tend to fight when they are put in a cage. Do not put more than five animals per cage. Mice older than 6 weeks are not recommended because mouse immune response to particulate antigens is significantly depressed with aging [13].
6. Polystyrene foam racks of the 50 mL centrifuge tubes can serve as dissection board.
7. Do not use tissue-culture treated dishes because these dishes will enhance cell adherence. Following this protocol, BMDC are the semi-adherent population that you can harvest by simple suspension. If you perform this experiment with tissue-culture

treated cells, the BMDC population will adhere to the plate and will not be distinguished from adherent fibroblasts.

8. If heat-inactivated FBS is not available, you can inactivate the serum by immersing the FBS bottle in 56 °C water bath for 30 min. To do that, a control water bottle with identical beginning temperature must be co-immersed to monitor the raise in temperature using suspending thermometer. Begin timing as soon as the temperature reaches 56 °C. Heat inactivation is not necessary for most cell cultures. On the contrary, it may adversely affect cell growth if done improperly. It is also less critical with FBS as compared with with fetal calf serum (FCS). In any case, the serum used, whether FBS or FCS, must be tested for endotoxin.
9. Purification of B and T cells from splenocytes cell suspension can be done by treatment with a lysis buffer (156 mM NH_4Cl, 10 mM $KHCO_3$, 100 μM EDTA) followed by nylon wool purification that can be assembled in the lab. From our experience, commercial isolation kits are more reproducible and give cleaner cell population.
10. Tetrazolium compounds used in cell viability assay are usually 3-(4,5-dimethylthiazol-2-yl)-2,5-diphenyltetrazolium bromide (MTT), 3-(4,5-dimethylthiazol-2-yl)-5-(3-carboxymethoxyphenyl)-2-(4-sulfophenyl)-2*H*-tetrazolium (MTS), 2,3-bis-(2-methoxy-4-nitro-5-sulfophenyl)-2*H*-tetrazolium-5-carboxanilide (XTT), or water soluble tetrazolium (WST) salts series [14]. MTT reduction produces insoluble formazan crystals that require further solubilization with DMSO or isopropyl alcohol. On the other hand, reduction of MTS, XTT, or WST series produces formazan products that are directly soluble in culture medium [15]. Tetrazolium reagents are unstable in light so make sure to reduce light exposure during work.
11. This antibiotic is added to culture medium in order to select cells that are stably transfected with neomycin resistance gene. The concentration used in this protocol is 500 μg/mL. However, you can titrate up to 1 mg/mL.
12. Dissolving PLGA in organic solvents may take around 30 min. To enhance this, weigh the needed amount and keep at room temperature for 30 min in autoclaved glass vial before pouring the organic solvent on it. PLGA tends to stick to the vial wall so try to lower the weighed PLGA with a small spatula to the bottom of the vial. Wash any sticking remnant with the amount of organic solvent poured on PLGA.
13. We often put the beaker in ice during secondary emulsification step in order to reduce heat generation. Excessive heat can adversely affect drug encapsulation as well as particle size. Carefully, rotate the beaker or vial around the immersed

sonication tip but be careful not to accidentally touch the tip with your fingers. The sonication tip should not touch the vial's or beaker's walls.

14. NPs suspension must be diluted in the range of 0.0001–1 % (v/v) to be measure by DLS.
15. The measured particle size is based on the particle-occupying volume rather than scattering intensity. Volume size distribution assumes unimodal homogenous distribution of particles. If your sample contains two size populations, you should employ intensity size distribution.
16. It is not uncommon to get different size measurement results between DLS and SEM because of the different size-detection principles. However, any discrepancy should not be vast.
17. Make sure not to remove the top of the femur. Carefully cut the tip of the bone and do not go closer to the middle so you do not lose or infect the cells. As you flush the bone, the color will change from dark red to light pale color. Keep flushing until the color does not get any lighter.
18. Withdrawing and supplying culture medium must be through slow pipetting at the edge of the dish to avoid disturbing the cells because BMDC may mature just by mechanical agitation.
19. Be careful when changing the needles not to poke your fingers. If the suspension is jammed in the syringe, it means there is a chunk of aggregated cells stuck in syringe tip. Slowly move the plunger back and forth to breakdown aggregates.
20. The fluorescent-tag choice is based on the desired flow cytometry analysis, e.g., if two-colored dot plot is sought for CD3 and CD4, you can choose anti-CD3 conjugated with a fluorophore that is detected on FL1 channel such as fluorescein isothiocyanate (FITC) and anti-CD4 conjugated with a fluorophore that is detected on FL2 channel such as phycoerythrin (PE) or FL3 channel such as peridinin chlorophyll (PerCP). FL2–FL3 compensation is hard sometimes depending on the fluorophore and the flow cytometer. Compensation is more critical with three-color analysis. In such case, do not hesitate to ask for the service of a flow cytometry technician.
21. The cell line must be tested for mycoplasma.
22. To get a feel of how the real data of in vivo antitumor immunity by PLGA NP vaccine would look like, you may see (Fig. 4).

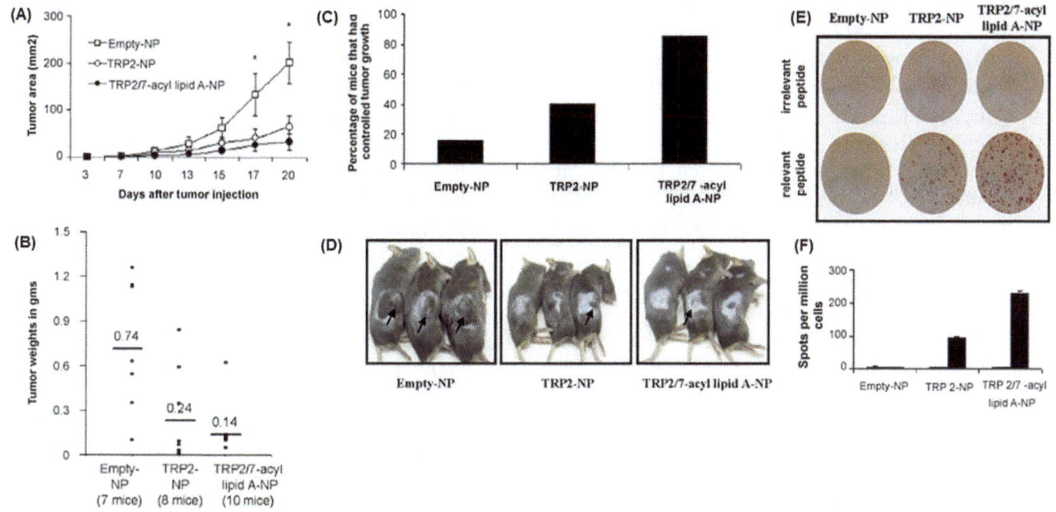

Fig. 4 In vivo antitumor immunity by PLGA NP vaccine. (**a**) Tumor growth chart showing significant reduction of tumor mass following vaccination with tyrosinase related protein 2 (TRP2)-loaded NP with or without immune modulator (7-acyl lipid-A) as compared to empty NP. (**b**) Scatter plot shows tumor weights of individual mice within each group. (**c**) Percentage of mice with controlled tumor growth (weight less than 0.3 g) in each group. (**d**) Tumor mass observed at study endpoint in each vaccination group. (**e**) Detection of IFN-γ secreted from antigen-specific $CD8^{+}$ T cells ex vivo by ELISPOT assay. (**f**) Bar graph represents number of spots per million cells. The correlation between tumor growth and lymphocyte activation is noted. However, extrapolation of such response to another species is not definitive. The figure was adopted and modified with permission from [11]

Acknowledgment

This work was supported by King Abdullah Institute for Nanotechnology and the Deanship of Scientific Research, King Saud University, Riyadh, Saudi Arabia.

References

1. Schuster M, Nechansky A, Kircheis R (2006) Cancer immunotherapy. Biotechnol J 1 (2):138–147. doi:10.1002/biot.200500044
2. Hamdy S, Alshamsan A, Samuel J (2009) Nanotechnology for cancer vaccine delivery, Nanotechnology in drug delivery. Springer, New York, pp 519–543
3. Bolhassani A, Safaiyan S, Rafati S (2011) Improvement of different vaccine delivery systems for cancer therapy. Mol Cancer 10:3. doi:10.1186/1476-4598-10-3
4. Fan Y, Moon JJ (2015) Nanoparticle drug delivery systems designed to improve cancer vaccines and immunotherapy. Vaccines 3 (3):662–685. doi:10.3390/vaccines3030662
5. Li W, Wei H, Li H, Gao J, Feng SS, Guo Y (2014) Cancer nanoimmunotherapy using advanced pharmaceutical nanotechnology. Nanomedicine 9(16):2587–2605. doi:10.2217/nnm.14.127
6. Hamdy S, Haddadi A, Hung RW, Lavasanifar A (2011) Targeting dendritic cells with nano-particulate PLGA cancer vaccine formulations. Adv Drug Deliv Rev 63(10–11):943–955. doi:10.1016/j.addr.2011.05.021
7. Elamanchili P, Lutsiak CM, Hamdy S, Diwan M, Samuel J (2007) "Pathogen-mimicking" nanoparticles for vaccine delivery to dendritic cells. J Immunother 30(4):378–395. doi:10.1097/CJI.0b013e31802cf3e3

8. Ali OA, Huebsch N, Cao L, Dranoff G, Mooney DJ (2009) Infection-mimicking materials to program dendritic cells in situ. Nat Mater 8(2):151–158. doi:10.1038/nmat2357
9. Lutz MB, Kukutsch N, Ogilvie AL, Rossner S, Koch F, Romani N, Schuler G (1999) An advanced culture method for generating large quantities of highly pure dendritic cells from mouse bone marrow. J Immunol Methods 223 (1):77–92
10. Hamdy S, Elamanchili P, Alshamsan A, Molavi O, Satou T, Samuel J (2007) Enhanced antigen-specific primary CD4+ and CD8+ responses by codelivery of ovalbumin and toll-like receptor ligand monophosphoryl lipid A in poly(D, L-lactic-co-glycolic acid) nanoparticles. J Biomed Mater Res A 81(3):652–662. doi:10.1002/jbm.a.31019
11. Hamdy S, Molavi O, Ma Z, Haddadi A, Alshamsan A, Gobti Z, Elhasi S, Samuel J, Lavasanifar A (2008) Co-delivery of cancer-associated antigen and Toll-like receptor 4 ligand in PLGA nanoparticles induces potent CD8+ T cell-mediated anti-tumor immunity. Vaccine 26(39):5046–5057. doi:10.1016/j.vaccine.2008.07.035
12. Weinstein Y, Ran S, Segal S (1984) Sex-associated differences in the regulation of immune responses controlled by the MHC of the mouse. J Immunol 132(2):656–661
13. Kishimoto S, Tsuyuguchi I, Yamamura Y (1969) Immune responses in aged mice. Clin Exp Immunol 5(5):525–530
14. Mosmann T (1983) Rapid colorimetric assay for cellular growth and survival: application to proliferation and cytotoxicity assays. J Immunol Methods 65(1–2):55–63
15. Riss TL, Moravec RA, Niles AL, Benink HA, Worzella TJ, Minor L (2004) Cell viability assays. In: Sittampalam GS, Coussens NP, Nelson H et al (eds) Assay guidance manual. Eli Lilly & Company and the National Center for Advancing Translational Sciences, Bethesda, MD

Chapter 16

Designing Multicomponent Nanosystems for Rapid Detection of Circulating Tumor Cells

Shashwat S. Banerjee, Vrushali Khobragade, and Jayant Khandare

Abstract

Detection of circulating tumor cells (CTCs) in the blood circulation holds immense promise as it predicts the overall probability of patient survival. Therefore, CTC-based technologies are gaining prominence as a "liquid biopsy" for cancer diagnostics and prognostics. Here, we describe the design and synthesis of two distinct multicomponent magnetic nanosystems for rapid capture and detection of CTCs. The multifunctional Magneto-Dendrimeric Nano System (MDNS) composed of an anchoring dendrimer that is conjugated to multiple agents such as near infrared (NIR) fluorescent cyanine 5 NHS (Cy5), glutathione (GSH), transferrin (Tf), and iron oxide (Fe_3O_4) magnetic nanoparticle (MNP) for simultaneous tumor cell-specific affinity, multimodal high resolution confocal imaging, and cell isolation. The second nanosystem is a self-propelled microrocket that is composed of carbon nanotube (CNT), chemically conjugated with targeting ligand such as transferrin on the outer surface and Fe_3O_4 nanoparticles in the inner surface. The multicomponent nanosystems described here are highly efficient in targeting and isolating cancer cells thus benefiting early diagnosis and therapy of cancer.

Key words Cancer diagnosis, Circulating tumor cell, Nanosystem, Multicomponent, Chemical conjugation

1 Introduction

Cancer is the second leading cause of death worldwide and metastasis causes more than 90 % of deaths in cancer patients [1]. Cancer metastasizes due to the migration of tumor cells from the primary site and spread to other parts of the body, via lymph system or bloodstream, where they form a secondary tumor [1]. Circulating tumor cells (CTCs) are imperative biomarkers for examining cancer prognosis as well as a real-time diagnosis and detecting them supports monitoring of drug resistance during the anticancer treatment and in clinical trials [2–4]. However, the detection of CTCs from blood has been challenging because of their extreme low occurrence (10–100 per mL) among a high number (10^9 cells per mL) of hematologic cells in blood. Thus, to efficiently obtain CTCs from

Reema Zeineldin (ed.), *Cancer Nanotechnology: Methods and Protocols*, Methods in Molecular Biology, vol. 1530,
DOI 10.1007/978-1-4939-6646-2_16, © Springer Science+Business Media New York 2017

peripheral blood, various platforms have been developed such as immunomagnetic beads, microfluidic-based platforms, and microfilter devices [1, 5, 6–14]. At present, CellSearch® technology (Veridex, LLC, Raritan, NJ, USA) is the only FDA approved technology for enumeration of CTCs from cancer patients. This technology relies on the immunomagnetic separation of cells based upon their expression of cell surface antigens, such as epithelial cell adhesion molecule (EpCAM). However, most of these approaches encounter drawbacks of slow capture, prolonged processing and less efficacy [15].

Here, we describe the methods for synthesis of two different immunomagnetic separation-based nanosystem platforms namely MDNS [16] and a CNT based magnetic microrocket system (Tf-CNT-Fe_3O_4) [17] for specific targeting and rapid isolation of CTCs (Fig. 1). The MDNS nanosystem consists of five functional components: (1) transferrin (Tf), to specifically target transferrin receptors (TfRs) overexpressing cancer cells (2) iron oxide (Fe_3O_4) nanoparticles for magnetic isolation, (3) imaging probe cyanine 5 *N*-hydroxysuccinimide (Cy5 NHS) to enable high-resolution imaging of the isolated CTCs, (4) fourth generation (G4) dendrimers to facilitate simultaneous attachment of multiple functional groups (e.g., Tf, Fe_3O_4 nanoparticles and Cy5) and also to increase the dispersibility of the nanosystem, and (5) glutathione (GSH) to act as a multifunctional reactive linker. This versatile MDNS system exhibited: (1) rapid (~5 min) and efficient (~80 %) capture of TfR^+ cancer cells from an artificial CTC-like suspension, (2) magnetic

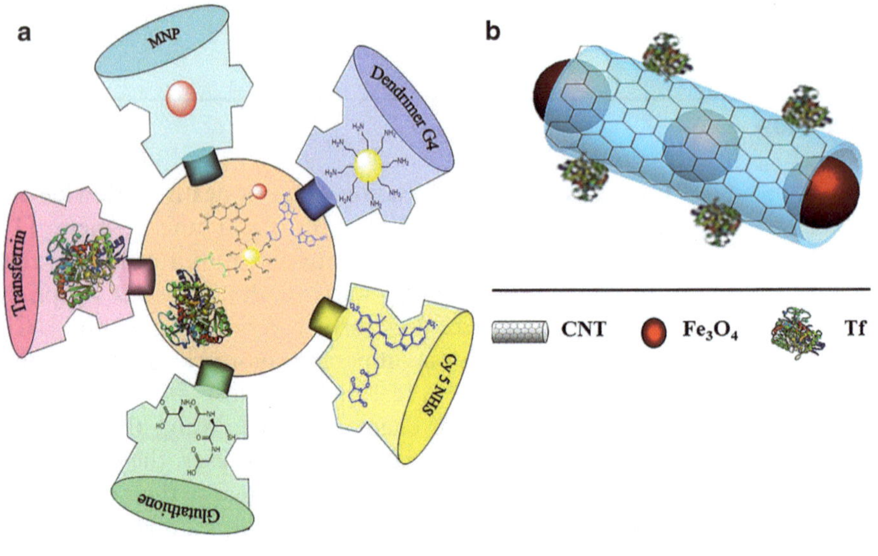

Fig. 1 Schematic illustration of (**a**) MDNS is designed by using multi-components, such as PAMAM G4 dendrimer, Tf, iron oxide nanoparticles, and imaging probe cyanine 5 (reproduced from [16]) and (**b**) Tf-CNT-Fe_3O_4 nanosystem is designed by using multi-components, such as CNT, iron oxide nanoparticles, and Tf (reproduced from [17])

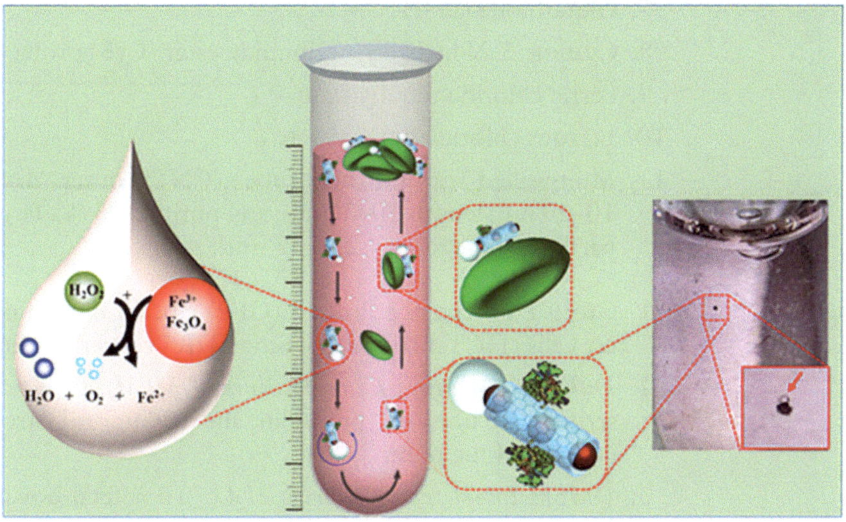

Fig. 2 Self-propulsion and CTC capture mechanism for the Tf-CNT-Fe_3O_4 microrocket. *Left* side *inset* shows the formation of O_2 bubble and Fe^{2+} due to Fe^{3+} reduction by the surrounding H_2O_2 which propels Tf-CNT-Fe_3O_4 microrocket. *Right* side *inset* shows Tf-CNT-Fe_3O_4 microrocket adhered with O_2 bubble (indicated by the *red arrow*) that influences upward motion (reproduced from [17])

isolation of the captured cells from peripheral blood cells and (3) subsequent high-resolution imaging. While the microrocket system is fabricated by conjugating three functional components: (1) CNT, (2) iron oxide (Fe_3O_4), and (3) the Tf ligand (Tf) (Fig. 2). The microrocket platform possesses unique advantages such as: (1) instantaneous propellant motion of microparticles (downward and upward) due to the formation of O_2 bubbles which helps in rapid recognition and capture (~5 min) of TfR^- overexpressing (TfR^+) cancer cells, (2) specific targeting ability due to presence of Tf ligand, (3) magnetic isolation of the captured cells owing to the presence of Fe_3O_4 nanoparticles, and (4) large surface area and internal volume allows multiple components to be loaded onto the nanotube.

2 Materials

2.1 Chemicals

1. Poly(amidoamine) (PAMAM)-G4-NH_2 dendrimer (M_w. 14214.7 Da, 64 end groups, 10 wt.% in methanol)
2. *N*-(3-dimethylaminopropyl)-*N*-ethylcarbodiimide hydrochloric acid (EDC.HCl)
3. Succinic anhydride
4. *N*,*N*-diisopropyl ethylamine (DIPEA)
5. Transferrin (Tf)
6. 4-(dimethylamino)pyridine (DMAP)

7. Glutathione (GSH)
8. Cyanine 5 *N*-hydroxysuccinimide ester (Cy5) probe
9. Ferric chloride tetrahydrate
10. Ferrous chloride hexahydrate
11. Multiwalled carbon nanotube (CNT; outer diameter of 10–20 nm; length 10–30 μm; and purity >95 %), Fe_3O_4 nanoparticle (average size: 23 ± 7 nm).

2.2 Biologicals

1. Green Fluorescence Protein (GFP) labeled human colon cancer cells (HCT 116) or any other TfR^+ cancer cell line.
2. *Dulbecco's Modified Eagle Medium (DMEM)*: 10 % fetal bovine serum, 100 unit/mL penicillin, and 100 μg/mL streptomycin in DMEM medium.
3. *DMEM complete media with H_2O_2*: 10 % fetal bovine serum, 100 unit/mL penicillin, 100 μg/mL streptomycin, 4 % hydrogen peroxide (H_2O_2) in DMEM medium (*see* **Note 1**).
4. *Roswell Park Memorial Institute medium (RPMI) media*: 10 % fetal bovine serum, 100 unit/mL penicillin, and 100 μg/mL streptomycin in DMEM medium.
5. Whole blood from healthy volunteer, heparinized vacutainer tubes, Ficoll-Hypaque solution, sterile PBS 1×, sterile 15 and 50 mL tubes, sterile 25 mL pipettes, sterile pipette, Neubauer chamber or hemocytometer, trypan blue (*see* **Note 2**).
6. MDNS, Tf-CNT-Fe_3O_4, magnet (with a surface magnetization of 6000 G).

3 Methods

3.1 Synthesis of MDNS

3.1.1 Synthesis of PAMAM G4 Dendrimer-Cy5 Conjugate

1. Dry 500 μL of 10 wt. % PAMAM-G4-NH_2 dendrimer solution in methanol to obtain 50 mg of PAMAM G4 NH_2 in a vial.
2. Dissolve 50 mg of PAMAM G4 NH_2 in 2.5 mL of ultrapure water and add 400 μL of 1000 ppm Cy5 NHS in water along with 100 μL of 1000 μg/mL DIPEA.
3. Adjust the final solution pH to 7.8. Stir the reaction mixture continuously at room temperature for 24 h.
4. Purify the reaction mixture by gel filtration through Sephadex G-10 with >700 molecular weight cut off size (*see* **Note 3**) to remove the unreacted Cy5 NHS.
5. Dry the product at room temperature under vacuum.

3.1.2 Synthesis of PAMAM G4 Dendrimer-Cy5-GSH Conjugate

1. Dissolve 5.4 mg GSH in 1.0 mL of ultrapure water and activate the carboxyl group of GSH for 1 h using 3.5 mg of EDC.HCl and DMAP as catalysts (*see* **Note 4**).

2. Mix the reaction mixture with the PAMAM G4 dendrimer-Cy5 (35 mg) conjugate previously dissolved in 1.0 mL of ultrapure water.
3. Continue stirring the reaction mixture at room temperature for 24 h.
4. Purify the conjugate by both membrane dialysis followed by Sephadex G-10 column with >700 molecular weight cut off size to remove the unreacted GSH.
5. Dry the reaction mixture at room temperature under vacuum.

3.1.3 Conjugation of Transferrin Succinate (TfS) with PAMAM G4 Dendrimer-Cy5-GSH

1. First convert Tf to TfS by reacting with succinic acid using EDC.HCl coupling.
2. Dissolve 10 mg of TfS in 2 mL of ultrapure water and add 30 mg of the PAMAM G4 dendrimer-Cy5-GSH (30 mg) conjugate.
3. Add EDC.HCl to the reaction mixture (adding the same number of moles of EDC.HCl as TfS) and constantly stir at room temperature for 4 h.
4. The reaction time is limited to 4 h to avoid any possible intramolecular cross linking.
5. Purify the reaction mixture by membrane dialysis followed by Sephadex G-10 column with >700 molecular weight cut off size to remove unreacted EDC.HCl and dry at room temperature under vacuum.

3.1.4 Synthesis of Fe_3O_4 Nanoparticles

1. To prepare Fe_3O_4 magnetic nanoparticles (MNP), first dissolve ferric and ferrous chlorides (molar ratio 2:1) in water at a concentration of 0.3 M iron ions.
2. Chemically precipitate at 25 °C under vigorous stirring by adding ammonium hydroxide till the pH of the solution attains 10.
3. The precipate is then washed several times with deionized water and ethanol,
4. Finally dry in a vacuum oven at 70 °C.

3.1.5 Anchoring of Fe_3O_4 with PAMAM G4 Dendrimer-Cy5-GSH-TfS Conjugate (MDNS)

1. Heat the precipitates at 80 °C on a water-bath for 30 min, then wash several times with ultrapure water and ethanol, and finally dry in a vacuum oven at 70 °C.
2. Then disperse 5 mg of Fe_3O_4 nanoparticles in 0.15 mL of ultrapure water and 0.05 mL of methanol.
3. Sonicate for 15 min and then mix with 22 mg of G4 dendrimer-Cy5-GSH-TfS conjugate dissolved in 1.8 mL of ultrapure water and again sonicate the suspension for 2 h.

4. Isolate MDNS by magnetic separation to remove unreacted TfS, Cy5, PAMAM G4 dendrimer, and PAMAM G4 dendrimer-Cy5-GSH-TfS conjugate.
5. Wash MDNS with repeated cycles of excess deionized water, and dry under vacuum.

3.2 Synthesis of Tf-CNT-Fe_3O_4

3.2.1 Functionalization of CNT (AO-CNT)

1. Add 5 mg CNTs to concentrated HCl in a screw top vial.
2. Sonicate for 2 h with the vial sealed and ensure that the exterior of the vial does not contain any concentrated HCl. Also ensure that the vial has airspace above the solution to avoid any popping of the vial.
3. Then keep the solution standing for 24 h at room temperature.
4. Dilute the solution with deionized water and filter through Whatman 41 filter paper and collect the treated CNT using a spatula.
5. Sonicate the CNTs collected from filter paper in 2 mL of 98 % H_2SO_4:65 % HNO_3 (v/v 3 : 1) for 1.5 h.
6. Dilute the mixture with 25 mL of distilled water and filter. Collect the CNTs off of the filter paper using a spatula. Dry the treated CNTs at room temperature under vacuum and sonicate in a mixture of 98 % H_2SO_4/H_2O_2 (v/v 4:1) for 10 min and then keep standing for 2 h.
7. Wash the mixture thoroughly with deionized water, filter and dry under vacuum at room temperature.

3.2.2 Synthesis of CNT-Fe_3O_4 Microparticle

1. Mix 2 mg CNTs (AO-CNT) with 0.5 mL ethylene glycol (M. Wt. 62.07) and 1 mL deionized water.
2. Add $FeCl_3{\cdot}6H_2O$ and $FeCl_2{\cdot}4H_2O$ (molar ratio 2:1 and concentration of 0.3 M iron ions) to the mixture and sonicate for 2 h, followed by vigorous stirring for 4 h.
3. Afterward, adjust the pH value to ~10 using concentrated NH_3 solution. Isolate the resulting CNT-Fe_3O_4 microparticles by magnetic separation, wash with deionized water and dry overnight under vacuum.

3.2.3 Conjugation of Tf with CNT-Fe_3O_4

1. Dissolve 2 mg of Tf in 2 mL of ultrapure water and add 1 mg of the CNT-Fe_3O_4 to it.
2. Add EDC.HCl to this reaction mixture (adding the same number of moles of EDC.HCl as Tf) and stir constantly at room temperature for 4 h.
3. Limit the reaction time to 4 h to avoid any possible intramolecular cross linking.

4. Isolate the resulting Tf conjugated CNT-Fe_3O_4 microparticles by magnetic separation.
5. Wash with deionized water and dry at room temperature under vacuum.

3.3 Isolation of Human Peripheral Blood Mononuclear Cells (hPBMC)

1. Collect blood from a subject in a sterile heparinized blood-collection tube.
2. Add 15 mL of Ficoll-Hypaque solution in a sterile 50 mL test tube. Mix blood and phosphate buffered saline PBS in 1:1 proportion in a separate sterile 50 mL test tube.
3. Overload this blood-PBS mixture on to 15 mL of Ficoll-Hypaque solution.
4. Centrifuge at 1500 RCF for 40 min at 18 °C.
5. After centrifugation remove the upper layer containing plasma and platelets with a sterile pipette.
6. Transfer the white-colored buffy coat layer containing hPBMCs into a fresh tube using a sterile pipette.
7. Wash this buffy layer with 20 mL PBS twice at the interval of 5 min.
8. Finally resuspend it into complete RPMI 1640 culture media.
9. Count the cells using Neubauer chamber or hemocytometer and trypan blue exclusion test for viability of cells.

3.4 Spiking of hPBMC with Green Fluorescence Protein (GFP) Labeled Human Colon Cancer Cells (HCT 116)

1. Culture GFP labeled HCT116 cells in complete DMEM culture media and incubate at 37 °C.
2. After 24 h of incubation, count numbers of cells per mL of media under the microscope using trypan blue exclusion test for viability of cells.
3. To prepare synthetic CTC samples, mix GFP labeled HCT116 cells and hPBMC in (HCT116:hPBMC 1:50, 1:200, 1:1000, 1:2000, 1:10000, 1:100000), respectively.

3.5 Detection of CTCs Using MDNS and Capture of Cancer Cells from Synthetic CTC Samples

1. Mix and incubate the artificial CTC sample with 100 μg/mL MDNS for 5 min at room temperature.
2. Expose it to a magnetic field for 1 min or till the cell pellet is separated due to strong magnetic field.
3. Separate the cell pellet from rest of the cell suspension containing hPBMCs and uncaptured cancer cells (Fig. 3).
4. Wash the captured cell pellet using DMEM complete media and resuspend it in the media.
5. Visualize both captured and uncaptured cell fraction under the microscope and count the cells using ImageJ cell counter plugin.

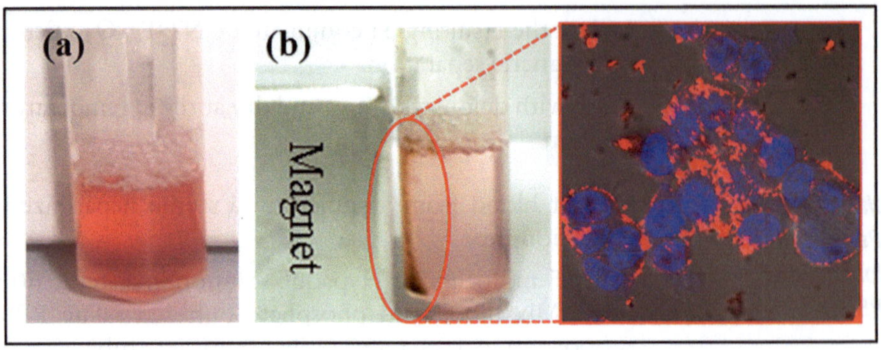

Fig. 3 (**a**) The synthetic CTC sample having HCT116 (TfR^+) cells and hPBMCs (TfR^- blood cells in 1:50 ratio. (**b**) MDNS captured and magnetically isolated HCT116 cells (*red circle*) from synthetic CTC sample. *Right* side figure *inset* shows localization of MDNS particles on the cell membrane confirming the rapidity and specificity of the MDNS–cell interaction after just 5 min of exposure

6. Calculate the capture efficiency of MDNS system by the formula as mentioned in note.

3.6 Detection of CTCs Using Tf-CNT-Fe_3O_4 Nanosystem and Capture of CTCs from Synthetic CTC Samples

1. Seed 2×10^5 cells/mL of HCT116-GFP labeled cells on glass coverslips in 35 mm culture dishes.
2. Incubate at 37 °C for 24 h; add 1×10^6 cells per ml in DMEM complete media with 4 % H_2O_2 (*see* **Note 1**).
3. Transfer the cells in NMR tube (*see* **Note 5**) and treat them with 500 μg/mL of Tf-CNT-Fe_3O_4 for 5 min.
4. Expose the NMR tube containing the cells treated with the material to the strong magnet for isolation of immuno-labeled cells.
5. One minute after exposure to the strong magnetic field, remove the rest of the cell suspension containing uncaptured cancer cells to a separate tube in order to separate the cell pellet formed.
6. Resuspend the captured cell pellet in 500 μL PBS.
7. Visualize the captured and uncaptured fraction of GFP labeled HCT116 cells under the fluorescence microscope and count the number of cells using ImageJ cell counter plugin.
8. Calculate the capture efficiency of MDNS system by the formula mentioned in **Note 6**.
9. Figure 4 shows the magnetically isolated GFP-labeled HCT116 cells (green) as well as number of cells captured by MDNS and Tf-CNT-Fe_3O_4 nanosystems.

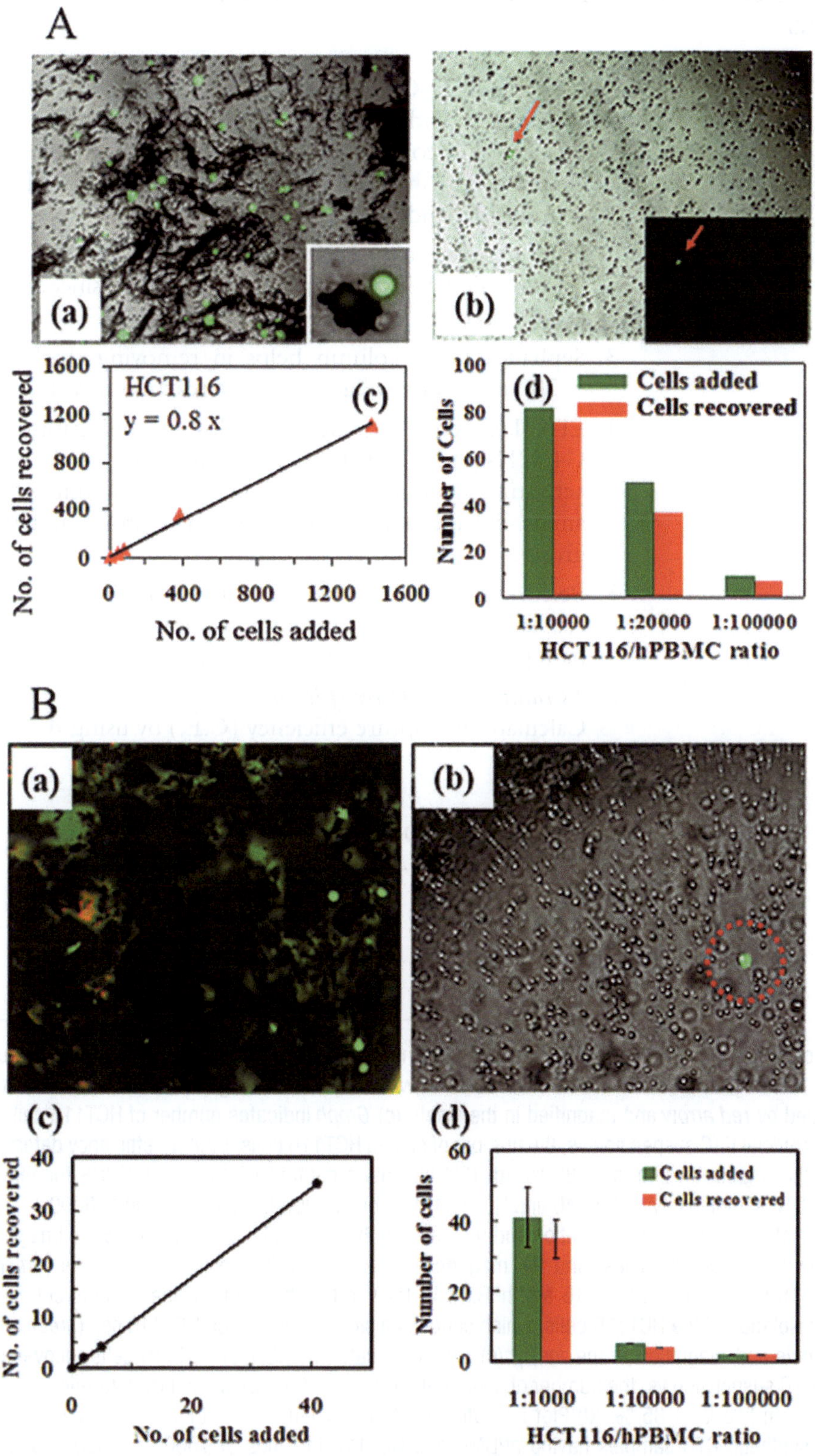

Fig. 4 (*A*) (**a**) Image of MDNS captured (*black* particles) and magnetically isolated GFP-labeled HCT116 cells (*green*) from an artificial CTC suspension of HCT116 and hPBMC in 1:10^3 ratio. The *inset* is magnified image of

4 Notes

1. Presence of H_2O_2 helps in propulsion of Fe_3O_4 nanoparticles as it reacts with Fe^{3+} in Fe_3O_4 to generate Fe^{2+} and O_2 bubbles. The formation of O_2 bubbles propels the nanoparticles resulting in motion. Furthermore, the speed of micro-rocket is dependent on H_2O_2 concentration.
2. During isolation of hPBMC add 15 mL of Ficoll-Hypaque solution slowly in a sterile 50 mL test tube since the solution is very viscous.
3. Sephadex G-10 column helps in removing small molecules > 700 molecular weight from the reaction mixture.
4. EDC.HCl coupling method helps in conjugating PAMAM G4–NH_2 with GSH. EDC.HCl is generally used as a carboxyl activating agent for the coupling of primary amines to yield an amide linkage between the carboxylic-group and the amine group.
5. Performing CTC capture experiments in NMR tube is beneficial as it is easier to capture the motion of the Tf-CNT-Fe_3O_4 nanoparticles using high magnification camera.
6. *Estimation of capture efficiency*
   Calculate the capture efficiency (C.E.) by using the equation:

$$\text{C.E.} = N_C/(N_C + N_U)$$

   Where, N_C is number of captured cells, N_U is number of uncaptured cells.

Fig. 4 (continued) such single cell isolated using magnet and captured by MDNS. (**b**) Image of the residual cell fraction after magnetic isolation of the HCT116 cells, which contains a single GFP labeled HCT116 cell (*green*, as indicated by *red arrow* and magnified in the inset). (**c**) *Graph* indicates number of HCT116 cells recovered from the artificial CTC suspension vs. the number of spiked HCT116 cells. Capture efficiency determined using slope of the regression line is ~ 80 %. (**d**) Plot indicating capture efficiency of MDNS for three different synthetic CTC samples having hPBMC and HCT116 in ratios of 10000:1, 20000:1 and 100000:1, respectively. Green indicates initial cell concentration and red denotes the final cell concentration. (*B*) (**a**) Image of Tf-CNT-Fe_3O_4 captured (*black* particles) and the magnetically isolated GFP labeled HCT116 cells (*green*) from an artificial CTC suspension of HCT116 and hPBMC in 1:10^3 ratio. (**b**) Image of the residual cell fraction after magnetic isolation of the HCT116 cells, which contains a single GFP labeled HCT116 cell (*green*, as indicated by *red circle* and magnified in the *inset*). (**c**) Graph indicates number of HCT116 cells recovered from the artificial CTC suspension vs. the number of spiked HCT116 cells. Capture efficiency determined using slope of the regression line is ~ 85 %. (**d**) Plot indicating capture efficiency of Tf-CNT-Fe_3O_4 microrocket for three different synthetic CTC samples having hPBMC and HCT116 in ratios of 1000:1, 10000:1, and 100000:1, respectively. *Green* indicates initial cell concentration and *red* denotes the final cell concentration

References

1. Hanahan D, Weinberg RA (2011) Hallmarks of cancer: the next generation. Cell 144 (5):646–674. doi:10.1016/j.cell.2011.02.013
2. Cohen SJ, Punt CJ, Iannotti N, Saidman BH, Sabbath KD, Gabrail NY, Picus J, Morse M, Mitchell E, Miller MC, Doyle GV, Tissing H, Terstappen LW, Meropol NJ (2008) Relationship of circulating tumor cells to tumor response, progression-free survival, and overall survival in patients with metastatic colorectal cancer. J Clin Oncol 26(19):3213–3221. doi:10.1200/JCO.2007.15.8923
3. Hayes JD, McMahon M (2006) The double-edged sword of Nrf2: subversion of redox homeostasis during the evolution of cancer. Mol Cell 21(6):732–734. doi:10.1016/j.molcel.2006.03.004
4. Danila DC, Heller G, Gignac GA, Gonzalez-Espinoza R, Anand A, Tanaka E, Lilja H, Schwartz L, Larson S, Fleisher M, Scher HI (2007) Circulating tumor cell number and prognosis in progressive castration-resistant prostate cancer. Clin Cancer Res 13 (23):7053–7058. doi:10.1158/1078-0432.CCR-07-1506
5. Wang S, Wang H, Jiao J, Chen KJ, Owens GE, Kamei K, Sun J, Sherman DJ, Behrenbruch CP, Wu H, Tseng HR (2009) Three-dimensional nanostructured substrates toward efficient capture of circulating tumor cells. Angew Chem Int Ed Engl 48(47):8970–8973. doi:10.1002/anie.200901668
6. Racila E, Euhus D, Weiss AJ, Rao C, McConnell J, Terstappen LW, Uhr JW (1998) Detection and characterization of carcinoma cells in the blood. Proc Natl Acad Sci U S A 95 (8):4589–4594
7. Krivacic RT, Ladanyi A, Curry DN, Hsieh HB, Kuhn P, Bergsrud DE, Kepros JF, Barbera T, Ho MY, Chen LB, Lerner RA, Bruce RH (2004) A rare-cell detector for cancer. Proc Natl Acad Sci U S A 101(29):10501–10504. doi:10.1073/pnas.0404036101
8. Galanzha EI, Shashkov EV, Kelly T, Kim JW, Yang L, Zharov VP (2009) In vivo magnetic enrichment and multiplex photoacoustic detection of circulating tumour cells. Nat Nanotechnol 4(12):855–860. doi:10.1038/nnano.2009.333
9. Sha MY, Xu H, Natan MJ, Cromer R (2008) Surface-enhanced Raman scattering tags for rapid and homogeneous detection of circulating tumor cells in the presence of human whole blood. J Am Chem Soc 130 (51):17214–17215. doi:10.1021/ja804494m
10. He W, Wang H, Hartmann LC, Cheng JX, Low PS (2007) In vivo quantitation of rare circulating tumor cells by multiphoton intravital flow cytometry. Proc Natl Acad Sci U S A 104(28):11760–11765. doi:10.1073/pnas.0703875104
11. Adams AA, Okagbare PI, Feng J, Hupert ML, Patterson D, Gottert J, McCarley RL, Nikitopoulos D, Murphy MC, Soper SA (2008) Highly efficient circulating tumor cell isolation from whole blood and label-free enumeration using polymer-based microfluidics with an integrated conductivity sensor. J Am Chem Soc 130(27):8633–8641. doi:10.1021/ja8015022
12. Scarberry KE, Dickerson EB, Zhang ZJ, Benigno BB, McDonald JF (2010) Selective removal of ovarian cancer cells from human ascites fluid using magnetic nanoparticles. Nanomedicine 6(3):399–408. doi:10.1016/j.nano.2009.11.003
13. Myung JH, Gajjar KA, Saric J, Eddington DT, Hong S (2011) Dendrimer-mediated multivalent binding for the enhanced capture of tumor cells. Angew Chem Int Ed Engl 50(49):11769–11772. doi:10.1002/anie.201105508
14. Zheng X, Cheung LS, Schroeder JA, Jiang L, Zohar Y (2011) A high-performance microsystem for isolating circulating tumor cells. Lab Chip 11(19):3269–3276. doi:10.1039/c1lc20331b
15. Cristofanilli M, Reuben J, Uhr J (2008) Circulating tumor cells in breast cancer: fiction or reality? J Clin Oncol 26(21):3656–3657. doi:10.1200/JCO.2008.18.0356, author reply 3657–3658
16. Banerjee SS, Jalota-Badhwar A, Satavalekar SD, Bhansali SG, Aher ND, Mascarenhas RR, Paul D, Sharma S, Khandare JJ (2013) Transferrin-mediated rapid targeting, isolation, and detection of circulating tumor cells by multifunctional magneto-dendritic nanosystem. Adv Healthc Mater 2(6):800–805. doi:10.1002/adhm.201200164
17. Banerjee SS, Jalota-Badhwar A, Zope KR, Todkar KJ, Mascarenhas RR, Chate GP, Khutale GV, Bharde A, Calderon M, Khandare JJ (2015) Self-propelled carbon nanotube based microrockets for rapid capture and isolation of circulating tumor cells. Nanoscale 7 (19):8684–8688. doi:10.1039/c5nr01797a

Chapter 17

Fluorescence and Bioluminescence Imaging of Orthotopic Brain Tumors in Mice

Emilie McKinnon, Alfred Moore, Suraj Dixit, Yun Zhu, and Ann-Marie Broome

Abstract

Optical imaging strategies, such as fluorescence and bioluminescence imaging, are non-invasive, in vivo whole body imaging techniques utilized to study cancer. Optical imaging is widely used in preclinical work because of its ease of use and cost-friendliness. It also provides the opportunity to study animals and biological responses longitudinally over time. Important considerations include depth of tissue penetration, photon scattering, absorption and the choice of light emitting probe, all of which affect the resolution (image quality and data information) and the signal to noise ratio of the image. We describe how to use bioluminescence and fluorescence imaging to track a chemotherapeutic delivery nanocarrier conjugated with a fluorophore to determine its localization in vivo.

Key words Bioluminescence, Fluorescence, In vivo imaging, Glioblastoma, Optical imaging

1 Introduction

Optical imaging strategies, such as fluorescence and bioluminescence imaging, are non-invasive, in vivo whole body imaging techniques utilized to study cancer. Both modalities are based on the detection of photons emitted from either the organism, as in bioluminescence imaging, or from a fluorophore, as in fluorescence imaging. Photon concentrations up to picomolar and femtomolar are detectable by whole animal-imaging systems [1]. Optical imaging is widely used in preclinical work because of its ease of use and cost-friendliness. It also provides the opportunity to study animals and biological responses longitudinally over time. Important considerations include depth of tissue penetration, photon scattering, absorption and the choice of light emitting probe, all of which affect the resolution (image quality and data information) and the signal to noise ratio of the image.

Bioluminescence is the emission of light photons from an animal, which in some organisms is a naturally occurring event.

Reema Zeineldin (ed.), *Cancer Nanotechnology: Methods and Protocols*, Methods in Molecular Biology, vol. 1530,
DOI 10.1007/978-1-4939-6646-2_17,

This phenomenon has been exploited by researchers to study different molecular processes in cells and whole organisms. Cells are genetically engineered to express a bioluminescent reporter enzyme (e.g., firefly luciferase) and are subsequently treated with the enzyme's substrate (e.g., luciferin), which results in the release of photons upon catalysis [1]. Bioluminescence imaging techniques emit photons in the visible light range, which inherently suffer from poor tissue penetration, making this technique currently only suitable for small animal imaging [2]. One major advantage of bioluminescence imaging is the absence of background signal, or noise. This is because animals inherently do not express luciferase. In this chapter, we outline the use of bioluminescent imaging to determine the tumor burden in an orthotopic mouse model of glioblastoma.

Fluorescence is the emission of a photon from a fluorophore after excitation by a laser. Different fluorophores absorb and emit photons at different wavelengths influencing tissue penetration and, consequently, the signal to noise (SNR) ratio, making the choice of fluorophore a critical design parameter. Fluorophores that emit light in the far red (>650 nm) or Near Infra-Red (NIR) range are optimal for in vivo imaging due to better tissue penetration and reduced scattering effects. The choice of excitation source is also important as fluorophores are only able to absorb photons at a specific wavelength. Table 1 illustrates which type of filters is optimal for a handful of commonly used fluorophores in small animal imaging. Unlike in bioluminescence, fluorescence imaging does suffer from autofluorescence. Hair, blood, and tissues can be excited by the same source as the fluorophore and consequently also emit photons, reducing the contrast of the image [3] (Fig. 1). Most new fluorescence imagers work with band pass filters to restrict the wavelengths of both excitation and emission light to ameliorate the contribution of autofluorescence to the signal. Often, background noise is quantified by measuring the fluorescence arising from the animal before the introduction of any fluorophores, which can then be used to unmix the autofluorescence signal in subsequent imaging steps from the true fluorescence signal. As an example, we describe how to use fluorescence imaging to track a chemotherapeutic delivery nanocarrier conjugated with a fluorophore to determine its localization in vivo.

In vivo whole body imaging is an invaluable tool when developing new cancer drugs. In this chapter, we elaborate step by step on how we combine bioluminescence and fluorescence imaging techniques to study the delivery of drug particles to an orthotopic glioblastoma in a mouse. First, genetically altered tumor cells expressing the luciferase enzyme are injected into mice brains. After 7 days (average), the mice are injected with luciferin and the tumor burden can be determined by a bioluminescence imaging system. When the tumors are of the appropriate size, approximately 1–3 cm, we first determine autofluorescence by imaging the mice (prior to the injection of the nanocarriers) on both the ventral and

Table 1
Excitation and emission wavelengths from commonly used fluorophores

Fluorophore			Maestro filter set name					
Name	Excitation (NM)	Emission (NM)	Yellow	Orange	Red	Deep Red	NIR	ICG
705 nm QDot®	<650	705	X					
800 nm QDot®	<750	800	X					
Alexa Fluor®680	679	702		X				
Alexa Fluor®700	700	719			X			
Alexa Fluor®750	750	779					X	
DyLight™ 680	692	712		X				
DyLight™ 755	754	776					X	
Cy5.5™	675	695		X				
Cy7™	743	805					X	
ICG	800	850						X

Maestro Filter Set Name	Excitation Filter (Range)	Emission Filter	Acquisition Settings*
White	Neutral attenuator	Transparent glass filter	500 to 800 in 10 nm steps
Yellow	595 nm (576 to 621 nm)	635 nm longpass	630 to 800 in 10 nm steps
Orange	605 nm (586 to 631 nm)	645 nm longpass	640 to 820 in 10 nm steps
Red	635 nm (616 to 661 nm)	675 nm longpass	670 to 900 in 10 nm steps
Deep Red	661 nm (641 to 686 nm)	700 nm longpass	700 to 950 in 10 nm steps
NIR	704 nm (684 to 729 nm)	745 nm longpass	740 to 950 in 10 nm steps
ICG	735 nm (700 to 770 nm)	790 nm longpass	780 to 950 in 10 nm steps

Colors indicate appropriate Maestro filter sets for imaging, with the ideal filter marked with an X. (Modified from Caliper Life Sciences filter selection guide)

dorsal sides with overlapping sets of filters (primarily orange and red filters). The example used herein is of mice treated with drugs conjugated with a Dylight 680 fluorophore. After the intravenous tail vein injection of the nanocarrier, the animals are longitudinally imaged at 1, 3, 6, and 24 h time points to acquire the fluorescence signal and this is correlated to the location of the nanocarriers and their relative intensity. The mice are euthanized after the 24 h time point and subsequently all the organs are harvested and imaged post mortem. It is important to note that the results arising from these techniques are either qualitative or relative to another image. Currently, it is not possible to exactly quantify the amount of fluorescence arising from the underlying tissues [4]. Furthermore, keep in mind that both bioluminescence and fluorescence imaging techniques are planar imaging modalities, meaning that they create two-dimensional topographic images, superimposing the signal(s) arising from the underlying tissues.

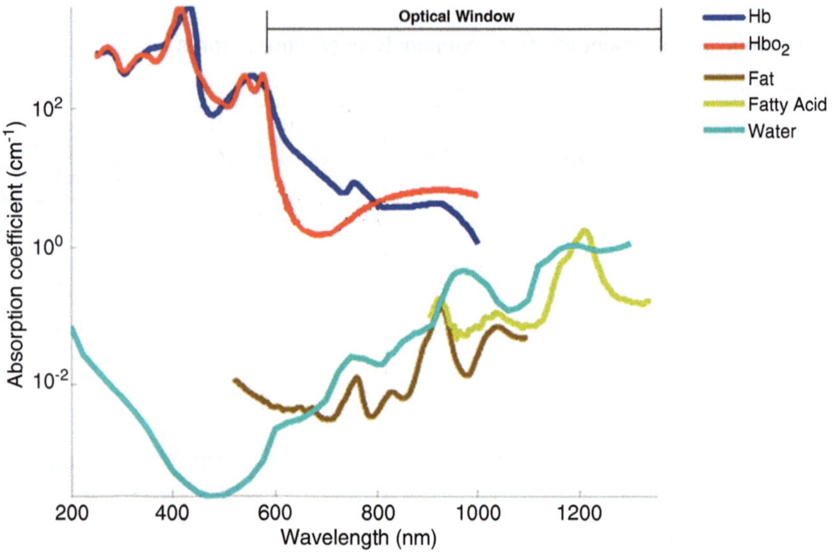

Fig. 1 Absorption spectra of major biological tissue components. Optical window indicates the part of the spectrum where a minimal amount of autofluorescence is encountered and in vivo imaging is optimal. *Hb* Hemoglobin, *HbO*$_2$ Oxyhemoglobin (Modified from Bo Wang et al., 2010 [6] with permission from Optical Society of America.)

2 Materials

1. U87-MG glioblastoma cell line (American Type Culture Collection, ATCC).
2. 2–3 % (v/v) isoflurane.
3. 150 μg/ml D-luciferin.
4. Bioluminescence imager: PerkinElmer IVIS 200 spectrometer (PerkinElmer, MA).
5. Fluorescence imager: PerkinElmer Maestro EX imaging System (PerkinElmer, MA), software version 3.0.

3 Methods

3.1 Make U87MG Luciferase Stable Cell Line

1. Electroporation of U87-MG using Bio-Rad GenePulser Xcell (BioRad, CA).
   Condition: Voltage 250 V, Capacitance: 500 UF, mammalian luciferase reporter expression vector pGL4.50 (Promega, WI): 30 μg added in four million of cells in 0.4 ml of growth media without fetal bovine serum (FBS).
2. After electroporation, plate cells in 100 mm dish and treat cells with antibiotic selection hygromycin B at 100 μg/ml after 72 h. Change with fresh media every 3 days.

3. Cell colonies will form in 2 weeks. Pick each clone for positive selection of the luciferase gene and transfer them to 24-well plate.
4. Using an in vitro bioluminescence assay, identify positive clone (s) and continue to amplify the selected clones for stable cell line propagation.

3.2 Athymic Nude Orthotopic Glioblastoma Animal Model

1. Use U87 cells that are nearly (70–80 %) confluent.
2. Trypsinize cells (0.05 % trypsin) for 3–5 min at 37 °C. Stop enzymatic activity with 10 ml cold medium.
3. Centrifuge cells 3 min at 1690 RCF.
4. Resuspend cells in 10 ml cold phosphate buffered saline (PBS) and count cells on hemacytometer. Centrifuge.
5. Repeat wash and centrifuge (if necessary to concentrate).
6. Resuspend cells in PBS to final cell count of 100,000 cells per μl. Keep on ice.
7. Administer 0.10 cc (cubic centimeter) of Buprenorphine (0.1 mg/kg) to athymic nude mouse (NIH Cr; Nu:Nu), subcutaneously, as a preemptive analgesia.
8. Anesthetize the animal with 0.25 cc ketamine–xylazine cocktail in the gut. Position the animal on its ventral surface (belly) on the stage of the stereotactic injection apparatus. Position the head using ear prongs and the tooth bar (keep superior head surface parallel to the work bench).
9. If needed, 1 % (v/v) isoflurane can be administered to the animal through a nose cone during surgery to prolong the anesthesia.
10. Wipe scalp with 70 % (v/v) ethanol. Using a scalpel, make an incision to the right of the midline. Clear away fascia and muscle with scraping motion of scalpel and cotton swabs.
11. Make a small opening in the skull 2 mm to the right of the bregma, just anterior to the suture line using a drill with a 0.7 mm burr.
12. Rinse a blunt 10 μl Hamilton syringe with sterile saline and keep filled with saline until used (remove air bubbles). Eject saline and fill syringe with 2 μl of cell suspension and place in syringe holder. Lower syringe until needle tip is at brain surface.
13. Lower needle to 4 mm and back off to 3 mm to make a cell pocket. Hold for 1 min.
14. Inject 1 μl of cells per minute, with small depressions of the syringe plunger every 15 s. Hold position for 3 min after injection. Total cell injection: 200,000 cells.

15. Remove the needle slowly over the course of 3 min, by raising 1/3 mm every 20 s (do not lift plunger). Rinse syringe immediately twice with saline and refill with saline.
16. Close burr hole in the skull with bone wax and then seal the incision with Vet Bond (3 M Animal Care Products, MN).
17. Allow animal to recover under heating lamp (or on thermo regulated heating pad) in new, separate cages. Monitor mouse until it awakens from anesthesia.
18. When finished, rinse syringe for storage—twice with saline and refill with saline. Then, rinse with PBS three times, double distilled H_2O twice, and ethanol twice. Store in sealed box.
19. Once animal awaken from anesthesia, be sure that it has Diet Gel (Clearh20, ME) in the cage in addition to dry food in the food rack and a full water bottle. Each animal will be isolated and housed individually overnight to allow for initiation of healing time. If the mice are doing well the following day, they can be housed two to a cage. Immediately monitor for fighting or aggression. If this occurs, separate animals into their own individual cages.
20. Assess animal health daily post-implantation and record observations.
21. Animals are ready for experimental procedures within 9 days after orthotopic implantation.

3.3 Synthesis of Platelet Derived Growth Factor (PDGF): Targeted Dylight 680 Conjugated Micelle-Encapsulated Temozolomide (TMZ)

1. Micelle encapsulation of TMZ (MTMZ) was carried out as described by Miller et al. [5].
   (a) Weigh 0.5 mg of TMZ and add 20 μl of dimethyl sulfoxide (DMSO); sonicate solution until TMZ is dissolved.
   (b) Add 2.5 mg of polyethylene glycol-phosphoethanolamine (PEG-PE) and 0.5 mg of PHC in the scintillation vial containing TMZ.
   (c) Add 2 ml of chloroform to the vial and sonicate the mixture for 1 h at room temperature.
   (d) Evaporate chloroform to complete dryness in a vacuum oven at room temperature (approximately 4–5 h).
   (e) Heat the pellet to 80 °C on a hot gun until the pellet becomes gel-like or shiny.
   (f) Add 1 ml of PBS buffer (pH 7.4, 37 °C) to the pellet and sonicate for 30 min until solution is clear.
   (g) Centrifuge the aqueous solution of micelles for 10 min at 7500 × *g* at room temperature. Discard any precipitate after the centrifugation. Repeat this process three times.
   (h) Syringe filter the aqueous supernatant using a 0.22 μm filter.

(i) Take the UV–vis absorption of the sample to determine the concentration of TMZ ($\lambda = 325$ nm, epsilon = 8.98/(μM cm).

(j) For size measurements, sonicate the sample again for 1 h at room temperature and filter it through a 0.22 μm filter and use 100 μl in the vial before taking the dynamic light scattering measurements.

2. For fluorophore conjugation, MTMZ solution is added to NHS (N-hydroxysuccinimide) Dylight 680 (ratio calculated to cover 30 % of available amines on the micelle surface).
   (a) Add PBS buffer (pH 7.2) to the solution.
   (b) Incubate at room temperature for 1 h.
   (c) Remove excess fluorophore by using a 10 K molecular weight cut off (MWCO) ultracentrifugal device three times.

3.4 In Vitro Bioluminescence Imaging: Imaging Standard Curve to Correlate Number of Cells to Tumor Size

1. Seed increasing cell numbers of the human glioma cell line implanted into the mouse, in this case U87-MG onto tissue culture plates.
2. Expand cells until they are between 70 and 90 % confluent in the wells.
3. Start the IVIS 200 program and initialize the system. (This can take several minutes). Wait for the light on the screen to switch from red to green indicating that the camera has reached the appropriate temperature of −83 °C.
4. Pre-image plates with the photograph option to determine correct field of view (either 13.4 or 22.7 cm depending on the plate size) (*see* **Note 1**).
5. Add D-luciferin (potassium salt) to the wells at a final concentration of 150 μg/ml.
6. Image serially at 1-min intervals until the luminescence signal peaks (≅10 min) and begins to decline (*see* **Note 2**). Imaging of cells is done using auto exposure and medium binning (*see* **Note 3**).
7. Select the image with the maximum signal intensity of lumens/s (≅10 min for luciferin) by double clicking and go to region of interest (ROI) tools on the tool palette.
8. Choose the *Circular ROI* and draw a circle around the first well. The ROI needs to stay consistent over all measurements, so proceed by copying and pasting the drawn ROI to all the other wells. (When working with square shaped plates the grid ROI can also be used).

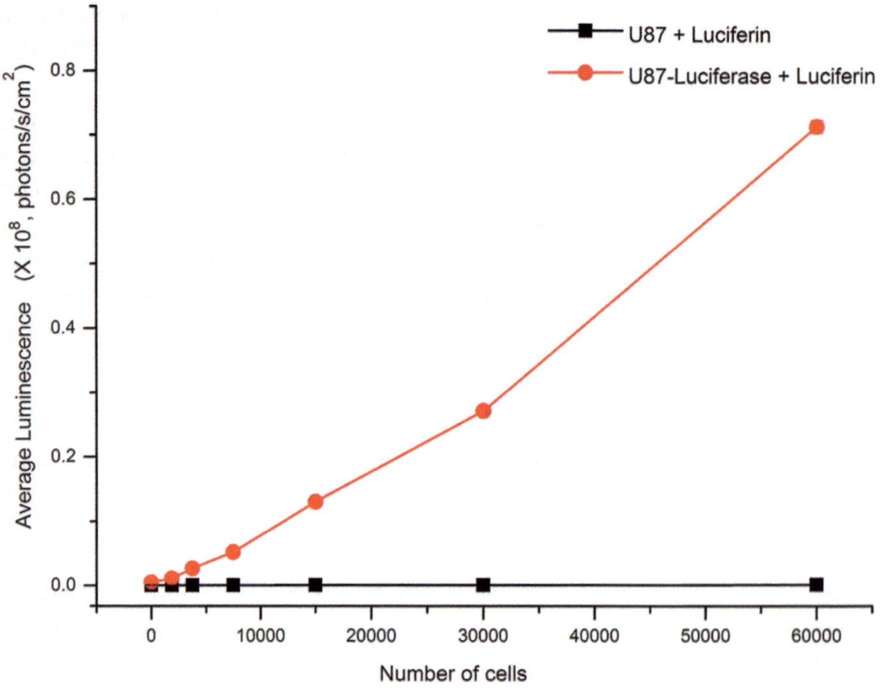

Fig. 2 Standard curve calculated using increasing amount of U87-MG cells expressing luciferase. Top two rows of plate are control cells not transformed with luciferase

9. Change the measuring units from counts to radiance (photons p/(s cm^2 sr)) in the upper left corner and click on measure ROIs.
10. Export data either in either .txt or .csv format for further processing in Microsoft Excel.
11. Create a standard curve plotting the amount of luminescence versus the number of cells using the bioluminescent results arising from the different tumor cell dilutions (amount of cells) (Fig. 2).

3.5 In Vivo Bioluminescence Imaging: Determine Tumor Burden

1. Inject mice orthotopically with luciferase-transfected cells and allow cells to grow (*see* **Note 4**).
2. Start the IVIS program and initialize the system. This can take a few minutes. Wait for the light on the screen to switch from red to green indicating that the camera has reached the appropriate temperature of −83 °C.
3. Anesthetize mice before imaging with inhalation anesthetic (isoflurane at 2–3 % (v/v) in oxygen) in an induction chamber.
4. Once animals are anesthetized, transfer animals to IVIS 200 imager. One to five animals can be imaged simultaneously.

5. Pre-image animals using the photograph option to determine binning and field of view (medium and C (13.4 cm) or D (22.7 cm) FoV) (*see* **Notes 1** and **3**).
6. Inject animals with D-luciferin (Intraperitoneal, 150 mg/kg) and image at 1 min after injection (*see* **Note 2**).
7. Continue imaging at 2–3 min intervals until the maximum signal has been measured and has initiated a decline (*see* **Notes 2** and **5**).
8. Select the image with the maximum amount of bioluminescence (≅10 min for luciferin) by double clicking and go to ROI tools on the tool palette.
9. Animals can be reimaged on subsequent days as the tumors grow by reinjecting luciferin on each day (*see* **Note 6**) (Fig. 3).
10. Choose the *Circular ROI* and draw a circle around the area of interest. The ROI needs to stay consistent over all measurements so it is best to do the analysis at the last day when the tumor is the largest. Determine luciferase activity by copying and pasting the same ROI to all the other time points.

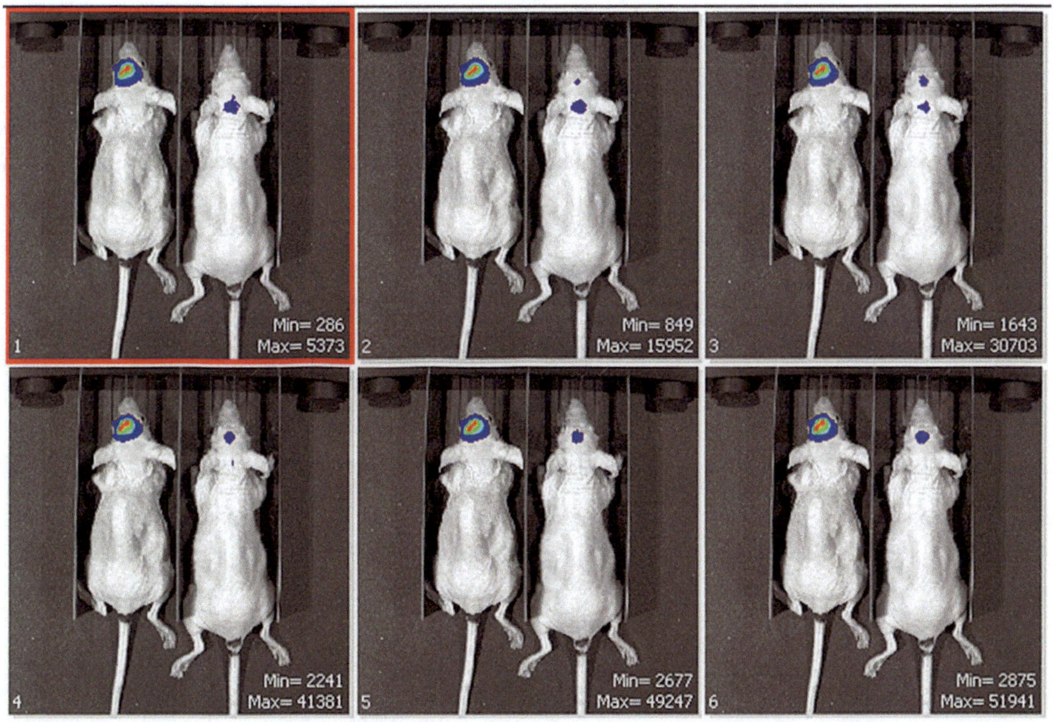

Fig. 3 Example of longitudinal bioluminescent imaging sequence. Mouse on the left contains implanted U87-luciferase cells in the brain. The mouse on the right was injected with regular U87-MG cells. The amount of bioluminescence increases with time (1, 4, 7, 10, 13, 16 min after injection with luciferin)

11. Change the measuring units from counts to radiance (photons p/(s cm^2 sr)) in the upper left corner and click on *Measure ROIs*.
12. Export data either in .txt or .csv format for further processing in Microsoft Excel.
13. Use the standard curve created in Subheading 3.4 to determine the number of tumor cells present in the animal.

3.6 In Vitro Fluorescence Imaging: Measure Spectrum of Conjugated Fluorophore

1. Start Maestro program on the computer and turn on the Maestro imaging device. (Start up can take up to 30 min.) Make sure the excitation lamp is "on" and the shutter is "off." Wait until the excitation lamps are warmed up and the light stabilizes. When imaging in vitro solutions the stage and chamber heating system can be turned "off" as it will dry out the suspension.
2. Prepare different concentrations (100–1000 nM) of conjugated fluorophore. (*see* **Note 7**).
3. Using a pipette, transfer a drop of each dilution onto a clean slide or saran wrap (Fig. 4a).
4. Put sample drops on the Maestro stage. First, acquire a white image by changing the filter to *White* (under *Filter* > *Wavelength* selection) and click *Acquire Mono.*
5. Next change the *Acquire Cubes* to the appropriate filters. For Dylight 680, use either the orange or the red filters (Table 1). Also set the binning and exposure time appropriately (*see* **Note 3**).

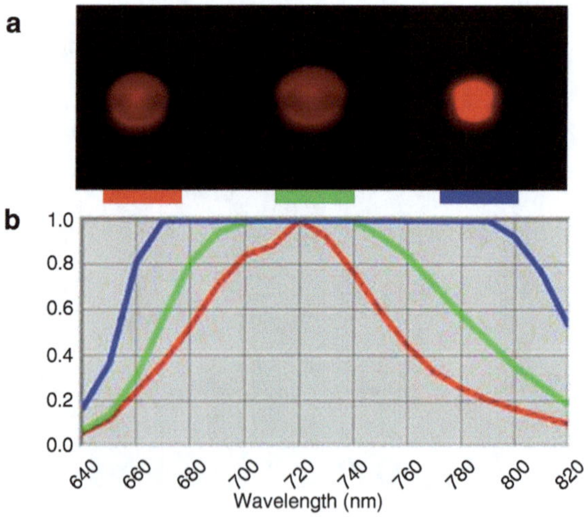

Fig. 4 (**a**) From *left* to *right*, dilutions of 100 (*red*), 500 (*green*), and 1000 (*blue*) nM MTMZ-Dylight 680. (**b**) Emission spectra measured from the different nanoparticle dilutions with and orange filter and 500 ms exposure time. At higher concentrations, the spectrum becomes more saturated

6. Click on *Load Cube* and open image acquired from conjugated fluorophore drops.
7. Click on the *Draw* icon next to Channel 1 and draw a line inside the drop.
8. Repeat **step 6** for the different concentrations of fluorophore and add spectra to different channels.
9. Choose the sharpest and most unsaturated spectrum for subsequent analysis and creation of the spectral library (Fig. 4b).
10. Save spectral library by clicking *File* > *Save Spectral Library.* Choose an appropriate name and folder.

3.7 In Vivo Fluorescence Imaging: Acquire Fluorescent Images

1. Start Maestro program on the computer and subsequently turn "on" the Maestro imaging device. (Start up can take up to 30 min.) Make sure the excitation lamp is "on" and the shutter is "off." Wait until the excitation lamps, chamber, and stage are warmed up and the light lamp stabilizes.
2. Anesthetize mice with 2–3 % isoflurane in medical grade oxygen in an induction chamber.
3. Clean stage and transfer mice to Maestro fluorescence imager platform stage. (Up to three animals can be imaged simultaneously.) Clicking on the *Live* button displays a live feed from the machine's interior platform.
4. Before the fluorophore is injected, the animals must be pre-imaged to determine background fluorescence. The filter set used for imaging will be determined depending on the fluorophore that is used, i.e., Dylight 680 is imaged using the orange (preferred) and red filter sets (Table 1). Use exposure times of 500, 1000, 2000, and 4000 ms at 2 × 2 binning (*see* **Note 3**).
5. After choosing the appropriate settings, click *Acquire Cube.* Image both the dorsal and the ventral sides (*see* **Note 8**). Save cube after each image is acquired (*File* > *Save Cube*).
6. For help with post analysis, also take an image with the white filter at 250 ms exposure at 1 × 1 binning (*Acquire Mono*).
7. Inject fluorophore either intravenously or intraperitoneally, depending on the model and kinetics of the fluorophore. Here, we injected the mice intravenously in the tail vein.
8. After injection repeat **step 3** with the same filter, exposure time, and binning settings.

3.8 Fluorescence Imaging Analysis: Create Spectral Library

1. Go to *Spectra* tab in the main Maestro window and click on *Import Spectra from Library.* Load spectrum of fluorophore saved in Subheading 3.6, **step 9**. Give the spectrum an appropriate name, color and spectrum number and click on transfer

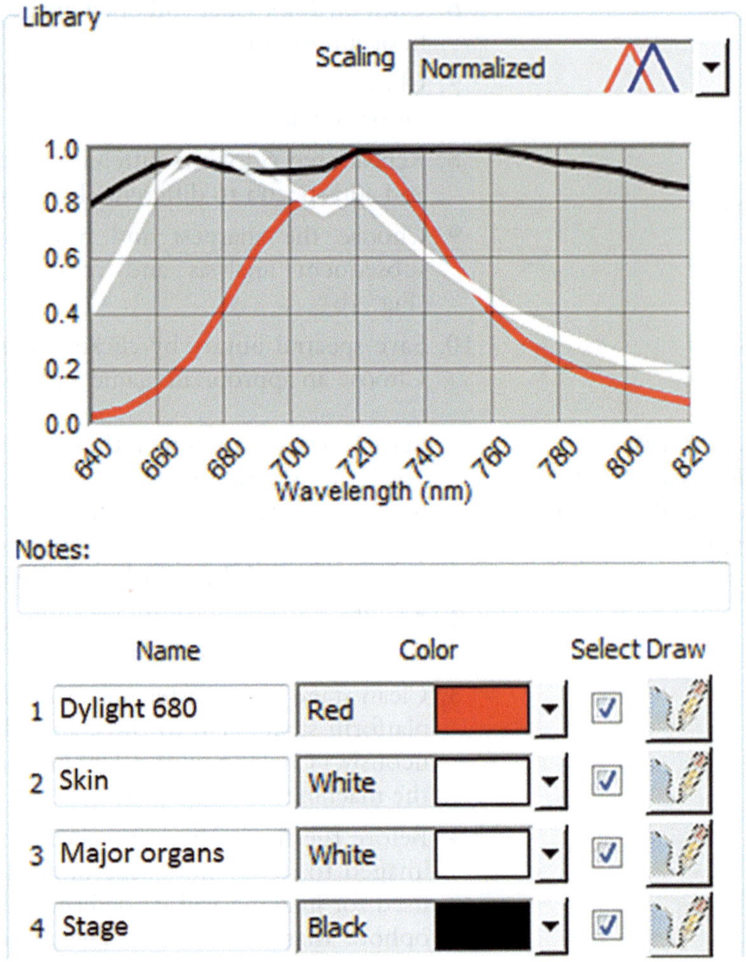

Fig. 5 Spectral library for athymic nude mouse before the injection of fluorophore. Channel 1 represents the spectra of the conjugated fluorophore. Channels 2 and 3 are autofluorescence spectra from the mouse and Channel 4 is the autofluorescence of the stage

to library (*see* **Note 9**). An example spectrum of the fluorophore Dylight 680 acquired with an orange filter is shown in Fig. 5.

2. Click on *Load Cube* and open the mouse pre-image. Choose the image acquired with the same filter as used for the fluorophore spectra in Subheading 3.8, **step 1**.
3. In the next step, identify the different autofluorescence channels (*see* **Note 10**) present in the pre-imaged animal. Click on *Real Component Analysis* [RCA] and a new window will appear. Next click on *Find Component Images.* Several images will appear; these are the different spectral components found by the component analysis (*see* **Note 11**). Click on the image

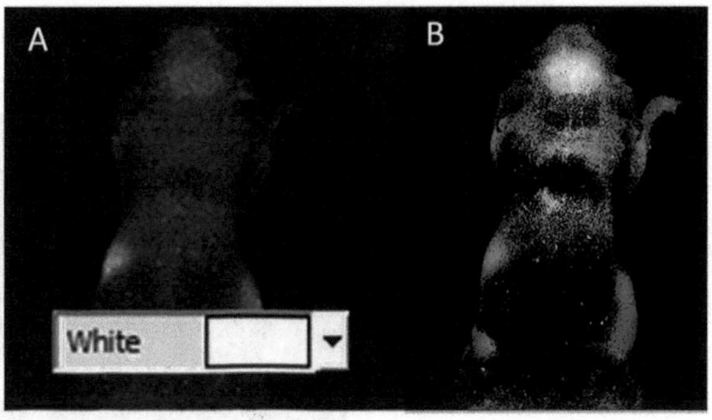

Fig. 6 (**a**) Example of channel after RCA analysis representing auto fluorescence arising from the kidney. Assign one color (e.g., *white*) to all background signals. (**b**) After unmixing, each channel in the spectral library is represented by an image representing the amount of signal coming from that specific channel. This is an example of a channel capturing signal coming from the major organs, the skull and the skin

boxes that appear to contain relevant autofluorescence channels, i.e., different organs, skin, eyes (Fig. 6a). Next click on *Find Spectra* (*see* **Note 12**). Give the channels an appropriate name (preimage_eyes, preimage_liver, ...) and assign them a spectrum number (*see* **Note 9**). Give all the autofluorescence channels the same color, for example white. Click on *Transfer to Library* and close the window (Fig. 5).

4. Reselect the fluorophore channel (most likely Channel 1), which is now unchecked and click *Unmix*. Different windows will open, which represent the amount of fluorescence present in each of the chosen channels. These images are represented in gray scale, which means the whiter the values; the higher the fluorescence. Looking at the highlighted areas will tell you which part of the animal are captured by which channel. Figure 6b shows an example of a channel that represents the autofluorescence from the brain/skull and the major organs. The window that has a border color matching the color chosen for the fluorophore channel represents the signal arising from the fluorophore. Because the pre-image animal has no fluorophore, this signal should be as close to zero as possible (*see* **Note 13**).
5. Open a *Compare Image* window (*Tools* > *Compare Images*) and drag the window that represents the fluorophore signal into one of the empty spaces of the Compare Image window (Fig. 7). This will give you an idea of the highest value of signal in the image (here, 0.00408). Our goal is to set this value as low as possible. Keep this *Compare Image* window open.
6. Save the spectral library by clicking *File* > *Save Spectral Library*. Choose an appropriate name and folder.

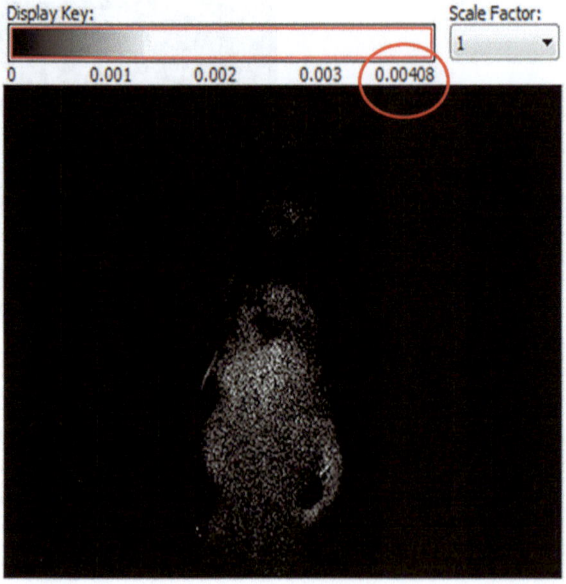

Fig. 7 "*Compare Image* window" quantifying the resulting background fluorescence present in a fluorophore channel. Some auto-fluorescence arising from the skin is still visible. The value *circled* in *red* is the maximum fluorescence present in the image which needs to be as low as possible

7. Save unmixed images for future reference by clicking *File* > *Save Image* > *Save All as Displayed*. Choose appropriate name and folder.

3.9 Image Analysis: Longitudinal Analysis of Fluorescence (Qualitative)

1. Click on *Load Cube* (or on *File* > *Open Cube*) and find the image that corresponds to the same animal, same filter and same exposure time used in Subheading 3.6.
2. If there is no spectral library present (from Subheading 3.6), load the correct spectral library by going to the *Spectra* tab in the main Maestro window and clicking on *Import Spectra from Library*.
3. Click on *Unmix*. Different windows will open, each of them represent the the amount of signal coming from the different channels in the spectral library made in Subheading 3.6.
4. If desired, save all images by clicking *File* > *Save Image* > *Save All Images*.
5. Drag fluorophore image (image with the border that corresponds to the fluorophore color) to the *Compare Image* window (Subheading 3.6, **step 5**) (*see* **Note 14**) to the next open spot and change the *Color Map* from gray to jet. This will make it easier to differentiate the intensity values in the images (*see* **Note 15**). Repeat **steps 1** and **3** for all available experimental time points (Fig. 8).

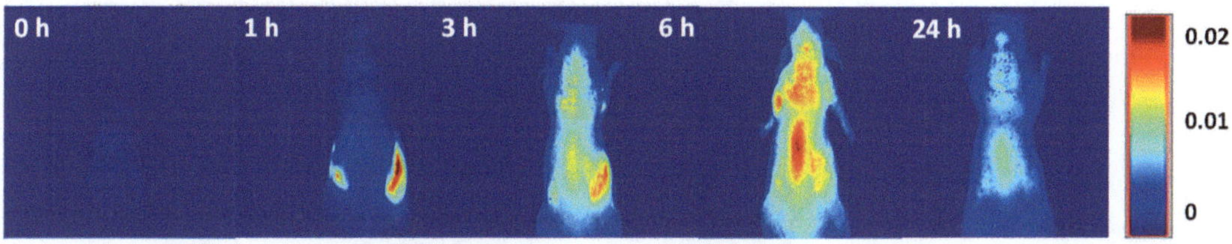

Fig. 8 Fluorescence hot map (before Injection up to 24 h after injection) of athymic nude mice implanted with U87-luciferase cells, injected with MTMZ. Time series shows the dispersion and break down of the drug particles

6. Keep *Compare Image* window open if you are doing a cross-sectional study (for example, when comparing targeted versus untargeted micelles).

3.10 Fluorescence Imaging Analysis: Longitudinal Analysis of Fluorescence (Quantitative)

1. Click on *Load Cube* (or on *File* > *Open Cube*) and find the image that corresponds to the first time point of the same animal, same filter and same exposure time used in Subheading 3.9.
2. If there is no spectral library present (from Subheading 3.9), load the correct spectral library by going to the *Spectra* tab in the main Maestro window and by clicking on *Import Spectra from Library.*
3. Click on *Unmix*. Different windows will open, each of them represent the amount of signal coming from the different channels in the spectral library made in Subheading 3.9.
4. Right-click on the image that contains the fluorescence from the fluorophore channel (border color corresponds to the fluorophore color in the spectrum) and click on *Keep Open*.
5. Repeat **steps 1–4** for all other study time points.
6. Click on the *Measure* tab on the left in the main Maestro window and click *Draw.*

   At the top of the tab, there are different ROIs to draw with (ellipse, rectangle, free hand). Draw an ROI over the region where you quantitatively want to measure the fluorescence. (It is possible to draw more than one ROI.)
7. Save the ROI by right clicking on the image and click on *Save Measurement Regions*. Name file with image and location.
8. Right click on the next study time point and choose the option *Load Measurement Region*. Select the region from **step** 7 (*see* **Note 16**).
9. Repeat **step 8** for all the study time points (*see* **Note 17**) (Fig. 9).
10. Save all images (with ROI) by clicking on *File* > *Save Image* > *Save All.*

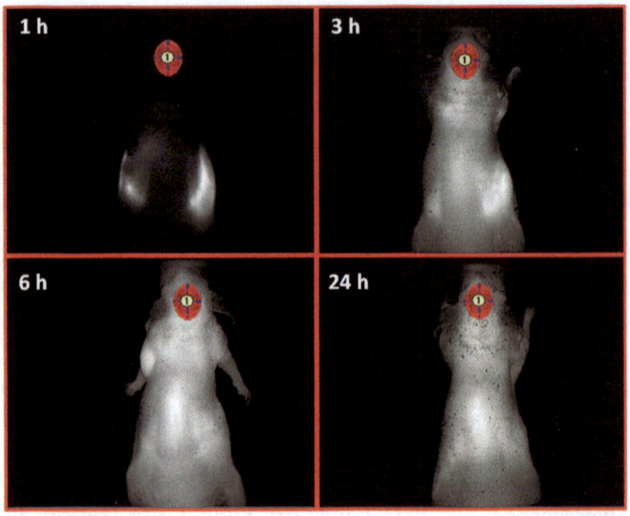

Fig. 9 Placement of elliptical region of interest used to quantify the amount of photons, which are emitted by the brain 1 h after injection up to 24 h after injection

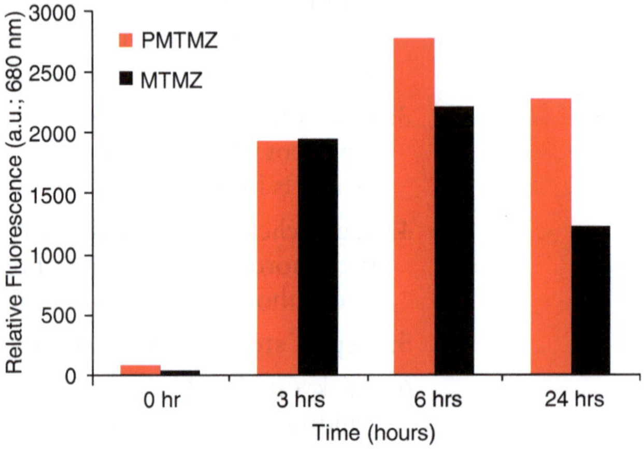

Fig. 10 Relative fluorescence from the brain between 0 and 24 h after drug injections. Amount of fluorescence in this case is compared between targeted (PMTMZ (platelet derived growth factor, micelle-encapsulated TMZ) and untargeted (MTMZ) (micelle-encapsulated TMZ) drug particles

11. Click on the image from the first study time point and then click on *Copy Measurements to Clipboard*.
12. Open your preferred data analysis program (for example, Microsoft Excel) and paste the measurements here.
13. Repeat **steps 11–12** for all time points.
14. Measurements include values such as total signal in the different ROIs and Average Signal (Fig. 10).

3.11 Fluorescence Imaging Analysis: Cross-Sectional Analysis of Fluorescence (Qualitative)

1. Repeat Subheading 3.9 for a second animal and drag the fluorophore intensity images to a new row in the same *Compare* window.

3.12 Fluorescence Imaging Analysis: Cross-Sectional Analysis of Fluorescence (Quantitative)

1. Repeat Subheading 3.10 for all other animals.

3.13 Fluorescence Imaging Analysis: Ex Vivo Measurements of Organ Fluorescence

1. Repeat the steps in Subheading 3.7 after harvesting the organs from the euthanized mouse to obtain fluorescence images of all the individual organs.
2. Use the steps in Subheading 3.8 to create a new spectral library for the organs. Organ autofluorescence needs to be determined from a sacked control animal that does not contain any fluorophore.
3. Load images of treated organs (by clicking *Load Cube*) and click *Unmix* to find the amount of fluorescence coming from the fluorophore.
4. If desired, save all images by clicking *File* > *Save Image* > *Save All Images.*
5. Drag fluorophore image (image with the border that corresponds to the fluorophore color) to a new *Compare Image* window (Subheading 3.8, **step 5**) (*see* **Note 14**) to the next open spot and change the color map from gray to jet. This will make it easier to differentiate the different intensity values in the images (*see* **Note 15**).
6. Repeat **steps 3** and **5** for all the different organs studied to obtain a qualitative comparison (Fig. 11).
7. Repeat steps in Subheading 3.10 to obtain quantitative fluorescence intensity measurements.

4 Notes

1. The field of view is dependent on the size of the object that you are imaging. Putting the camera further from the sample results in a wider field of view. When imaging bigger plates or more animals, a longer field of view is called for (Fig. 12).

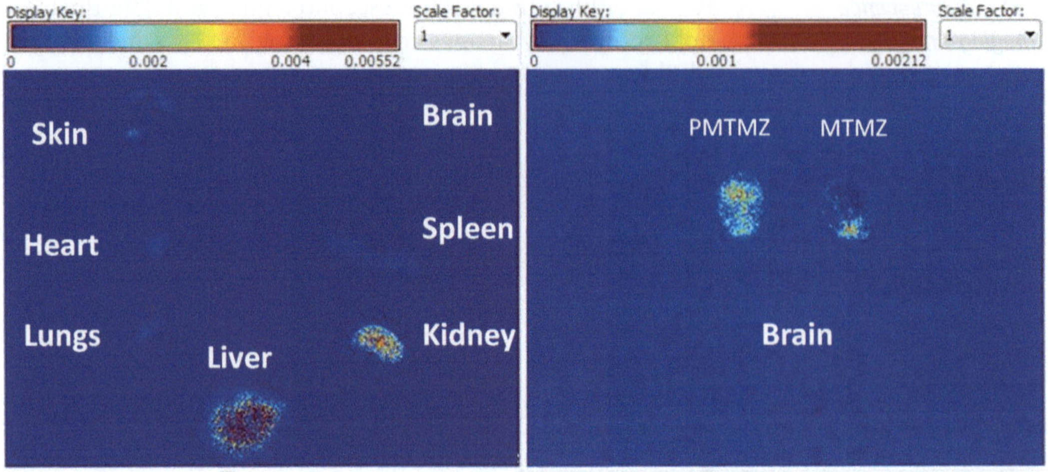

Fig. 11 *Left* Amount of fluorescence captured by the different major excised mice organs after euthanasia (24 h after drug injection). *Right* Fluorescence arising from the excised brain, the brain on the left was treated with a glioblastoma targeted drug particle, while the brain on the right was untargeted

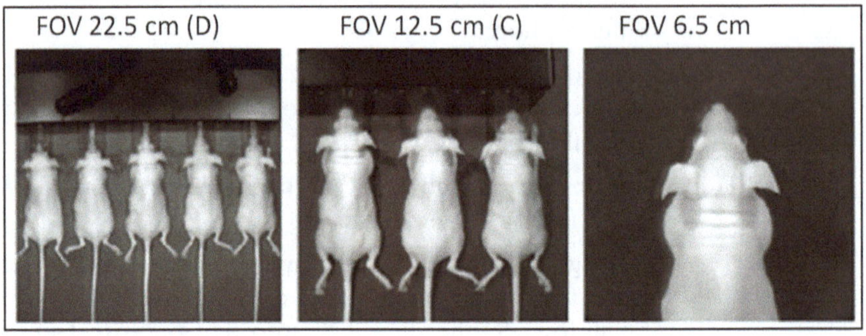

Fig. 12 Field of view options for whole animals on the PerkinElmer IVIS spectrum. Modified from PerkinElmer, IVIS Spectrum product note

2. Imaging can either be done manually by setting a timer and acquiring an image every minute or by setting up an imaging sequence (*Add and Acquire Sequence*). While setting up an imaging sequence, the number of segments and the time delay needs to be chosen appropriately. For example, 6 segments with a delay of 3 min will take a total of 6 images one at 3, 6, 9, 12, 15, and 18 min after the addition of luciferin (Fig. 3). When working with animals, the animals must be completely anesthetized before starting because for the entire duration of the imaging sequence, the door cannot be opened. Furthermore, only the first photograph taken is used for the projection of the luminescence so you will not be able to see if the mice changed positions.

3. Exposure time, binning and f/stop (lens aperture) are settings on the machine that control the sensitivity of the measurement. There is a fine balance between sensitivity and measuring noise. At higher exposure times, more photons are collected, but this diminishes throughput and increases the chances of measuring noise. Be aware that at very high exposure times, long exposure times can saturate the camera with lumens and no further differences can be measured. The lens aperture determines the amount of photons that reach the CCD camera. F/1 is a wide open lens which is the default setting for bioluminescent studies. Lastly, the amount of binning will determine the resolution of the image. Binning combines multiple pixels into a single pixel. Higher binning numbers increase the sensitivity of the image but simultaneously lower the resolution of the image and reduce the exposure time. The interplay between all these parameters will determine the quality of the final image. Using auto-exposure, the machine will try and determine the most optimal settings for the experiment. In general, start with an exposure time of 1 min. If the signal is too bright, lower the exposure time. If the signal is not detectable, increase the exposure time. Keep in mind that when making a comparison over multiple time points, the exposure time needs to be consistent. For this reason, more so in fluorescence imaging, images are acquired with more than one exposure time. This is because initially it is not known how long of an exposure time is needed to get a signal from a small amount of drugs (preferentially in the tumor). To prevent having to redo the experiment, acquire several different fluorescent images with exposure times ranging from 500 to 4000 ms.
4. Ideally, the tumor is between 1 and 3 cm in size. If the tumor is too small, there will not be enough vascularization for appropriate drug delivery and tumors above 3 cm in size are considered inhumane. Time between implantation and imaging is highly dependent on the type of tumor cell implanted. On average with glioblastoma U87-MG cells, we begin imaging at day 7 to determine the tumor size.
5. This step is dependent on the type of reporter gene used. When using luciferase, the bioluminescent activity usually peaks within 20 min after injection.
6. Exercise caution when reimaging your animals because a background signal can arise from residual luciferin within the mouse. Pre-imaging the animal becomes increasingly more important here.
7. As a general rule of thumb, start with the concentration that you hypothesize results in an appropriate drug delivery. From this concentration, both add and subtract a logarithm and

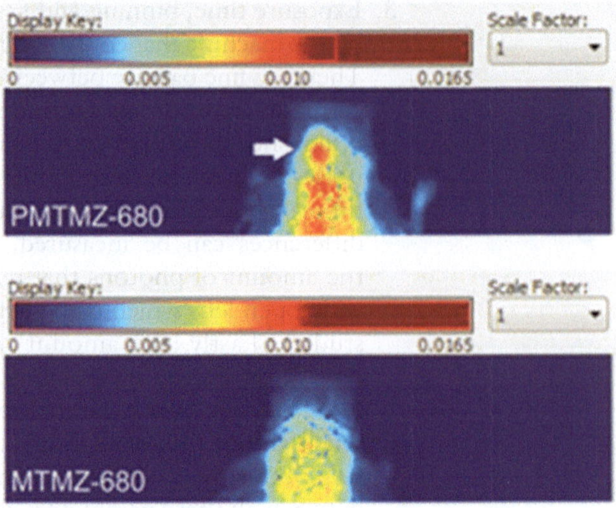

Fig. 13 Fluorescence hotmap from mice orthotopically implanted U87-luciferase cells, intravenously injected with either targeted or untargeted drug particles. Mice were covered with white paper to suppress the fluorescence arising from the rest of the body

determine the fluorescence from all three dilutions. First of all, this step will confirm that your particles are detectable by the instrument and allow you to determine the emitting spectrum. Furthermore, by determining the amount of fluorescence in each of the dilutions, the efficiency of conjugation can be assessed as well. For example, when 1 μM of particles results in only moderate fluorescence, it is a good indicator that the conjugation step was not optimal.

8. When studying drug delivery to the brain, we are often presented with a relatively low signal arising from the brain as compared compared to the signal coming from organs involved in drug elimination. To deal with this, we often acquire an additional image in which we cover up the body of the mouse with black paper and only measure the fluorescence coming from the head. Note, that in this case, you also need to pre-image the covered mouse to optimally determine the autofluorescence signal for accurate processing (Fig.13).
9. When transferring spectra to your library, make sure nothing is already stored under the spectrum number that you choose. The program will overwrite the spectra. For example, if you already have a fluorophore spectrum stored in Channel 1, make sure you start numbering your autofluorescence channels from Channel 2 and beyond.
10. There are two ways of identifying the different autofluorescence channels. We recommend the use of the RCA as

described in the Methods sections. Although when RCA fails, another possibility is to more precisely draw your own channels. Namely, you can fill in the channels yourself by clicking on the *Draw* icon (next to the channels on the left of the screen) and draw a line in the different areas that you think have different fluorescence spectra. When you are done, click *Unmix* and continue from Subheading 3.8, **step 4**.

11. On the top of the screen it says "You can click once for Signal and twice for background." Technically, this animal has no fluorescence, so the image only consists of background signals. However, the auto-fluorescence is most likely made up of different channels, as you can only choose one background channel, we will treat everything here as a signal.

12. *Find Spectra* will show you the different spectra arising from the signals that you chose. If some of the spectra overlap, it is better to choose one of the signals. These images represent the same fluorescence pattern and the program will have a hard time unmixing the signals in the following steps.

13. When there are parts of the image highlighted in the fluorophore channel, this signal needs to be removed. More channels need to be added, representing these channels that were captured in the fluorophore channel. This will remove them from this channel and put them in their respective autofluorescence channel. You can either go back to the RCA or click on the images that resembles the region that you are looking for. For example, if you see the stage and part of the skin light up in the fluorophore channel (Fig. 14a.), you need to go back to the RCA button and choose a signal that looks like the autofluorescence of the stage and/or skin. Another possible way of removing these channels is by clicking on the *Draw* icon of the next available channel to add a new channel. Here we can manually add a channel for skin and for the stage by drawing on them (Fig. 14b). Click *Unmix* again and see if the fluorophore channel is almost empty. Repeat these steps until you get a satisfactory result. Note that It will be very hard to remove all the background noise.

14. If you accidentally close the *Compare Image* window, reload the pre-image (*Load Cube*) and click *Unmix*. Drag the image corresponding to the fluorophore to the first box in the *Compare Image* window (*Tools* > *Compare Images*). This will be your reference point as this image represents native fluorescence in the fluorophore channel.

15. Note how the scale has changed to the highest value found in all the images and how the program rescales the images. The background noise becomes barely visible anymore because it has much lower values than the values inside the images that we

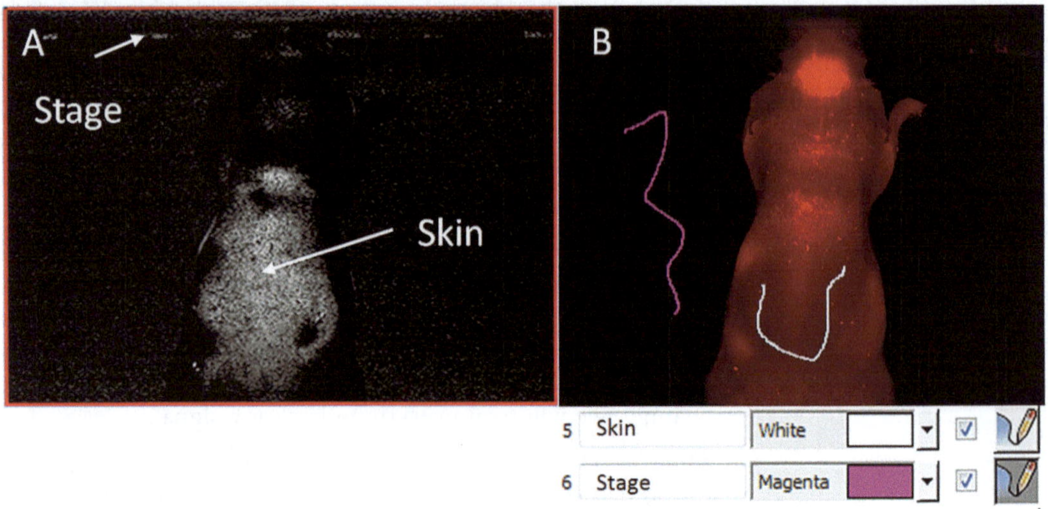

Fig. 14 (**a**) After unmixing, for each channel in the spectral library an image opens representing the amount of fluorescence captured by that channel. This figure shows fluorescence captured by the fluorophore channel before injection of the fluorophore. This channel is contaminated by autofluorescence of both skin and stage. In pre-injected animals this channel needs to be as close to zero as possible. (**b**) To remove fluorophore channel contamination assign extra channels to the spectral library for autofluorescence arising from background sources such as skin and stage

added. Sometimes an image has a spot with very high fluorescence, which will drastically change the scale. For example, sometimes the fluorescence at the injection site at time point 1 can overshadow high amounts of fluorescence at the later time points. When this occurs use a different compare image window (*Tools > Compare Images*) and remove the image at this time point.

16. The ROI can be moved by right clicking on the image and selecting the *Move Region* option. This may be necessary if the animals were placed on the exact same location between the different study time points.
17. Depending on the fluorescence intensity, sometimes the image does not display the full body contour, which can make it difficult to place your ROI. A possible solution is to change the contrast at the Display tab (for example, to −1). After placing the ROI, the original image contrast can be restored by clicking on *Restore to Default* (Fig. 15).

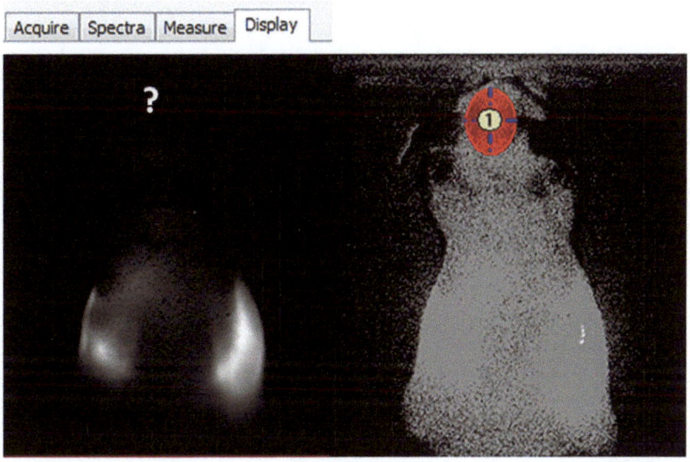

Fig. 15 When placing regions of interests, it is possible that not the whole animal is visible. Play with the image contrast under the *Display* tab to reveal the entire animal, simplifying the placement of the region of interest

References

1. Sandhu GS, Solorio L, Broome AM, Salem N, Kolthammer J, Shah T, Flask C, Duerk JL (2010) Whole animal imaging. Syst Biol Med 2 (4):398–421
2. Kelkar M, De A (2012) Bioluminescence based in vivo screening technologies. Curr Opin Pharmacol 12(5):592–600
3. Arranz A, Ripoll J (2015) Advances in optical imaging for pharmacological studies. Front Pharmacol 6:189
4. Leblond F, Davis SC, Valdés PA, Pogue BW (2010) Pre-clinical whole-body fluorescence imaging: review of instruments, methods and applications. J Photochem Photobiol B 98 (1):77–94
5. Miller K, Dixit S, Bredlau A, Moore A, McKinnon E, Broome AM (2016) Delivery of a drug cache to glioma cells overexpressing platelet-derived growth factor receptor using lipid nanocarriers. Nanomedicine 11(6):581–595
6. Wang B, Su JL, Amiran J, Litovsky SH, Smalling R, Emelianov S (2010) Detection of lipid in atherosclerotic vessels using ultrasound-guided spectroscopic intravascular photoacoustic imaging. Opt Express 18(5):4889–4897

Chapter 18

An Ultrasensitive Biosensing Platform Employing Acetylcholinesterase and Gold Nanoparticles

Dingbin Liu and Xiaoyuan Chen

Abstract

Enzyme-linked immunosorbent assay (ELISA) is a well-known strategy for biomarker detection with a color change, which can be seen by the naked eyes. However, the moderate sensitivity of conventional ELISA limits its applications in many cases where the concentrations of biomarker are very low, such as cancer diagnosis. Here we describe an ultrasensitive colorimetric assay based on acetylcholinesterase (AChE)-catalyzed hydrolysis reaction, whose products trigger the aggregation of gold nanoparticles (AuNPs), causing a distinct color change of the solution from red to purple. This enhanced colorimetric immunoassay offers extremely high sensitivity and specificity. In this study, we employed enterovirus 71 (EV71), the major cause of hand, foot, and mouth disease (HFMD), as a model to evaluate the analytical performance of the plasmonic immunoassay.

Key words Gold nanoparticles, Colorimetric immunoassay, Acetylcholinesterase, Magnetic beads, Signal amplification

1 Introduction

ELISA has received intense attention owing to its advantages such as high throughput detection and no requirement of sophisticated instruments. However, both the detection sensitivity and specificity of the commonly used clinical ELISAs are unable to fulfill the requirements for early diagnosis and monitoring of fatal diseases [1, 2]. For example, ELISA is the gold standard for cancer biomarker detection, whose detection limit is about 0.1 ng/mL. This value is generally higher than the concentrations of cancer biomarker in most serum samples especially at their early stages or after radical prostatectomy. Therefore, ELISA usually allows detection only after biomarker levels have already reached critical threshold concentrations, at which point the disease has already advanced markedly. Therefore, improvement of detection sensitivity as well as specificity is the key of cancer diagnostics. Over the past two decades, AuNP-based assays have drawn considerable research

Reema Zeineldin (ed.), *Cancer Nanotechnology: Methods and Protocols*, Methods in Molecular Biology, vol. 1530, DOI 10.1007/978-1-4939-6646-2_18, © Springer Science+Business Media New York 2017

interests owing to their distinct physical and optical properties [3]. For example, solutions containing mono-dispersed AuNPs display a ruby red color, while the presence of analytes can induce the formation of AuNP aggregates, thus leading to a red-to-blue color change [4]. The color change upon aggregation of AuNPs has been increasingly utilized for colorimetric sensing of biomarkers [5, 6]. Particularly, the extremely high extinction coefficients of AuNPs make them a perfect alternative to organic molecules (e.g., 3,3′,5,5′-tetramethylbenzidine, TMB), which generally serve as the substrate for the labeled enzymes in conventional ELISAs [7]. We therefore designed such an immunoassay by employing AuNPs to generate detection signals.

In our study, the AChE-induced aggregation of AuNPs and magnetic beads were integrated into the immunoassays to induce high signal amplification (Fig. 1). To do this, detection antibodies are conjugated with AChE, which catalyzes its substrate acetylthiocholine (ATC, an analog of acetylcholine) to generate thiocholine. Thiocholine can be adsorbed on the Au surface via Au-S bond and

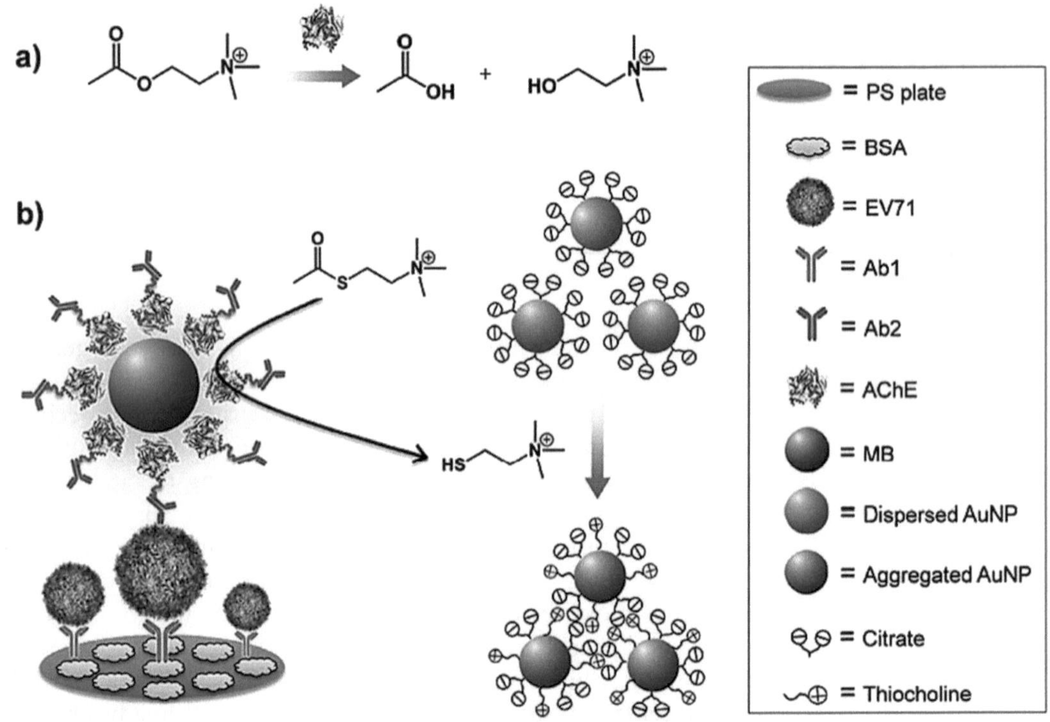

Fig. 1 The design of acetylcholinesterase (AChE)-catalyzed hydrolysis reaction for the colorimetric detection of EV71. (**a**) AChE catalyzes the hydrolysis of acetylcholine to generate acetate and choline. (**b**) Scheme of the improved sandwich ELISA format. EV71 is pulled down onto the polystyrene (PS) substrate by capture antibody (Ab1) and recognized by detection antibody (Ab2) which is conjugated with AChE on magnetic bead (MB). In the presence of acetylthiocholine (ATC) and citrate-covered AuNPs, AChE catalyzes the hydrolysis of ATC to generate thiocholine, thus inducing the aggregation of AuNPs via electrostatic interaction

cause aggregation of the citrate-capped AuNPs owing to the electrostatic interactions [8]. This aggregation event can be transformed into color change of the AuNP solution from red to purple. In addition, magnetic beads can load a large number of AChE. After the normal immunoassay operation, very small amount of analyte can thus be detected most likely due to the high density of AChE on magnetic beads where the AChE activity is still preserved. To evaluate the sensitivity and specificity of the plasmonic immunoassay, EV71 in clinically relevant samples was employed as a model and compared with polymerase chain reaction (PCR). This plasmonic immunoassay was further simplified and employed to detect *Treponema pallidum* antibodies [9].

2 Materials

Prepare all solutions using deionized water (Milli-Q grade, Millipore) with a resistivity of 18.2 MΩ-cm (at 25 °C). Prepare all reagents and store them at room temperature unless indicated otherwise. Diligently follow all waste disposal regulations when disposing waste materials.

1. 10 mg/mL N-hydroxysuccinimide-activated magnetic beads (NHS-MBs) with a diameter of around 1 μm (Fisher Scientific, Dallas, TX, USA).
2. Phosphate-buffered saline (PBS, 10×, pH 7.4): 1.37 M NaCl, 27 mM KCl, 100 mM Na_2HPO_4, and 20 mM KH_2PO_4.
3. PBST: PBS (1×, pH 7.4) containing 0.05 % Tween 20 (*see* **Note 1**).
4. Tris buffered saline: 50 mM Tris–HCl, 138 mM NaCl, 2.7 mM KCl, pH 8.0.
5. 1 mM ice-cold HCl solution: (*see* **Note 2**).
6. 100 mg/mL AChE: Weight 10 mg AChE and transfer to a 1 mL centrifuge tube. Add water to a volume of 0.1 mL. Store at −20 °C (*see* **Note 3**).
7. 100 mM NHS-activated azide: Dissolve 0.1 g NHS-activated azide in 2.6 mL dry DMSO before diluting in final reaction buffer. Store the as-prepared solution at −20 °C (*see* **Note 4**).
8. 100 mM NHS-activated dibenzocyclooctyl (DBCO): The procedure is similar to that for preparing NHS-activated azide, i.e., Dissolve 0.1 g NHS-activated DBCO into 1.54 mL dry DMSO. Store at −20 °C.
9. 3 mg/mL secondary anti-EV71 antibody (EV71-Ab2): Provided by the National Institute of Diagnostics and Vaccine Development in Infectious Disease in China.

10. A centrifugal filter device with a 30 K Nominal Molecular Weight Limit (NMWL).
11. AChE assay kit (*see* **Note 5**).
12. Prepare 100 mM methoxyl poly(ethyleneglycol) amine ($mPEG-NH_2$, MW = 2000) with dry DMSO.
13. 1 % (w/v) bovine serum albumin (BSA): Dissolve 1 g BSA in 100 mL PBS. Store at 4 °C.
14. 96-well polystyrene plates.
15. 3 mg/mL monoclonal primary anti-EV71 antibody (EV71-Ab1): Provided by the National Institute of Diagnostics and Vaccine Development in Infectious Disease in China.
16. 2.3 nM citrate-stabilized AuNPs with a diameter of 15 nm (*see* **Note 6**).
17. 1 M acetylthiocholine (ATC): Dissovle 289 mg ATC into 1 mL deionized water. Store at 4 °C (*see* **Note 7**).
18. 10^{11} copies/mL Cultured EV71 isolates: Provided by the National Institute of Diagnostics and Vaccine Development in Infectious Disease in China (*see* **Note 8**).
19. 1 M K_2CO_3 solution: Dissolve 138 mg K_2CO_3 into 1 mL deionized water.
20. 50 mM coating buffer: Dissolve the exactly pre-weighed carbonate–bicarbonate tablets with 50 mL deionized water and stir the solution for a few minutes. Make up to 100 mL with water and stir until full dissolution.
21. Human throat swab (HTS) samples: Collected from the hospitals in Xiamen of China (*see* **Note 9**).
22. 1 M Quenching buffer (Tris–HCl, pH 8): Dissolve the exactly pre-weighed powder in a pouch with 900 mL deionized water and stir the solution for several minutes. Make up to 1000 mL with water and stir until full dissolution.

3 Methods

Carry out all procedures at room temperature unless otherwise specified.

3.1 Conjugation of DBCO to Ab2

1. Prepare 100 mM NHS-activated DBCO by dissolving the compounds (0.1 g) in 1.54 mL dry DMSO before diluting in final reaction buffer.
2. Prepare 1 mg/mL EV71-Ab2 with PBS.
3. Dilute the as-prepared NHS-activated DBCO to be 10 mM using dry DMSO. Mix 33 μL of the resulted NHS ester with the 1 mg/mL EV71-Ab2 solution at a 50:1 mol ratio and allow them to be incubated at room temperature for 30 min.

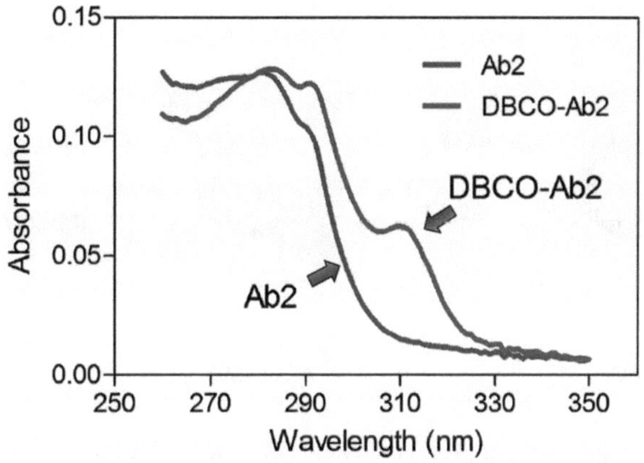

Fig. 2 UV–vis absorption spectra of purified EV71 detection antibody (Ab2, *blue line*) and that labeled with DBCO moieties (DBCO-Ab2, *green line*). The absorption band at 309 nm indicates the DBCO moieties on Ab2

4. Stop the reaction by adding quenching buffer to a final concentration of 50 mM Tris and allow the quenching reaction to proceed at room temperature for 5 min. Purify the resulting products with a centrifugal filter device (Amicon Ultra-0.5, Millipore) with a 30 K Nominal Molecular Weight Limit (NMWL).
5. The obtained products display a new absorption peak at around 309 nm (Fig. 2), which is attributed to the DBCO moieties on DBCO-Ab2 [10]. We can determine the number of DBCO on each Ab2 by means of the absorbance scan of the purified product. On the basis of the Beer-Lambert law,

$$\text{Number DBCO per Ab2} = \frac{A_{309}\text{DBCO} \times \varepsilon_{280}\text{Ab2}}{\varepsilon_{309}\text{DBCO} \times A_{280\text{C}}\text{Ab2}} \quad (1)$$

where A_{309} DBCO is the absorbance of DBCO-Ab2 at 309 nm; ε_{309} DBCO and ε_{280} Ab2 represent the extinction coefficients of DBCO (12,000 $M^{-1}cm^{-1}$) and Ab2 (204,000 $M^{-1}cm^{-1}$), respectively; A_{280C} Ab2 is the corrected absorbance of DBCO-Ab2 at 280 nm, which can be calculated by the equation A_{280C} Ab2 = A_{280} Ab2—(A_{309} DBCO × CF_{DBCO}), where A_{280} Ab2 is the absorbance of DBCO-Ab2 at 280 nm; CF_{DBCO} is the correction factor at 280 nm (1.089). In combination with the absorbance as shown in Fig. 2, the average number of DBCO per Ab2 was calculated to be 17.

3.2 Preparation of Ab2-AChE-MBs

Figure 3 shows the step-by-step procedure for the preparation of Ab2-AChE-MBs.

1. Place 100 μL of NHS-activated MBs (10 mg/mL) into a 1.5 mL microcentrifuge tube and remove the supernatant with a magnetic stand (*see* **Note 10**).

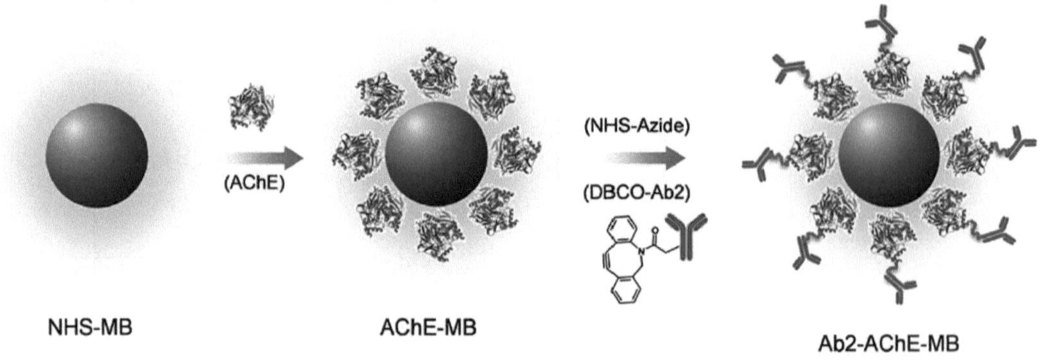

Fig. 3 Procedure of preparing Ab2-AChE-MB. AChE molecules are coated onto MB through NHS chemistry. The AChE-MB further reacts with NHS-azide, and then conjugates with DBCO-Ab2 via copper-free click chemistry to form Ab2-AChE-MB

2. Activate the purified NHS-activated MBs by adding ice-cold HCl solution (1 mM) to wash the beads.
3. Mix the activated beads with 100 μL of AChE (1.0 mg/mL) in PBS using a vortex for 30 s. Incubate the mixture for 2 h at room temperature on a rotator. During the first 30 min of the incubation, mix the solution using a vortex for 15 s every 5 min. For the remaining time, mix the solution using a vortex for 15 s every 15 min until the reaction was complete (*see* **Note 11**).
4. Once obtain the AChE-loaded MBs, measure the activity of the anchored AChE by using AChE assay kit. By means of the equation,

$$\text{AChE activity} = \frac{\text{OD}_{10\text{min}} - \text{OD}_{2\text{min}}}{\text{OD}_{\text{Cal}} - \text{OD}_{\text{H}_2\text{O}}} \times n \times 200(\text{U/L}) \tag{2}$$

where $\text{OD}_{10\text{min}}$ and $\text{OD}_{2\text{min}}$ are the OD_{412} values of the samples at 10 min and 2 min, respectively; OD_{Cal} and OD_{H2O} are the values of the calibrator and water at 10 min; n is the dilution factor, the activity of the anchored AChE was calculated to be 15.7 U/mL. Since covalent conjugation may cause some loss of enzyme activity, it is therefore necessary to calculate the remaining AChE activity after loading onto MBs. The theoretical AChE activity on MB was calculated to be 17.6 U/mL by subtracting the excess AChE from the added AChE. Therefore, 89.1 % (15.7/17.6 × 100 %) of the original AChE activity (1256 U/mg protein) was maintained after the conjugation and its activity was decreased to be 1119 U/mg protein. Based on this finding, the amount of the loaded AChE was calculated to be 14.03 μg/mL (=3.1 × 10^{13}AChE/mL). Since the concentration of MBs was roughly 10^9 particles/mL, we estimate the number of AChE per MB to be 31,000.

5. Add 10 μL of mPEG-NH_2 (MW = 2000, 100 mM) into 1 mL of the obtained AChE-MBs (1 mg/mL) to block the unreacted NHS ester. Incubate the mixture at room temperature for 2 h and purify the products with a magnetic stand.
6. In order to conjugate with DBCO-Ab2, modify the AChE-MBs with azide groups by adding 5 μL of NHS-activated azide (1 mM) into the obtained AChE-MB solution. Incubate the resulting solution at room temperature for 30 min and purify the products with a magnetic stand.
7. Mix the resulting azide-modified AChE-MBs (1 mL, 1 mg/mL) with the as-prepared DBCO-Ab2 (10 μL, 1 mg/mL) and incubate the resulting mixture at room temperature for 2 h. Collect the resulting Ab2-AChE-MBs puriy the product with a magnetic stand for further use.

3.3 Identification of AuNP-Based Probe

1. Optimize the pH value of the citrate-AuNPs (15 nm, 2.3 nM) to be around 8.0 by adding K_2CO_3 solution (1 mM) where AChE may hold maximal activity when reacting with its substrate [11] (*see* **Note 12**).
2. Add different concentrations of Ab2-AChE-MBs into the solutions composed of 100 μL of the as-prepared citrate-AuNPs (2.3 nM) and ATC (20 μM). The final concentrations of the beads are in the range from 1.0 to 20 × 10^3 particles/mL. Incubate the mixtures at room temperature for 10 min (*see* **Note 13**).
3. Collect the absorbance of the samples at 520 and 700 nm by a Synergy 2 Multi-Mode Microplate Reader every 1 min during the hydrolysis of ATC.
4. Figure 4 shows the plots of A_{700}/A_{520} (the ratio of absorbance at 700 and 520 nm) values versus the incubation time (0–10 min) for various concentrations of Ab2-AChE-MB. Within the incubation time, the A_{700}/A_{520} values increased except for the blank sample, whose A_{700}/A_{520} values had negligible changes.

3.4 AuNP-Based Colorimetric Immunoassay for EV71 Detection

Conduct the immunoassay detection in the commonly used 96-well polystyrene (PS) plates.

1. Add the anti-EV71 capture antibodies (Abl, 4 μg/mL) into the wells of the PS plate and incubate at 4 °C overnight.
2. After rinsing with PBS for three runs, add 1 % bovine serum albumin (BSA) into each well as blocking agent to minimize the nonspecific binding when conducting the immunoassay detection.
3. Add EV71-spiked PBS and HTS solutions respectively at concentrations ranging from 10^4 to 10^8 copies/mL, and Set the

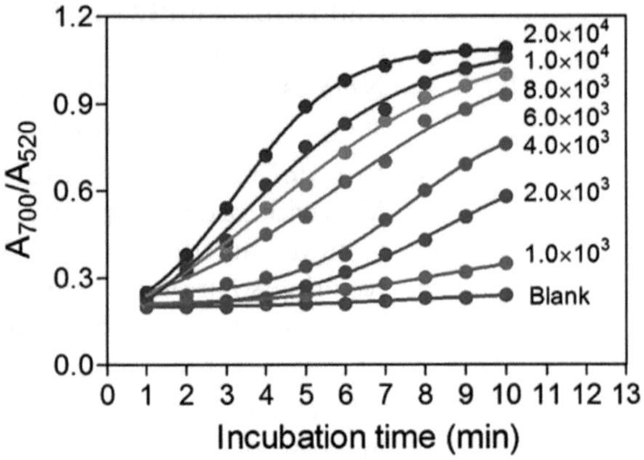

Fig. 4 Plots of A_{700}/A_{520} values of citrate-AuNP solutions incubated with ATC (20 μM) and different concentrations (1.0–20 × 10^3 particles/mL) of Ab2-AChE-MB versus incubation time (0–10 min). Collect the absorbance at 520 and 700 nm simultaneously every 1 min by a Synergy 2 Multi-Mode Microplate Reader. Set the citrate-AuNP solution incubated with ATC (20 μM) alone as the blank

PBS- only and HTS-only solutions as the blank. Keep the plate at 37 °C for 1 h and wash the wells with PBS for three runs.

4. Add 100 μL of Ab2-AChE-MB (0.1 mg/mL) solutions into each well, and incubate for 20 min. Add 200 μL of PBST into each well and rinse for three runs (*see* **Note 14**).
5. Add 100 μL of the mixture composed of ATC (20 μM) and citrate-AuNPs (15 nm, 2.3 nM) at pH = 8.0 into each well. Collect the absorbance at 520 and 700 nm by a Synergy 2 Multi-Mode Microplate Reader.
6. Calculate the A_{700}/A_{520} values for each sample, and compare the values among various concentrations of EV71 (*see* **Note 15**).

4 Notes

1. Dilute 100 mL of 10× concentrated PBS to 990 mL with deionized water and add 10 mL of 5 % Tween-20. Care should be taken to add Tween-20 solution, since it makes bubbles. PBST was used mainly as the diluent.
2. Dilute 1 mL of concentrated HCl (37 %, 12 M) to 12 mL with ice-cold water. 1 mL of the resulted HCl (1 M) was further diluted to 1 L by adding 999 mL ice-cold water. Finally, 1 mM of diluted HCl was achieved with pH 3.
3. To maintain the enzyme activity of AChE, it should be prepared with deionized water in a relatively high concentration (100 mg/mL), and store at −20 °C. When used, the

concentrated AChE can be diluted to the desired concentrations with PBS.

4. Since the NHS ester tend to degrade in the presence of water, dry DMSO was used to dissolve the NHS ester powder to a relatively high concentration (100 mM), so as to minimize the possible degradation. When used to react with amine derivatives, the concentrated NHS ester can be diluted to the desired concentrations with dry DMSO.
5. The working reagent was freshly prepared before the measurements. Ab2-AChE-MBs solutions were diluted to desired folds by using assay buffer. 10 μL of each solution was added into separate wells in a 96-well polystyrene plate, followed by adding 190 μL of working reagent into the wells and mixed thoroughly. Meanwhile, 200 μL of calibrator and 200 μL of H_2O were added into separate wells, respectively. The plate was placed in a plate reader to collect the optical density (OD) values at 412 nm at 2 and 10 min.
6. The commerically avalaible citrate-stabilized AuNPs are sensitive to enviromental conditions such as high salts and high/low temperature, under which the native AuNPs tend to aggregate. It should be avoided to contaminate the native AuNPs with PBS owing to its high ionic strength. Also note that the native AuNPs should be stored at 4 °C.
7. In aqueous solutions, ATC could be hydrolyzed into thiocholine and acetic acid. To minimize the nonspecific hydrolysis, ATC should be concentrated to a high concentration (1 M) and stored at 4 °C. Dilute the concentrated ATC solution to the desired concentrations when conducting the detection.
8. Cultured EV71 isolates (~10^{11} copies/mL) were diluted with Dulbecco's Modified Eagle's Medium (DMEM, GIBCO) to the desired concentrations. Care should be taken to handle the samples, since it possesses possible biosafety issues.
9. The clinical samples were prepared in DMEM and stored at −80 °C for further use. The handling of these samples followed all necessary safety precautions in BSL-2 laboratories.
10. To keep dispersity of the beads in the process of transport and storage, they are commonly stabilized by supernatants. The supernatants should be removed by a magnetic stand before activating the beads.
11. Owing to their big size, the magnetic beads tend to precipitate in the process of modification, thus the reaction should be conducted on a rotator. Importantly, the tube should be mixed using a vortex frequently in the whole process.
12. The original pH value of citrate-stabilized AuNPs solution is usually 4~5 because of the presence of citric acid. However, the

maximal activity of AChE is usually at pH 8. So it is necessary to adjust the pH value of the solution to around 8 by adding K_2CO_3 whose final concentration is 1 mM.

13. Long time of incubation of ATC in aqueous solutions may lead to degradation of ATC even in the absence of AChE, thereby it is necessary to set the citrate-AuNP solution incubated with ATC (20 μM) alone as the blank.
14. Rinsing the wells with 200 μL of PBST three times will help remove a bulk of the nonspecific adsorption of the beads.
15. By measuring the A_{700}/A_{520} value for various concentrations of EV71, we observed that the A_{700}/A_{520} values for both EV71-spiked PBS and HTS samples had a similar trend: increasing gradually from around 0.5 to 1.0 as the amount of EV71 added was increased.

Acknowledgment

We acknowledge the support from the National Natural Science Foundation of China (Grants 21475066 and 81401463), the Fundamental Research Funds for Central Universities (China), and the Intramural Research Program (IRP) of the National Institute of Biomedical Imaging and Bioengineering, National Institutes of Health.

References

1. Park JS, Cho MK, Lee EJ, Ahn KY, Lee KE, Jung JH et al (2009) A highly sensitive and selective diagnostic assay based on virus nanoparticles. Nat Nanotechnol 4:259–264
2. Rissin DM, Kan CW, Campbell TG, Howes SC, Fournier DR, Song L et al (2010) Single-molecule enzyme-linked immunosorbent assay detects serum proteins at subfemtomolar concentrations. Nat Biotechnol 28:595–599
3. Rosi NL, Mirkin CA (2005) Nanostructures in biodiagnostics. Chem Rev 105:1547–1562
4. Liu D, Qu W, Chen W, Zhang W, Wang Z, Jiang X (2010) Highly sensitive, colorimetric detection of mercury(II) in aqueous media by quaternary ammonium group-capped gold nanoparticles at room temperature. Anal Chem 82:9606–9610
5. Zagorovsky K, Chan WCW (2013) A plasmonic DNAzyme strategy for point-of-care genetic detection of infectious pathogens. Angew Chem Int Ed 52:3168–3171
6. Liu JW, Lu Y (2006) Fast colorimetric sensing of adenosine and cocaine based on a general sensor design involving aptamers and nanoparticles. Angew Chem Int Ed 45:90–94
7. De la Rica R, Stevens MM (2012) Plasmonic ELISA for the ultrasensitive detection of disease biomarkers with the naked eye. Nat Nanotechnol 7:821–824
8. Liu D, Wang Z, Jin A, Huang X, Sun X, Wang F et al (2013) Acetylcholinesterase-catalyzed hydrolysis allows ultrasensitive detection of pathogens with the naked eye. Angew Chem Int Ed 52:14065–14069
9. Nie XM, Huang R, Dong CX, Tang LJ, Gui R, Jiang JH (2014) Plasmonic ELISA for the ultrasensitive detection of treponema pallidum. Biosens Bioelectron 58:314–319
10. Marks IS, Kang JS, Jones BT, Landmark KJ, Cleland AJ, Taton TA (2011) Strain-promoted "click" chemistry for terminal labeling of DNA. Bioconjug Chem 22:1259–1263
11. Wang M, Gu XG, Zhang GX, Zhang DQ, Zhu DB (2009) Continuous colorimetric assay for acetylcholinesterase and inhibitor screening with gold nanoparticles. Langmuir 25:2504–2507

Part V

Nanotechnology-Based Therapies

Chapter 19

Gene Silencing Using Multifunctionalized Gold Nanoparticles for Cancer Therapy

Alexandra R. Fernandes and Pedro V. Baptista

Abstract

Multifunctionalized gold nanobeacons (Au-nanobeacon) combine, in a single and unique platform, targeting, detection and silencing providing an effective impact in clinics boosting cancer theranostics. Here, we describe a nano-integrated platform based on Au-nanobeacons able to detect and inhibit gene expression specifically in cancer cells. The surfaces of gold nanoparticles (AuNPs) are functionalized with targeting peptides to enhance tumor cell recognition and uptake, and with fluorescently labeled antisense DNA hairpin oligonucleotides to detect AuNPs. These oligonucleotides, upon recognition and hybridization to the target, open their structure resulting in separating apart the dye and the quencher allowing the fluorophore to emit light and to monitor the intracellular interactions of AuNPs with the target and the specific silencing of gene expression. This strategy allows inhibiting *KRAS* gene expression in colorectal carcinoma cell lines with no relevant toxicity for healthy fibroblasts. Importantly, this nano-integrated platform can be easily adapted to hybridize with any specific target thus providing real benefits for the diagnosis and treatment of cancer.

Key words Gold nanoparticles, Au-nanobeacon, Peptides, Gene silencing, Targeted delivery, Colorectal carcinoma cell lines, *KRAS*

1 Introduction

The fight against cancer has focused on the understanding of molecular and cellular events that lead to malignancy that can be used as molecular markers of disease, and eventually as targets for more precise and efficient chemotherapeutics, allowing to tackle cancer cell whilst sparing the healthy tissues. As such, one of the main challenges in cancer therapy has been the development of novel integrated systems capable of increasing the therapeutic index, which is only attained by improving the pharmacokinetic parameters of these drugs. Another issue has been the selectivity towards cancer cells and the precision of action. Ideally such systems ought to have increased circulating times in the blood stream without being detected and cleared by the immune system resulting

Reema Zeineldin (ed.), *Cancer Nanotechnology: Methods and Protocols*, Methods in Molecular Biology, vol. 1530,
DOI 10.1007/978-1-4939-6646-2_19,

in failed delivery to tumor cells, and should be able to simultaneously address disease diagnostics and treatment—theranostics. Nanotechnology has been addressing this challenge by offering a plethora of novel multifunctional nanodevices capable of bypassing biological barriers, specifically recognizing a desirable target and signaling it for effective gene silencing in cancer cells, thus reducing systemic toxicity and severe adverse side effects in healthy tissues [1–5]. AuNPs are prime nontoxic carriers for gene therapy due to their fine chemical properties and ease of surface modification with a multiplicity of ligands (e.g., targeting moieties, silencing moieties, or therapeutic loads) [6–10]. Nanotechnology and AuNPs in particular have put forward several unconventional strategies largely spinning around the concept of precision medicine to improve the limited therapeutic outcomes for several types of cancers [1].

Oligonucleotide-based therapeutics have been under clinical development since the early 90s and antisense DNA constitutes a powerful tool for specific posttranscriptional gene silencing [11–13]. The development of nanocarriers for antisense-oligonucleotide targeted delivery could have a positive contribution in cancer therapy minimizing toxicity and side effects [13]. In fact, we have previously demonstrated that AuNPs functionalized with a fluorophore-labeled hairpin-DNA (Au-nanobeacon) may be used as a theranostics approach in antisense DNA/RNA interference (RNAi) [6, 10, 14]. The ease of translation of this concept to any cellular target(s) of interest with the ability to monitor in real time their therapeutic effects in cancer cells will, thus, be of uttermost importance in the development of successful anti-cancer strategies [6, 10, 13, 14].

Ras monomeric GTPases are transduction molecules that regulate cell proliferation, survival, and differentiation [15]. KRAS is one of the most commonly activated oncogenes in human cancer, with 17–25 % of all human tumors harboring an activating *Kras* mutation [16]. Thus, the relevance of the KRAS oncogene in cancer maintenance and progression is well recognized together with its role in increasing resistance to conventional chemotherapies [17]. In this respect the search for KRAS-targeting therapies has long been high on the agenda of cancer therapeutics [17–19].

The protocol described here details the synthesis and characterization of a multifunctional Au-nanobeacon to detect and inhibit *KRAS* gene for a theranostic approach in colorectal carcinoma cells. The in vitro proof-of-concept may become a valuable tool in the lab to assist molecular studies and screening of cell targets, and might in the short term be extended to the clinics. The hairpin configuration and the proximity of the fluorophore to the AuNPs' surface quenches fluorescence emission, whereas recognition and hybridization to the KRAS mRNA restores fluorescence emission due to the opening of the hairpin allowing tracking the silencing in real time. The Au-nanobeacons may also be functionalized with targeting moieties (e.g., RGD peptide) for tumor specific targeting (Fig. 1).

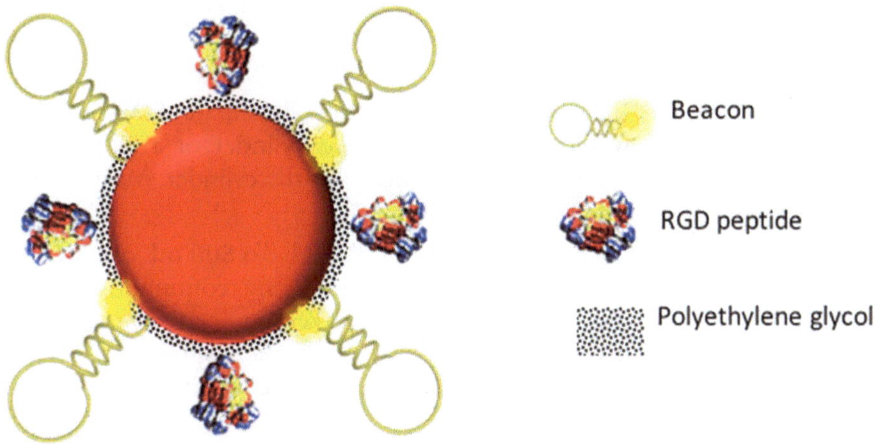

Fig. 1 Multifunctional Au-nanobeacons addressed in this protocol for specific detection and inhibition of *KRAS* gene in cancer cells

2 Materials

Prepare all solutions using ultrapure water (prepared by deionizing water to attain a sensitivity of 18 MΩ cm at 25 °C) and analytical grade reagents. Prepare and store all reagents at room temperature (unless indicated otherwise). Follow all waste disposal regulations when disposing of waste materials. Wear gloves in all the procedures.

2.1 Design of Beacon

Several tools to design and evaluate sequence stability are freely available from the web and may be used to assist hairpin assembly:

1. http://www.broadinstitute.org/rnai/public/seq/search
2. http://blast.ncbi.nlm.nih.gov/Blast.cgi
3. http://www.basic.northwestern.edu/biotools/oligocalc.html

2.2 Synthesis of Citrate Gold Nanoparticles

1. 1 mM gold(III) chloride trihydrate, hydrogen tetrachloroaurate ($HAuCl_4$). Add about 100 mL water to a 1-L graduated cylinder or a glass beaker. Weigh 339.79 mg $HAuCl_4$ and transfer to the cylinder. Make up to 1 L with water.
2. 38.8 mM sodium citrate tribasic dihydrate. Add about 100 mL water to a 1-L graduated cylinder or a glass beaker. Weigh 5.71 mg $HAuCl_4$ and transfer to the cylinder. Make up to 1 L with water.

2.3 Synthesis of PEGylated Gold Nanoparticles

1. 1 mg/mL SH-EG(8)-$(CH_2)_2$-COOH (alpha-Thio-omega-(propionic acid) octa(ethylene glycol)—PEG-COOH).

2. 1 mg/mL SH-$(CH_2)_3$-CONH-EG(6)-$(CH_2)_2$-N_3 (*N*-(20-azido-3,6,9,12,15,18-hexaoxoicosane)-4-mercaptobutanamide—PEG-N_3).
3. 0.028 % (w/v) Sodium dodecyl sulfate (SDS). Prepare 100 mL water to a 1 L graduated cylinder or a glass beaker. Weigh 0.28 g SDS and transfer to the cylinder. Make up to 1 L with water (*see* **Note 1**).
4. 2 M stock solution of NaOH. To 800 mL of water, slowly add 80 g of NaOH pellets, stirring continuously. As an added precaution, place the beaker on ice. When the pellets have dissolved completely, adjust the volume to 1 L with H_2O. Store the solution in a plastic container at room temperature (*see* **Note 2**).
5. Diethylpyrocarbonate (DEPC) (*see* **Note 3**).
6. DEPC-treated water. Add 0.1 mL DEPC for each 100 mL of water to be treated (i.e., 0.1 % (v/v) DEPC) and shake vigorously to bring the DEPC into solution. Incubate the solution at least 1 h at 37 °C. Autoclave at least 15 min to inactivate any traces of DEPC. Store at 4 °C until use (*see* **Note 3**).
7. 0.05 mg/mL of 5,5′-dithio-bis-(2-nitrobenzoic acid) (DTNB, Sigma, Cat. No. D8130). Prepare 1 mL water to a 1.5 mL microfuge tube. Weigh 0.05 mg DTNB and transfer to the microfuge tube.
8. 1 M dibasic sodium phosphate (Na_2HPO_4). Weight 14.2 g Na_2HPO_4 and adjust the volume to 100 mL with H_2O.
9. 1 M monobasic sodium phosphate (NaH_2PO_4). Weight 12 g Na_2HPO_4 and adjust the volume to 100 mL with H_2O.
10. 1 M phosphate buffer solution (pH 7): Mix 57.7 mL of 1 M Na_2HPO_4 and 42.3 mL of 1 M NaH_2PO_4. Sterilize by autoclaving and store at 4 °C until use.
11. 0.5 M phosphate buffer solution (pH 7): Add 100 mL of 1 M phosphate buffer solution and adjust the volume to 200 mL with H_2O. Sterilize by autoclaving and store at 4 °C until use.

2.4 Functionalization of PEGylated Gold Nanoparticles for Cancer Cell Targeting

1. Arginine-Glycine-Aspartic Acid (G-RGD-S)-Peptide (RGD peptide, MW 490.47 Da).
2. 25 mM 2-(*N*-morpholino)ethanesulfonic acid (MES) (pH 6.1). Dissolve 4.88 g MES in 800 mL of water. Adjust the pH to the desired value with 10 M NaOH. Bring up the volume to 1 L with water.
3. 1-ethyl-3-(3-dimethylaminopropyl)carbodiimide.
4. Sulfo-hydroxysuccinimide sodium salt (sulfo-NHS).
5. Pierce™ BCA Protein Assay Kit (Thermo Fisher Scientific, Cat. No. 23225).

Table 1
Thiol-DNA-hairpin Cy3 sequences

Nanobeacon	Sequence
Anti-*KRAS*	5′-AAACGCCAGCTAATTCAGAATCATTGCGTTT-3′
Non-sense	5′-TTTGCCCCGTTACTATTTGCACCACGGCAAA-3′

2.5 Synthesis of Gold Nanobeacons

1. Antisense gold Nanobeacon—a stem-looped oligonucleotide double labeled with 3′-Cy3 and 5′-Thiol-C6 (complementary to the KRAS target sequence) (*see* Table 1 for thiol-DNA-hairpin Cy3 sequence).
2. Nonsense gold Nanobeacon—a stem-looped oligonucleotide of unrelated sequence double labeled with 3′-Cy3 and 5′-Thiol-C6 (*see* Table 1 for thiol-DNA-hairpin Cy3 sequences).
3. 0.1 M dithiothreitol (DTT). Prepare 100 mL water to a 1-L graduated cylinder or a glass beaker. Weigh 15.43 g DTT and transfer to the cylinder. Make up to 1 L with water (*see* **Note 4**).
4. Ethyl Acetate.
5. Illustra™ NAP™-5 columns Sephadex™ G-25 DNA grade (GE Healthcare Life Sciences, Cat. No. 17-0853-02).
6. 10 mM phosphate buffer solution (pH 8): Mix 9.32 mM Na_2HPO_4 and 0.68 mM NaH_2PO_4. Sterilize by autoclaving and store at 4 °C until use.
7. 0.01 % (w/v) SDS. Prepare 100 mL water to a 1-L graduated cylinder or a glass beaker. Weigh 0.1 g SDS and transfer to the cylinder. Make up to 1 L with water (*see* **Note 1**).
8. 2 % (w/v) SDS. Prepare 100 mL water to a 1-L graduated cylinder or a glass beaker. Weigh 20 g SDS and transfer to the cylinder. Make up to 1 L with water (*see* **Note 1**).
9. 50 mM Sodium chloride (NaCl). Prepare 100 mL water to a 1-L graduated cylinder or a glass beaker. Weigh 2.922 g NaCl and transfer to the cylinder. Make up to 1 L with water.
10. 0.3 M NaCl. Prepare 100 mL water to a 1-L graduated cylinder or a glass beaker. Weigh 17.532 g NaCl and transfer to the cylinder. Make up to 1 L with water.
11. 0.5 M phosphate buffer solution (pH 7): Mix 288.55 mM Na_2HPO_4 and 211.45 mM NaH_2PO_4 to get a pH of 7.0. Sterilize by autoclaving and store at 4 °C until use.
12. AGE I solution: 2 % (w/v) SDS, 10 mM phosphate buffer (pH 8). Sterilize by filtration (0.22 μm) and store at 4 °C until use. Warm up to 25 °C before use.
13. AGE II solution: 1.5 M NaCl, 0.01 % (w/v) SDS, 10 mM phosphate buffer (pH 8). Sterilize by filtration (0.22 μm) and store at 4 °C until use. Warm up to 25 °C before use.

14. DEPC-treated water. *See* **item 6** under Subheading 2.3.
15. Ultrasound water bath.

2.6 Specificity Assays for Gold Nanobeacons

1. KRAS (NM_004985) Human cDNA ORF Clone (Origene, Cat. No. RC201958).
2. 1 M phosphate buffer solution (pH 7): Mix 57.7 mL of 1 M Na_2HPO_4 and 42.3 mL of 1 M NaH_2PO_4. Sterilize by autoclaving and store at 4 °C until use.
3. 10 mM of phosphate buffer (pH 7). Add 10 mL 1 M phosphate buffer solution (pH 7) and make up to 1 L with water.

2.7 In Vitro Gold Nanobeacons Delivery

1. Human cells to be transfected. A wide range of adherent cells (e.g., Human colorectal carcinoma HCT116 cell line (ATCC® CCL-247™)) can be used, and the choice of cells should take into consideration the desired gene silencing effect.
2. Dulbecco's modified Eagle's medium (DMEM).
3. 10 % heat inactivated fetal bovine serum (FBS).
4. 100 U/mL penicillin and 100 μg/mL streptomycin.
5. CO_2 cell culture incubator.

2.8 Silencing KRAS Expression with Antisense Au-Nanobeacons

1. Dulbecco's modified Eagle's medium (DMEM).
2. Phosphate-Buffered Saline (PBS) (10×) pH 7.4.
3. PBS (1×). Add 100 mL of PBS (10×) to a 1-L graduated cylinder or a glass beaker and make up to 1 L with water.
4. TRIsure® (Bioline, Cat. No. BIO-38033).
5. 75 % ethanol. Add 75 volumes of absolute ethanol to 25 volumes of DEPC-treated water. Store at −20 °C until use.
6. NZY First-Strand cDNA Synthesis Kit (NZYTEC, Cat. No. MB12501).
7. Primer forward and reverse for *KRAS* gene (Table 2).
8. Primer forward and reverse for rRNA18S5gene (Table 2) [20].
9. 5× HOT FIREPol® EvaGreen® qPCR Mix Plus (ROX) (Solis BioDyne; Cat. No. 08-24-00001).
10. Bio-Rad Protein Assay Kit I (Bio-Rad, Cat. No. 5000001).

Table 2
Sequence of forward and reverse primers used for *KRAS* and *rRNA18S5* genes amplification and size of the PCR product

Gene	Forward primer (5′–3′)	Reverse primer (5′–3′)	Size of PCR product (bp)
KRAS	TTGTGGACGAATATGATCCAA	TGACCTGCTGTGTCGAGAAT	100
rRNA18S5	GTAACCCGTTGAACCCCATT	CCATCCAATCGGTAGTAGCG	151

2.9 Cytotoxicity Evaluation

1. CellTiter 96® AQueous One Solution Cell Proliferation Assay (MTS) (Promega, Cat. No. G3582).
2. 96-well microplate reader.

2.10 Selective Targeting

1. Paraformaldehyde solution 4 % in PBS (Santa Cruz Biotechnology, Cat. No. CAS 30525-89-4).
2. ProLong® Gold Antifade Reagent with DAPI (Invitrogen, Cat. No. P-36931).
3. Primary Dermal Fibroblast Normal; Human, Neonatal (ATCC® PCS-201-010).
4. TrypLE™ Express (Thermo Fisher Scientific, Cat. No. 12605-010).
5. ImageJ software (downloaded from http://imagej.nih.gov/ij/).

3 Methods

Carry out all procedures at room temperature (RT) unless otherwise specified.

3.1 Nanobeacon Design

To attain excellent gene silencing effects it is crucial to use computational tools based on experimental data to increase the possibility of selecting effective target sequences, since not all sequences that are complementary to a given target mRNA are similarly effective. Algorithms and tools to design sequences such as that from the Whitehead Institute for Biomedical Research (http://sirna.wi.mit.edu/) or the Broad Institute (http://www.broadinstitute.org/rnai/public/seq/search) are an example. In order to analyze the specificity for the desirable target, avoiding cross homology, *BLAST* analysis should be performed (http://blast.ncbi.nlm.nih.gov/Blast.cgi). Secondary structures caused by self-complementary in the oligonucleotide sequence should be avoided and for that *OligoCalc* (http://www.basic.northwestern.edu/biotools/oligocalc.html) and *NUPACK* nucleic acid package (http://www.nupack.org/) may be used. *See* Table 1 for the sequences obtained.

3.2 Synthesis of Citrate Gold Nanoparticles

AuNPs are synthesized by the citrate reduction method described by Lee and Meisel [21]. Briefly:

1. Prepare aqua regia by mixing 3:1 concentrated HCl–HNO_3 in a large and open container in a fume hood (*see* **Note 5**).
2. Immerse in the freshly prepared aqua regia a 500 mL rounded bottom two-neck flask, magnetic stir bar, stopper, condenser, and a 250 mL Erlenmeyer for at least 15 min. Wash carefully all the glassware with filtered water.

3. Add 225 mL of a 1 mM $HAuCl_4$ into the rounded bottom two-neck flask and place the flask in the hot plate with respective adaptor.
4. Place the stirrer inside the flask, connect the condenser to one neck of the flask and place the stopper in the other neck. Put the flask on the hot plate to reflux while stirring.
5. When reflux begins, remove the stopper and add 25 mL of 38.8 mM sodium citrate solution. Place the stopper back into the rounded bottom two-neck flask. Allow the system to reflux for another 30 min (*see* **Note 6**).
6. Turn the system off.
7. Let the system to cool down to RT (23–25 °C) under stirring (protect from light).
8. The solution shall be transferred to a 250 mL Erlenmeyer flask with a ground glass cap. Characterize the synthesized citrate capped AuNPs by UV–visible Spectrophotometry and Transmission Electron Microscopy (TEM) [6] (*see* **Note 7**).
9. Calculate the AuNPs concentration via Lambert–Beer equation using the absorbance and the molar absorptivity of the AuNPs (typical Surface Plasmon Resonance peak at 520 nm (*see* **Note 8**).
10. The AuNPs are stable for several months at RT (stored in a glass container previously treated with aqua regia) (*see* **Note 9**).

3.3 Synthesis of PEGylated-Gold Nanoparticles

Functionalization of citrate AuNPs (at 25 % saturated surface) is carried out using equal amounts of two bifunctional spacers (PEG) with a thiol end to bond covalently to the AuNP. The other functional group at the other end is either an azide group (SH-$(CH_2)_3$-CONH-EG(6)-$(CH_2)_2$-N_3(PEG-N_3)) or a carboxylic groups (SH-EG(8)-$(CH_2)_2$-COOH (PEG-COOH)) for the other spacer. These end groups can act as substrates for 1-Ethyl-3-(3-dimethylaminopropyl)-carbodiimide (EDC)/*N*-Hydroxysuccinimide (NHS) coupling reactions (*see* **Note 10**).

1. Mix 41.7 mL of a 12 nM stock solution of citrate AuNPs (final concentration, 10 nM) with 150 μL of a 1 mg/mL stock solution of PEG-N_3 (final concentration, 7 μM) and 150 μL of a 1 mg/mL stock solution of PEG-COOH (final concentration, 7 μM) in an aqueous solution of SDS (0.028 %). Incubate for 10 min.
2. Add 625 μL of a 2 M stock solution of NaOH (final concentration of 25 mM) and incubate the mixture for 16 h at RT.
3. Centrifuge the mixture to remove the excess of PEG that did not bind to citrate AuNPs (14,000 × *g* for 30 min at 4 °C) (*see* **Note 11**).

4. Remove the supernatant (*see* **Note 12**) and resuspend the precipitate in DEPC-treated water.
5. Determine the concentration of the PEGylated AuNPs using the same methodology as described in Subheading 3.2 (**step 9**).
6. Calculate the amount of thiolated chains attached per AuNP based on the Ellman's assay using the following procedure: mix 100 μL of phosphate buffer 0.5 M (pH 7) with the appropriate amount of stock solutions of PEG for each concentration and add water to a final volume of 300 μL to be used as a concentration standard for generating a calibration curve; Mix 200 μL of the supernatant retrieved in **step 5** with 100 μL of phosphate buffer 0.5 M (pH 7); Add 7 μL of 0.05 mg/mL DNTB to both of these mixtures and incubate for 15 min at room temperature (RT); Take a UV–visible absorption spectrum (300–600 nm) of each of the mixtures and record the absorbance values at 412 nm (*see* **Note 13**).

3.4 Functionalization of PEGylated AuNPs for Targeting Cancer Cells

PEGylated AuNPs are functionalized with Arg-Gly-Asp (RGD peptide) amino acid sequence by EDC/NHS coupling reaction between the carboxylated spacer and the amine terminal group of the RGD peptide [13]. Functionalization can be performed with other peptides of interest (e.g., TAT peptide [22]).

1. For a 200 μL reaction: Incubate 20 nM of PEGylated AuNPs and RGD (final concentration of 0.5 mM) with 6 mM sulfo-*N*-hydroxysulfosuccinimide sodium salt and EDC in 25 mM MES buffer pH 6.1 for 16 h at RT.
2. Centrifuge the mixture (14,000 × *g* for 30 min at 4 °C) to remove the excess of unbound RGD peptide.
3. The supernatants are recovered and tested for protein concentration using the BCA Protein Assay Kit following the manufacturer specifications.
4. To determine the RGD coverage on PEGylated AuNPs@RGD subtract the amount of RGD in the supernatant to the amount of RGD added in **step 1**.

3.5 Synthesis of Gold Nanobeacons

Two different sequences of nanobeacons were prepared: a nanobeacon anti-KRAS (detects and inhibits *KRAS* mRNA) and a nanobeacon nonsense (designed to not hybridize with any target within the genome) (Table 1 for thiol-DNA-hairpin Cy3 sequences). Briefly:

1. Mix the thiolated oligonucleotides with DTT to attain a final concentration of 0.1 M. Incubate for at least 2 h at 4 °C.
2. Extract one volume (100–500 μL) of thiolated oligonucleotide with two volumes of ethyl acetate. Mix thoroughly.

3. Centrifuge (5 min at 21,000 × *g*) and discard the upper organic phase.
4. Repeat **steps 2** and **3** two more times.
5. Purify the mixture through a desalting NAP-5 column (eluent—10 mM phosphate buffer (pH 8)).
6. Quantify the purified oligonucleotide by UV–visible spectroscopy (*see* **Note 14**).
7. Mix the determined volume of the purified oligonucleotides with 10 nM of PEGylated AuNPs@RGD (prepared in Subheading 3.4) to result in a 1:100 PEGylated AuNPs@RGD–oligonucleotide ratio.
8. Add AGE I solution to the mixture to achieve a final concentration of 10 mM phosphate buffer (pH 8) and 0.01 % (w/v) SDS.
9. Sonicate the AuNPs mixture for 10 s (in an ultrasound bath) and incubated for 20 min at RT.
10. Add a specific volume of AGE II solution (final concentration of 10 mM phosphate buffer (pH 8), 0.3 M NaCl, 0.01 % (w/v) SDS) to the AuNPs mixture in order to increase the ionic strength of the solution sequentially (50 mM NaCl increments). After each increment, the AuNPs mixture is sonicated (10 s) and incubated at RT for 20 min before the next increment.
11. Leave the solution to rest for 16 h at RT.
12. Centrifuge the Au-nanobeacons (20 min, 21,000 RCF). There should be an oily precipitate at the bottom of the microfuge tube. Remove a fixed amount of supernatant and store it. Redisperse the precipitate in the same volume of DEPC-treated water (*see* **Note 15**).
13. Repeat **step 12** two more times.
14. Prepare a calibration curve (designated as calibration curve A within the range: 0.1–10 μmol of oligonucleotide) by mixing an appropriate amount of fluorescent oligonucleotide with AGE I and AGE II solutions to obtain a final volume of 100 μL (final concentration of 10 mM phosphate buffer (pH 8), 0.3 M NaCl and 0.01 % (w/v) SDS).
15. Prepare a second calibration curve (designated as calibration curve B; range 0.1–2.5 μmol of the oligonucleotide) by mixing an appropriate amount of fluorescent oligonucleotide with DEPC-treated water.
16. Take the fluorescence spectra of each of the mixtures for calibration curve A and B. Then take the spectra for the supernatants recovered in **steps 12** and **13** (*see* **Note 16**).
17. Determine the area under the curve from the emission spectra. Determine the amount of fluorescent oligonucleotide that is

present in each supernatant (use calibration curve A for the supernatant recovered in **step 12** and calibration curve B for the supernatants recovered in **step 13**).

18. Calculate the amount of oligonucleotides present at the surface of the Au-nanobeacon (subtract the results from **step 17** from the amount of oligonucleotides added in **step** 7.
19. Characterize the Au-nanobeacons by determining the hydrodynamic radius using Dynamic Light Scattering (DLS) and the surface charge through Zeta Potential [6].
20. Store the Au-nanobeacons at 4 °C in the dark (no loss of fluorescence signal or signs of aggregation at least for 3 months).

3.6 Specificity Assays for Gold Nanobeacons

1. For the detection of specific target add 5 nM of complementary KRAS target (Sigma) to 2.5 nM of nanobeacon anti-KRAS and to 2.5 nM of nanobeacon nonsense (negative control) in 10 mM of phosphate buffer pH 7.
2. Incubate the reactions for 120 min at 37 °C while recording the fluorescence intensity every 2 min at an excitation wavelength of 550 nm for Cy3-labeled gold nanobeacons in a microplate reader (*see* **Note 17**).

3.7 In Vitro Gold Nanobeacon Delivery

1. Colorectal carcinoma cell line (HCT116) are grown in DMEM supplemented with 10 % heat inactivated fetal bovine serum, 100 U/mL penicillin and 100 μg/mL streptomycin and maintained at 37 °C in 5 % CO_2.
2. Cells are seeded at a density of 1×10^5 cells/well in 24-well plates (prepare replicate plates to collect RNA after incubating with anti-sense or non-sense beacons for 0, 24, 48, and 72 h) and grown for 24 h prior to incubation with the Au-nanobeacons.
3. Check the cell density using an inverted optical microscope. Cells must be 50–80 % confluence at the incubation time with Au-nanobeacons.

3.8 Silencing KRAS Expression with Antisense Au-Nanobeacons

1. Incubate cells with 30 nM of Antisense Au-nanobeacons for *KRAS* silencing in DMEM Medium. Shake well to ensure even distribution of nanoparticles in the well (*see* **Note 18**).
2. After 24, 48 and 72 h, wash cells with 500 μL of 1× PBS.
3. Assess gene silencing effects by extracting total RNA to use for reverse-transcriptase quantitative PCR (RT-qPCR).
4. Extract total RNA using any suitable method. We describe here the protocol that we are currently using based on the single step method developed by Chomczynski and Sacchi [23].

5. Isolate Total RNA from HCT116 cell lines incubated with or without the Au-nanobeacons using TRIsure® (use 1 mL of TRIsure per 5 × 10^6 cells).
6. Lyse cells with 1 mL of TRIsure® and pass the lysate several times through a pipette tip and vortex.
7. Incubate samples for 5 min at RT.
8. Add 0.2 mL of chloroform (per 1 mL of TRIsure® used). Shake vigorously by hand for 15 s.
9. Incubate samples for 2–3 min at RT. Centrifuge samples (25,000 × *g* for 15 min at 4 °C) (*see* **Note 19**).
10. Transfer the aqueous phase to another microfuge tube. Precipitate the RNA with 0.5 mL of isopropyl alcohol (per 1 mL of TRIsure® used).
11. Incubate samples for 10 min at RT and centrifuge (25,000 × *g* for 10 min at 4 °C).
12. Wash the pellet with 75 % ethanol (add 1 mL of ethanol per 1 mL of TRIsure® used). Vortex samples and centrifuge (9000 × *g* for 5 min at 4 °C).
13. Air-dry the pellet for 10 min and dissolve in 25–50 μL of DEPC-treated water by pipetting the solution up and down and incubating for 10 min at 55 °C.
14. Store RNA at −80 °C or proceed with cDNA synthesis.
15. Synthesize cDNA using NZY First-Strand cDNA Synthesis Kit (according to the manufacturer specifications) using 500 ng of total RNA.
16. Perform RT-qPCR using primers described in Table 2. *rRNA18S5* was used as a reference gene. For each set of primers, briefly (20 μL final volume): mix 4 μL (1×) of 5× HOT FIREPol EvaGreen qPCR Mix Plus (Solis BioDyne), 10 ng/μL of cDNA template, and $MgCl_2$ and primers mix according to Table 3. Add PCR water to a final volume of 20 μL. At least three independent reactions should be processed in a thermocycler following the program described in Table 4.

Table 3
Concentrations of magnesium chloride and forward and reverse primer mixtures used for RT-qPCR of *rRNA18S5* and *KRAS* genes

Gene	$MgCl_2$ (mM)	Forward and reverse primers mix (pmol/μL)
KRAS	3.5	0.08
rRNA18S5	2	0.1

Table 4
RT-qPCR program used to amplify *rRNA18S5* and *KRAS* genes

	KRAS		*rRNA18S5*		
	Temperature (°C)	Time	Temperature (°C)	Time	Cycles
Initial denaturation	95	15 min	95	3 min	1
Denaturation	95	15 s	95	15 s	45
Annealing	50	15 s	59	20 s	
Extension	72	15 s	72	20 s	
Final extension	72	3 min	72	3 min	1

17. Gene expression is determined using the $2^{-\Delta\Delta CT}$ method as described in [20]. Briefly, the Ct values from each sample (exposed to antisense Au-nanobeacon or Nonsense Au-nanobeacon) are normalized with the respective Ct values of housekeeping gene *rRNA18S5 obtaining a* ΔCt value. The ΔCt values from the antisense Au-nanobeacon are normalized with the ΔCt values from the Nonsense Au-nanobeacon obtaining the respectives ΔΔCt values. The mean ± SEM of the biological replicates is calculated. The final $2^{-\Delta\Delta CT}$ value representing the gene expression level of *KRAS* gene is calculated (Fig. 2).

3.9 Measuring KRAS Fluorescence from Cell Lysates

1. Lyse cells (e.g., osmotic shock by incubating in 100 μL of water and sonicate for 5 min).
2. Pipette the cell lysate several times and vortex the mixture to ensure cell disruption. Keep lysates on ice (*see* **Note 20**).
3. Centrifuge cell lysates (25,000 × *g* at 4 °C for 5 min).
4. Remove the microfuge tubes from the centrifuge. The supernatant should be clear. Recover supernatants.
5. Measure fluorescence using 100 μL of supernatant in a spectrofluorimeter (*see* **Note 16**).
6. Determine the total protein concentration of each sample using the BCA assay (Subheading 3.4) (*see* **Note 21**).
7. All the KRAS fluorescence values should be normalized to the protein concentration. The normalized fluorescence values for each sample should be normalized for the untreated controls to determine percent of *KRAS* gene silencing.

3.10 Cytotoxicity Evaluation

1. After 0, 24, 48 and 72 h of HCT116 cell incubation in the presence or absence of each Au-nanobeacon formulation, cell viability was evaluated with the CellTiter 96® AQueous Non-Radioactive Cell Proliferation Assay and performed accordingly with [24]. The CellTiter 96® AQueous Assay is composed of a

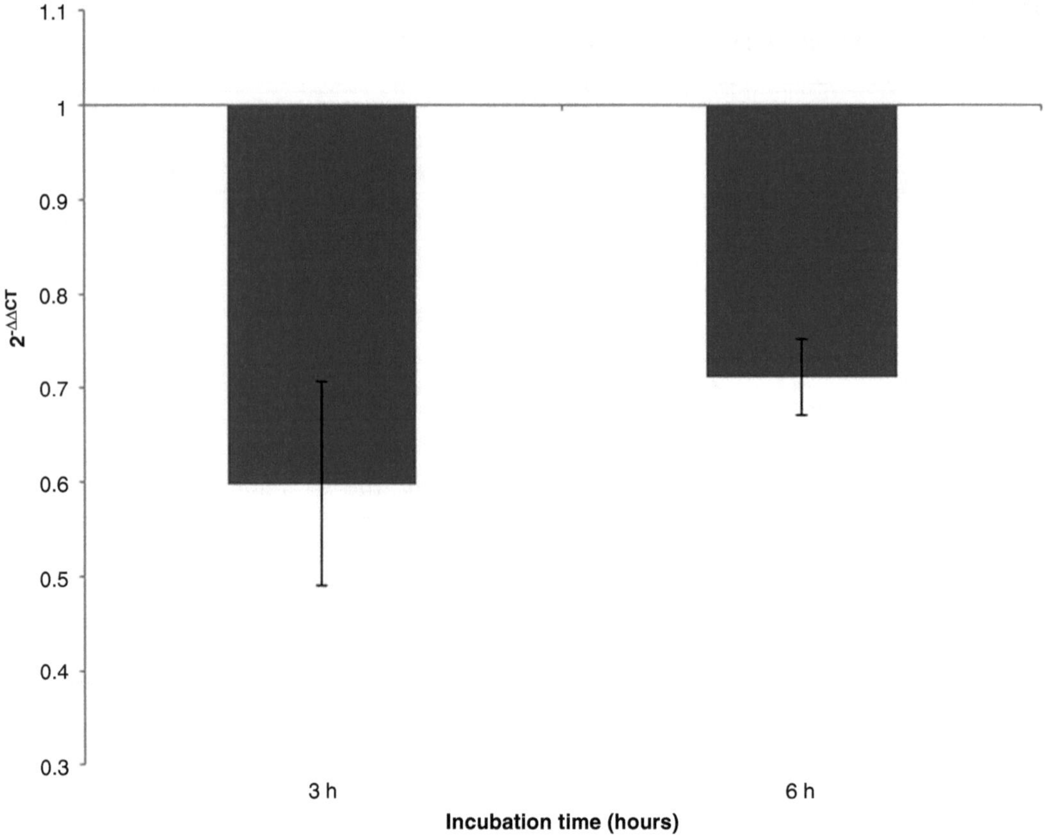

Fig. 2 Silencing of *KRAS* gene expression in HCT116 cell line after incubation in the presence of Antisense Au-nanobeacon for 3 and 6 h. $2^{-\Delta\Delta CT}$ values were normalized with the respective Ct values of housekeeping gene *rRNA18S5* and with samples exposed to Nonsense Au-nanobeacon. Data are the mean ± SEM of four biological replicates

solution of MTS and an electron coupling reagent (phenazine-methosulfate, PMS). MTS is bioreduced by dehydrogenase enzymes found in metabolically active cells into a formazan product that is soluble in tissue culture medium. Briefly,

2. Thaw the CellTiter 96® AQueous One Solution Reagent. It should take approximately 90 min at RT or 10 min in a water bath at 37 °C.
3. Pipet 20 μL of CellTiter 96® AQueous One Solution Reagent into each well of the 96-well assay plate containing the samples in 100 μL of culture medium.
4. Incubate the plate at 37 °C for 1 h in a humidified, 5 % (v/v) CO_2 atmosphere.
5. Record the absorbance at 490 nm using a 96-well microplate reader. The quantity of formazan product measured at 490 nm is directly proportional to the number of viable cells in culture.

3.11 Examination of Selective Targeting Using Fluorescence Microscopy

1. HCT116 cells and fibroblasts primary cultures are seeded at a concentration of 1 × 10^5 cells/well in 24-well plates on glass slides in 500 mL of DMEM with 10 % heat-inactivated fetal bovine serum and maintained at 37 °C 5 % CO_2.
2. Following exposure to different Au-nanobeacons for 0, 24, 48 and 72 h, HCT116 cell line and Fibroblasts cultures preparations are washed with 1× PBS and readily fixed with 4 % (v/v) paraformaldehyde in 1× PBS1 for 15 min at RT.
3. After three washing steps with 1× PBS, glass slide preparations are mounted in ProLong® Gold Antifade Reagent with DAPI to allow for nuclear staining.
4. Immunofluorescent images of HCT116 cell line and Fibroblasts primary cell culture are acquired using a confocal fluorescence microscope and a digital camera.
5. Cell count and fluorescence quantification is performed for all the conditions (*see* **Note 16**).
6. Cell number count and fluorescence quantification data is assessed through ImageJ software.

3.12 Examination of Selective Targeting Using Flow Cytometry

Fluorescence may also be assessed by Flow cytometry. Briefly,

1. Seed HCT-116 cells and fibroblasts primary culture separately on 35 mm plates at a concentration of 1 × 10^5 cells/well in 2000 μL of DMEM with 10 % heat-inactivated fetal bovine serum and culture at 37 °C 5 % CO_2.
2. Following exposure to Au-Nanobeacons (0, 24, 48 and 72 h), cells are washed with 1× PBS.
3. Extract cells by trypsinization and transfer to 2 mL microfuge tubes (*see* **Note 22**).
4. Cell samples were analyzed by flow cytometry on an Attune® Acoustic Focusing Flow Cytometer (Life Technologies, Carlsbad, California), through the acquisition of at least 10,000 events for each experimental condition.

4 Notes

1. *!CAUTION*. Wear mask when you are handling it. SDS is a respiratory tract irritant.
2. *!CAUTION* Wear gloves and mask when you are handling it. NaOH can cause chemical burns and may induce permanent blindness if it contacts eyes. Dissolution of NaOH is highly exothermic, which can cause breakage of glass containers and the resulting heat may cause heat burns or ignite flammables. Prepare this solution with extreme care in plastic beakers.

3. *!CAUTION.* Be careful when handling DEPC; it is combustible, unstable—readily decomposes, incompatible with strong oxidizing agents, strong acids, strong reducing agents, strong bases, ammonia. DEPC will react with primary amines and cannot be used directly to treat Tris buffers. DEPC is highly unstable in the presence of Tris buffers and decomposes rapidly into ethanol and CO_2. Residual DEPC must always be eliminated from solutions or vessels by autoclaving or heating to 100 °C for 15 min.
4. *!CAUTION.* DTT is an eye irritant.
5. *!CAUTION.* Be extremely careful when preparing and working with *aqua regia*. Wear goggles and gloves at all times, and perform all the experiment in a fume hood. *Aqua regia* should be freshly prepared and should never be stored in a closed vessel. Closed *aqua regia* containers may explode. Safe disposal should be performed by careful dilution and neutralization.
6. The initial pale yellow color of the Au(III) solution should become immediately colorless and then progressively change to deep red (Au(III) ions are reduced to Au(I) and when the solution becomes saturated of Au(I) atoms, they start to precipitate in the form of AuNPs). The citrate acts as capping and stabilizing agent covering the AuNPs' surface avoiding its aggregation [25].
7. The AuNPs produced should be red, have an average diameter of 14.0 nm (between 13 and 15 nm) and spherical under TEM [6].
8. Do not exceed an absorbance of 2 (avoid deviations to the Lambert–Beer law). Sample dilution should be considered when the measured absorbance exceeds 2. Take this dilution into consideration when calculating the original stock concentration.
9. Do not freeze the nanoparticles.
10. Since only 25 % of the AuNP is saturated with the PEG layer, the incorporation of additional thiolated components (e.g., a desired thiolated DNA-hairpin-Cy3) is possible.
11. A clear supernatant and an oily red precipitate should be observed after centrifugation.
12. Preserve the supernatant for subsequent analysis.
13. To determine the amount of PEG molecules bonded to the AuNPs' surface use the calibration curve to calculate the amount of PEG in the supernatant and subtract this value from the amount added to the AuNPs solution.
14. Use the extinction coefficient at 260 nm provided by the oligonucleotide manufacturer or calculate it through one of

the many available online tools (e.g., http://www.basic.northwestern.edu/biotools/oligocalc.html)) for quantification.

15. Be careful and do not disturb the precipitate while removing the supernatant. This can result in major losses of Au-nanobeacons and contamination of the supernatant with Au-nanobeacons.
16. Use a quartz cuvette for measuring fluorescence and the appropriate excitation, detection wavelengths and their respective slits (i.e., for Cy3 excite the fluorophore at 550 nm, collect the emission at 570 nm and use 5 nm slits).
17. Hybridization of the DNA hairpin to a complementary target (i.e., Kras mRNA) restores fluorescence emission due to the Au-nanobeacons' conformational reorganization (the fluorophore and the quencher to part from each other), yielding a quantitative response (increase fluorescence with time). The nonsense nanobeacon does not hybridize with any target and will not produce a quantitative response and no fluorescence increase with time will be observed.
18. Carry out a titration series of the various concentrations of fluorescent oligonucleotide functionalized on the AuNPs' surface to identify the most effective sequence and the lowest possible concentration that still generates the desired level of knockdown.
19. The sample will separate into three phases: (1) a pale green phenol–chloroform phase, (2) an interphase, and (3) a colorless upper aqueous phase (contains the RNA).
20. All cell lysates will be further used to quantify the total protein using the BCA assay.
21. The total protein concentration of each sample may also be measured using the Bradford assay [26].
22. Samples can be stored at 4 °C for up to 2 h. If analysis to be performed after longer time, then it is recommended to fix the cells by resuspending them in 0.5–1 mL PBS containing paraformaldehyde to a final concentration of 4 % (v/v) (10 min at 37 °C) and washing them 3× with PBS and storing them at 4 °C.

Acknowledgments

The authors acknowledge financial support from Fundação para a Ciência e Tecnologia/Ministérios da Ciência e do Ensino Superior (FCT/MCES)—UCIBIO (project UID/Multi/04378/2013 and cofinanced by ERDF under PT2020 Partnership Agreement POCI-01-0145-FEDER-007728).

References

1. Baptista PV (2014) Gold nanobeacons: a potential nanotheranostics platform. Nanomedicine (Lond) 9:2247–2250
2. Cabral RM, Baptista PV (2014) Anti-cancer precision theranostics: a focus on multifunctional gold nanoparticles. Expert Rev Mol Diagn 14:1041–1052
3. Baptista PV (2014) Nanodiagnostics: leaving the research lab to enter the clinics? Diagnosis 1:305–309
4. Gil PR, Parak WJ (2008) Composite nanoparticles take aim at cancer. ACS Nano 2:2200e5
5. Peer D, Karp JM, Hong S, Farokhzad OC, Margalit R, Langer R (2007) Nanocarriers as an emerging platform for cancer therapy. Nat Nanotechnol 2:751e60
6. Conde J, Rosa J, de la Fuente JM, Baptista PV (2013) Gold-nanobeacons for simultaneous gene specific silencing and intracellular tracking of the silencing events. Biomaterials 34:2516–2523
7. Conde J, Ambrosone A, Sanz V, Hernandez Y, Marchesano V, Tian F, Child H, Berry CC, Ibarra MR, Baptista PV, Tortiglione C, de la Fuente JM (2012) Design of multifunctional gold nanoparticles for in vitro and in vivo gene silencing. ACS Nano 6:8316–8324
8. Ghosh P, Han G, De M, Kim CK, Rotello VM (2008) Gold nanoparticles in delivery applications. Adv Drug Deliv Rev 60:1307e15
9. Conde J, Doria G, Baptista P (2012) Noble metal nanoparticles applications in cancer. J Drug Deliv 2012:751075
10. Conde J, Larguinho M, Cordeiro A et al (2014) Gold-nanobeacons for gene therapy: evaluation of genotoxicity, cell toxicity and proteome profiling analysis. Nanotoxicology 8:521–532
11. Modarresi F, Faghihi MA, Lopez-Toledano MA, Fatemi RP, Magistri M, Brothers SP, van der Brug MP, Wahlestedt C (2012) Inhibition of natural antisense transcripts in vivo results in gene-specific transcriptional upregulation. Nat Biotechnol 30:453–459
12. Fichou Y, Ferec C (2006) The potential of oligonucleotides for therapeutic applications. Trends Biotechnol 24:563–570
13. Moreno PMD, Pêgo AP (2014) Therapeutic antisense oligonucleotides against cancer: hurdling to the clinic. Front Chem 2:87
14. Rosa J, Conde J, de la Fuente JM, Lima JC, Baptista PV (2012) Gold-nanobeacons for real-time monitoring of RNA synthesis. Biosens Bioelectron 36:161–167
15. Jančík S, Drábek J, Radzioch D, Hajdúch M (2010) Clinical relevance of KRAS in human cancers. J Biomed Biotechnol 2010:150960
16. Kranenburg O (2005) The KRAS oncogene: past, present, and future. Biochim Biophys Acta 1756:81–82
17. Brito H, Martins AC, Lavrado J, Mendes E, Francisco AP, Santos SA et al (2015) Targeting KRAS oncogene in colon cancer cells with 7-Carboxylate indolo[3,2-b]quinoline tri-alkylamine derivatives. PLoS One 10:e0126891
18. Wang JH, Newbury LJ, Knisely AS, Monia B, Hendry BM, Sharpe CC (2012) Antisense knockdown of Kras inhibits fibrosis in a rat model of unilateral ureteric obstruction. Am J Pathol 180:82–90
19. Arrington AK, Heinrich EL, Lee W, Duldulao M, Patel S, Sanchez J, Garcia-Aguilar J, Kim J (2012) Prognostic and predictive roles of KRAS mutation in colorectal cancer. Int J Mol Sci 13:12153–12168
20. Luís DV, Silva J, Tomaz AI, de Almeida RFM, Larguinho M, Baptista PV, Martins LMDRS, Silva TFS, Borralho PM, Rodrigues CMP, Rodrigues AS, Pombeiro AJL, Fernandes AR (2014) Insights into the mechanisms underlying the anti-proliferative potential of a Co(II) coordination compound bearing 1,10-phenanthroline-5,6-dione: DNA and protein interaction studies. J Biol Inorg Chem 19:787–803
21. Lee PC, Meisel D (1982) Adsorption and surface-enhanced Raman of dyes on silver and gold sols. J Phys Chem 86:3391–3395
22. Sanz V, Conde J, Hernández Y, Baptista PV, Ibarra MR, de la Fuente JM (2012) Effect of PEG biofunctional spacers and TAT peptide on dsRNA loading on gold nanoparticles. J Nanoparticles Res 14:917 (9 pages)
23. Chomczynski P, Sacchi N (1987) Single-step method of RNA isolation by acid guanidinium thiocyanate-phenol-chloroform extraction. Anal Biochem 162:156–159
24. Silva TFS, Martins LMDRS, Guedes da Silva MF, Fernandes AR, Silva A, Borralho PM, Santos S, Rodrigues CMP, Pombeiro AJL (2012) Cobalt complexes bearing scorpionate or pyrazole ligands: synthesis, characterization and applications as in vitro tumour-inhibitors. Dalton Trans 41:12888–12897
25. Sperling RA, Parak WJ (2010) Surface modification, functionalization and bioconjugation of colloidal inorganic nanoparticles. Philos Trans A Math Phys Eng Sci 368:1333–1383
26. Bradford MM (1976) A rapid and sensitive method for the quantitation of microgram quantities of protein utilizing the principle of protein-dye binding. Anal Biochem 72:248–254

Chapter 20

Generation of Dose–Response Curves and Improved IC50s for PARP Inhibitor Nanoformulations

Paige Baldwin, Shifalika Tangutoori, and Srinivas Sridhar

Abstract

Poly(ADP-ribose) polymerase (PARP) inhibitors that target DNA damage repair pathways in cancer cells are increasingly attractive for treating several cancers. Determining the half maximal inhibitory concentration (IC50) of these molecular inhibitors in cell lines is crucial for further dosing for in vivo experiments. Typically these in vitro assays are conducted for 24–72 h; however, PARP inhibitors exhibit cytotoxicity based on the inability to repair DNA damage and thus the accumulation of deleterious mutations takes place over longer times. Therefore, in order to determine a relevant dose response, the time frame of the assay must be modified to account for the time required for the cells to exhibit effects from the treatment. Here, we describe two techniques for generating both short- and long-term dose–response curves for both free PARP inhibitors and nanoparticle formulations of these drugs.

Key words IC50, PARP inhibitors, Short-term, Long-term, Doubling time

1 Introduction

IC50 values, the concentration of an inhibitor required to reduce cellular response by 50 %, are widely published for most drugs and typically used in the planning of more in depth in vitro drug studies. However, these values depend on cell line, drug, time frame, and the type of assay conducted [1, 2]. Currently, molecularly targeted therapies are a major area of research in development of personalized cancer treatments. Molecular therapeutics differ from standard chemotherapeutics in that they do not simply kill cells, but interact with a specific target leading to a downstream effect [3]. Thus, in order to determine the applicability of these drugs, they must be tested in large panels of cell lines with different genomic profiles to elicit sensitivity and potential resistance mechanisms [4].

Poly(ADP-ribose) Polymerase (PARP) plays an important role in a number of DNA repair pathways, and has thus become a prime target of inhibition [5]. PARP inhibitorsPoly(ADP-ribose) Polymerase nhibitors (PARPi) exploit the concept of synthetic lethality

Reema Zeineldin (ed.), *Cancer Nanotechnology: Methods and Protocols*, Methods in Molecular Biology, vol. 1530,
DOI 10.1007/978-1-4939-6646-2_20, © Springer Science+Business Media New York 2017

by selectively targeting cancer cells with defective DNA repair pathways, promoting the accumulation of single- and double-strand breaks eventually leading to cell death [6, 7]. The typical 24–72 h viability assessments are therefore, not relevant for determining the IC50 values of such drugs in which the cytotoxicity is a downstream effect of the drug target. By increasing the length of the assay the cells will replicate multiple times and those which are sensitive to the drug treatment will accumulate genotoxicity eventually halting proliferation and leading to cell death. The effect here is similar to studying radiation effects where the clonogenic assay is used to determine efficacy of radiation treatment in vitro [8].

Lipid based nanoformulations of the PARP inhibitors Olaparib and Talazoparib have been developed by us with the goal of enhancing the bioavailability of the drugs, thereby increasing the tumor accumulation and efficacy in vivo. Dose response and IC50 values are crucial for ensuring that the nanoformulations offer the same potency in vitro as the free drugs. Here we detail a short-term high throughput manner of determining IC50s for cell line sensitivity, and a long-term method to provide an accurate dose response for comparison of free drug and nanoformulations.

The short-term assay involves determining the population doubling time, and seeding an appropriate amount of cells to ensure that cells could be treated for four doubling cycles without cell death occurring because of over confluence and lack of nutrients. The long-term assay is a 14-day colony formation assay in which cells are treated with nanoparticles or free drug twice weekly to maintain drug exposure over the length of the assay [9]. The nanoparticles are PEGylated (i.e., functionalized with polyethylene glycol or PEG), which allows them to evade recognition by the immune system and therefore reduce clearance by the reticuloendothelial system and enhance the circulation time in vivo [10]. PEGylated particles also may not be taken up by the cells as quickly as that of the free drugs, therefore the 14-day assay provides enough time to ensure the particles are being taken up and that the drug has enough time to generate DNA damage and cell death.

2 Materials

1. Cell lines to be tested with their corresponding cell culture media.
2. Tissue culture treated 6- and 96-well plates.
3. CellTiter 96® AQueous One Solution Cell Proliferation Assay, or other commercial assay to measure cell metabolic activity.
4. Plate reader.
5. 1 % (w/v) crystal violet dye.

6. 10 % (v/v) formalin.
7. Olaparib, Selleck Chemicals.
8. NanoOlaparib, a lipid based nanoformulation composed of particles with an average diameter of 100 nm, Sridhar Laboratory, Northeastern University.
9. GraphPad Prism, http://www.graphpad.com/scientific-software/prism/

3 Methods

3.1 Determine Doubling Time of Cells

1. Seed the inner wells of five 96-well plates with 500, 1000, 2000, 4000, and 8000 cells per well. You will have two rows per cell density. Plate 1 should have 100 μL of media per well, while plates 2–5 should have 200 μL of media per well (*see* **Note 1**).
2. Allow plate 1 to equilibrate for 1 h before measuring cell viability using cell metabolism. Using Promega Cell Titer 96 AQueous One Solution, briefly add 20 μL of reagent to each well and incubate plate for 1–4 h at 37 °C and 5 % CO_2. Measure the absorbance at 490 nm in a microplate reader (*see* **Notes 2** and **3**).
3. Measure cell viability at 24, 48, 72, and 96 h after the original seeding time. Briefly, mix 20 μL of reagent with 100 μL of media for each well, and incubate for the same length of time as in **step 3** before measuring absorbance at 490 nm (*see* **Note 4**).
4. Utilize the reading from plate 1 to generate a standard curve correlating absorbance to number of cells. Use this curve to extrapolate the number of cells at each density for each time point.
5. Plot cell density against time for each starting density and fit each curve using exponential regression. The population doubling time can be calculated by $t_d = \ln(2)/\mu_{net}$, where μ_{net} can be calculated from $Y = ae^{(\mu net \times t)}$ where t_d is the population doubling time, μ_{net} is net specific growth rate, a is the initial cell concentration, t is time in hours, and Y is the cell concentration at time t.

3.2 Short-Term IC50 Generation

1. Seed the inner wells of two 96-well plates at the appropriate seeding density as determined from the doubling time calculation (*see* **Note 5**).
2. The following day remove all media, and treat cells with a range of doses of free drug and nanoparticles. Concentrations will vary based on the drug potency; for the PARP inhibitor Olaparib, cells were treated with 0–100 μM free Olaparib or NanoOlaparib (*see* **Note 6**).

3. Allow cells to incubate with the drug treatments for four doubling cycles.
4. Measure cell viability by mixing 20 μL of reagent with 100 μL of media for each well. Prepare enough of this solution to add it to all treated wells as well as six empty wells, which will serve as blanks (*see* **Note 7**).
5. Incubate both plates for 1–4 h at 37 °C and 5 % CO_2. Measure the absorbance at 490 nm in a microplate reader.
6. Determine percent cell viability at each concentration. Plot percent viability versus log[concentration] and fit using a four parameter logistic regression. Software such as GraphPad Prism can be used, and will provide the IC50 value in the results tab.

3.3 Long-Term IC50 Generation

1. Seed three 6-well plates in duplicate with cell densities ranging from 50 to 2000 cells per well. Three plates will be used for free drug and three for testing nanoparticles. The first two sets of wells will be controls, and the remaining seven will have increasing drug concentrations. The number of cells seeded will increase as the drug concentration increases (*see* **Note 8**).
2. Remove media and wash each well with PBS after cells have attached, 4–6 h post seeding.
3. Treat each well with either Olaparib or NanoOlaparib in increasing concentrations.
4. Replace the media in each well twice a week for 2 weeks (*see* **Note 9**).
5. On day 14 wash with PBS and add formalin to fix the cells. Add crystal violet stain directly to the formalin, and allow to sit for 30 min.
6. Wash each plate three times with water to remove any excess crystal violet, and allow plates to dry overnight.
7. Count all colonies that contain more than 50 cells (*see* **Note 10**).
8. Using the cell counts for the two control wells, determine the plating efficiency (PE).

   PE = (number of colonies counted)/(number of cells seeded) Percent cell viability (PCV) should be calculated as follows: PCV = (number of colonies counted/number of cells seeded) × PE.
9. Plot data and fit curve in the same manner as **step 6** of Subheading 3.2 to determine the IC50.

4 Notes

1. Use only the inner 60 wells to ensure no evaporation of media from the outer wells.

2. There are a number of commercial assays available for measuring cell viability. These assays can be used to measure viability according to the protocol provided.
3. For the CellTiter 96® AQueous One Solution Cell Proliferation Assay the reagent changes color as it interacts with viable cells. The color change is more prominent over time, therefore, it is crucial to note down the time the cells were treated with the reagent and the exact time in which the plate is read in the plate reader.
4. Length of exposure to the CellTiter reagent is crucial; therefore, on each subsequent day incubate plates for the exact length of time as the calibration curve.
5. Optimal seeding density is a subjective choice. You need to consider the length of four doubling cycles and if the controls will bypass the linear range of the detection assay at that time. Typically choose the lowest seeding density with the fastest doubling time.
6. Treat cells from lowest to highest drug concentrations to ensure no contamination by higher concentrations. If you are comparing a nanoformulation to the free drug treat them completely separately so as to minimize risk of error.
7. Blanks are wells with no cells but with the reagent and media mixture. This will provide the baseline reading for no viable cells. Without subtracting out blanks, wells with no viable cells will still show some viability.
8. The seeding densities for this assay are in a range, which may need to be optimized before the final assay is conducted. Control wells usually should have between 50 and 250 cells. The lowest drug concentrations will have similar densities, while the high concentrations can have more cells. If you find that at high concentrations you are seeing no colonies you want to increase the seeding density to 100 times the control wells. If you are still seeing no colonies after 14 days then there is 0 % viability.
9. Prepare fresh nanoparticle/drug dilutions before each media replenishing to ensure treatment with active drug.
10. Colonies are only counted if they have more than 50 cells. There are a number of computer programs which can count or aid in the counting process, but be sure that each colony is at least 50 cells. Colonies are not to be overlapping, if so they cannot be counted. This must be taken into account for choosing seeding density.

Acknowledgments

This work was supported by W81XWH-14-1-0092 and NSF-DGE-0965843.

References

1. Hatzis C, Bedard PL, Birkbak NJ et al (2014) Enhancing reproducibility in cancer drug screening: how do we move forward? Cancer Res 74:4016–4023. doi:10.1158/0008-5472.CAN-14-0725
2. Riss TL, Niles AL, Minor L et al (2004) Cell viability assays. Assay guidance manual. Assay Guid Man 1–23. doi:10.1016/j.acthis.2012.01.006
3. Collins I, Workman P (2006) New approaches to molecular cancer therapeutics. Nat Chem Biol 2:689–700. doi:10.1038/nchembio840
4. Scherf U, Ross DT, Waltham M et al (2000) A gene expression database for the molecular pharmacology of cancer. Nat Genet 24:236–244. doi:10.1038/73439
5. Rouleau M, Patel A, Hendzel MJ et al (2010) PARP inhibition: PARP1 and beyond. Nat Rev Cancer 10:293–301. doi:10.1038/nrc2812
6. Ashworth A (2008) A synthetic lethal therapeutic approach: poly(ADP) ribose polymerase inhibitors for the treatment of cancers deficient in DNA double-strand break repair. J Clin Oncol 26:3785–3790. doi:10.1200/JCO.2008.16.0812
7. Farmer H, McCabe N, Lord CJ et al (2005) Targeting the DNA repair defect in BRCA mutant cells as a therapeutic strategy. Nature 434:917–921. doi:10.1038/nature03445
8. Franken NAP, Rodermond HM, Stap J et al (2006) Clonogenic assay of cells in vitro. Nat Protoc 1:2315–2319
9. Shen Y, Rehman FL, Feng Y et al (2013) BMN 673, a novel and highly potent PARP1/2 inhibitor for the treatment of human cancers with DNA repair deficiency. Clin Cancer Res 19:5003–5015. doi:10.1158/1078-0432.CCR-13-1391
10. Van Vlerken LE, Vyas TK, Amiji MM (2007) Poly(ethylene glycol)-modified nanocarriers for tumor-targeted and intracellular delivery. Pharm Res 24:1405–1414. doi:10.1007/s11095-007-9284-6

Chapter 21

Artificial Antigen-Presenting Cells for Immunotherapies

Alyssa L. Siefert, Tarek M. Fahmy, and Dongin Kim

Abstract

Artificial antigen-presenting cells (aAPCs) overcome many of the limitations of biologically based adoptive immunotherapy protocols. While these acellular systems can be designed with a variety of parameters, including material type, diameter, and proliferative signals for T cells, we outline methods to formulate and characterize a comprehensive polymeric microparticle aAPC platform. These aAPCs, which can be reproducibly fabricated in large quantities, efficiently stimulate antigen-specific T cell activation and proliferation by both paracrine cytokine signals and engagement of T cell surface proteins.

Key words Polymer, Microparticle, aAPC, Immunotherapy, Paracrine delivery, PLGA

1 Introduction

Adoptive immunotherapy, in which tumor-specific T cells are activated and expanded by antigen-presenting cells (APCs) presenting tumor antigens and co-stimulatory signals, is a promising strategy to fight cancer. However, the process of stimulating T cells using natural APCs, such as patient-derived dendritic cells pulsed with antigen, is costly, time- and resource-intensive, and unpredictable. Therefore, cleverly engineered acellular artificial antigen-presenting cells (aAPCs) hold tremendous promise for cancer immunotherapy. Several types of acellular aAPC platforms presenting ligands like T-cell-activating antibodies and peptide-major histocompatibility-complexes (pMHC) have been tested. aAPC systems assayed include novel liposomal and polymeric formulations, and modification of commercially available iron oxide or latex micro- and nanoparticles [1] (Fig. 1).

Successful aAPCs initiate tumor-specific adaptive immunity by delivering signals to T cells in a physiologically relevant manner. In natural interactions between APCs and T cells, three signals are delivered in the immunological synapse formed by pMHC on APCs and T cell receptors (TCR) on T cells. APC signals delivered to T cells are pMHC, costimulatory ligands CD80 and CD86 that ligate

Reema Zeineldin (ed.), *Cancer Nanotechnology: Methods and Protocols*, Methods in Molecular Biology, vol. 1530,
DOI 10.1007/978-1-4939-6646-2_21, © Springer Science+Business Media New York 2017

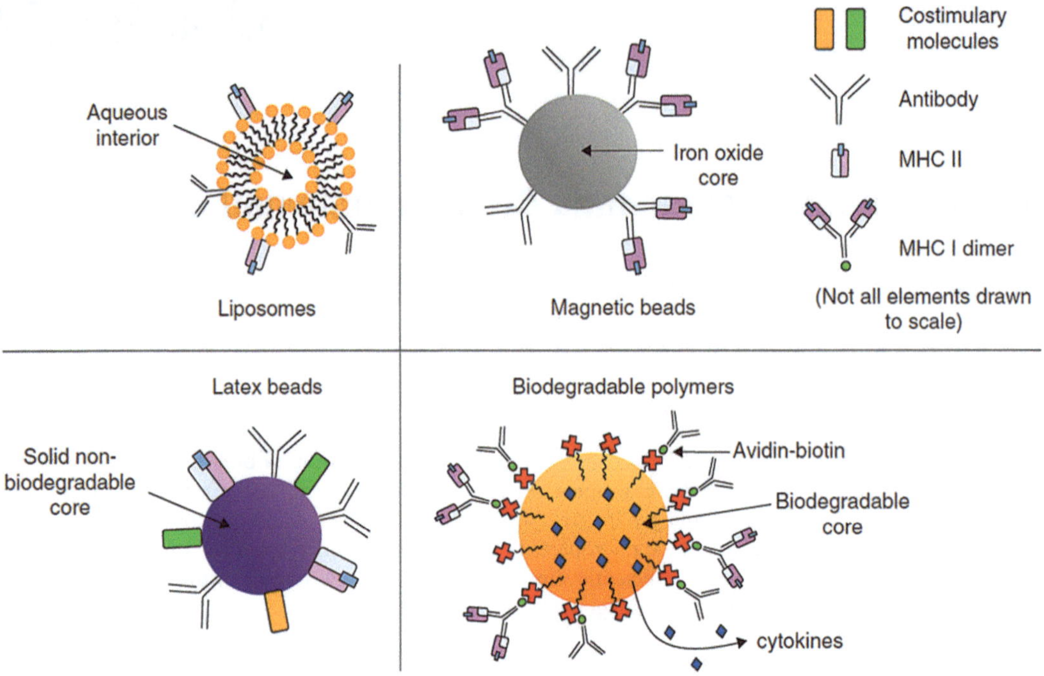

Fig. 1 Four types of acellular aAPCs. Research strategies generally include the addition of peptide-MHC complexes and activating antibodies to the surfaces of spherical acellular particles. Adapted from [1]

T cell surface protein CD28, and proliferative cytokines secreted in a paracrine fashion (Fig. 2).

Numerous factors must be considered when choosing and optimizing aAPCs. Many aAPCs are fabricated from biocompatible, aliphatic polymer poly(lactic-co-glycolic) acid (PLGA) because of its extensive clinical use, favorable safety profile, and sustained release of encapsulated payloads [3]. Others have optimized paramagnetic iron-dextran nanoparticles, termed nano-aAPC, surface-presenting pMHC and anti-CD28 antibodies, which are the first in class to activate naïve T cells, which have a higher activation threshold than antigen-experienced T cells [4]. This recent advance is notable because nanoparticles are more suitable for in vivo immunotherapy than microparticles, due to size-mediated favorable trafficking and biodistribution [4]. Further work into aAPC development has shown that particle geometry is an important design parameter, as ellipsoid PLGA microparticles activated CD8+ T cells to a greater extent, both in vitro and in vivo against melanoma, than spherical microparticles with constant particle volume and antigen [5]. Additionally, surface properties of aAPC platforms, such as roughness, can enhance immunotherapeutic effects. This effect was elegantly demonstrated by the finding that aAPCs, a composite of carbon nanotubes and polymer nanoparticles, efficiently expanded antigen-specific T cells using a 1000-fold less IL-2 than clinical standards [6].

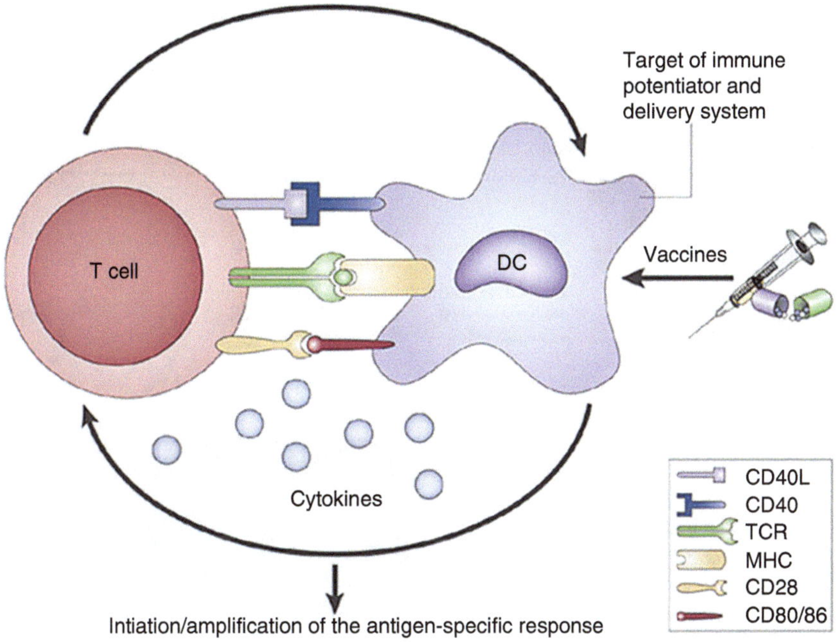

Fig. 2 Schematic of natural interaction between T cell and APC, showing the three signals necessary for durable adaptive immunity. Adapted from [2]

Initial attempts to engineer aAPCs relied on delivering pMHC and costimulation to cells, along with added soluble cytokines to cell culture media, but they faced problems such as acute toxicity and cytokine withdrawal. These limitations motivated Steenblock and colleagues to develop a flexible aAPC platform [7] that includes the three signals necessary for adaptive immunity in a biodegradable microparticle platform (Fig. 3).

We choose to focus on this comprehensive PLGA microparticle platform based on its relative ease and low cost of manufacturing, high potential for clinical translation, and reproducible results. Importantly, the diffusion kinetics between microparticles and cells are characteristic of in vivo interactions [8]. The properties of PLGA micro- and nano-particles depend on several formulation factors, including fabrication technique, solvent volatility and miscibility, polymer molecular weight (MW), encapsulant properties, and drug–polymer ratio [9].

Techniques to formulate particles include single emulsion (oil-in-water), double emulsion (water-in-oil-in-water), nanoprecipitation, and phase separation. Emulsion processes involve first dissolving the PLGA polymer in a volatile organic solvent, followed by addition of encapsulant in an aqueous phase to create a solution in which energy, in the form of sonication or stirring, is added to form droplets. The solvent is then removed from the emulsion, which is often stabilized, by extraction or evaporation, and oil

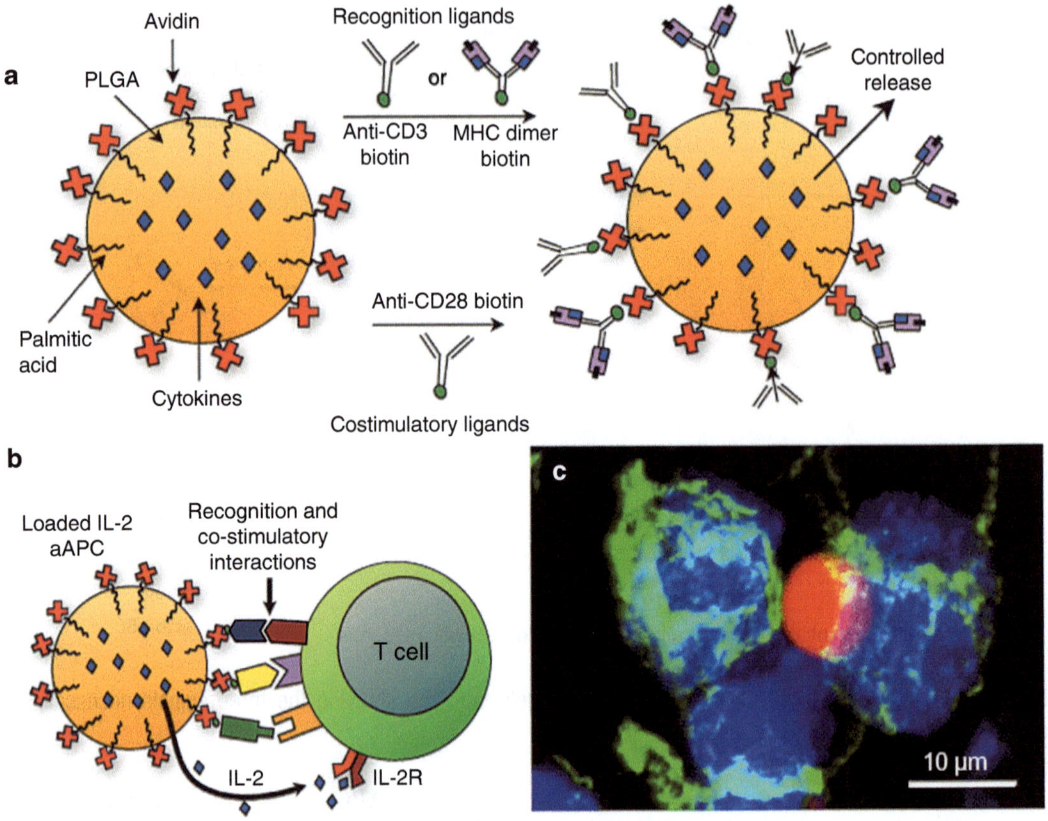

Fig. 3 PLGA aAPC schematic, showing surface ligand coupling via addition of biotinylated antibodies to avidin-coated microparticles (**a**), and subsequent interactions with T cells (**b**). Different keys in (**b**) illustrate various interactions between a T cell and an aAPC. Engineered aAPCs trigger T cell receptors and surface proteins and deliver paracrine IL-2 to activate T cells. Schematic interactions are confirmed by microscopy images showing rhodamine-B-encapsulating aAPCs (*red*) creating physiologically relevant immune synapses with T cells (nuclei in *blue*, cytoskeleton in *green*) (**c**). Adapted from [7]

droplets harden and are collected by filtration, sieving, or centrifugation. The resulting hardened emulsions are particles that can be washed and lyophilized to create a shelf-stable, dry product [9]. The components of designed particles, arranged on a polymeric matrix, are (1) pMHC complexes to confer antigen specificity to T cells, (2) costimulatory molecules, including but not limited to antibodies against CD3 and CD28, to activate T cells, and (3) soluble cytokines to further differentiate and proliferate antigen-specific T cells.

2 Materials

Use ultrapure water and analytical grade reagents to prepare solutions at room temperature (unless otherwise noted). Follow proper waste disposal regulations.

2.1 PLGA Microparticles

1. PLGA 50/50 inherent viscosity 0.59 dL/g.
2. 2 % (w/v) sodium deoxycholate.
3. NHS-palmitate.
4. Poly(vinyl) alcohol (PVA), 2.5 %.
5. Recombinant human (rh) Interleukin 2 (IL-2).
6. 10 μg/mL biotinylated anti-mouse CD3ε.
7. Biotinylated peptide-loaded MHC-K^b-Ig dimers (obtained as a generous gift from Jonathan Schneck, Johns Hopkins University) [10].
8. 10 μg/mL biotinylated anti-mouse CD28.
9. Avidin.
10. Palmitic acid.
11. Sodium deoxycholate.
12. Pierce BCA Assay.

2.2 T Cell Stimulation Experiments

1. Ammonium-Chloride-Potassium (ACK) Lysing buffer.
2. CD8+ negative selection kit.
3. ELISA kits to quantify bioactive IFN-γ and IL-2.
4. Complete RMPI tissue culture medium: RPMI 1640 supplemented with FBS (10 %), L-glutamine (1 %), HEPES buffer (1 %), nonessential amino acids, 2-ME (0.1 %), and penicillin (2 %), and stored at 4 °C before use.

3 Methods

Unless otherwise specified, procedures are performed at room temperature and pressure.

PLGA microparticles, adapted from [11], are formulated with IL-2 encapsulated and avidin on the surface for attachment of pMHC and antibodies against CD28 and/or CD3. First, avidin-palmitate is prepared for incorporation into microparticles. After formulation, microparticles are characterized by procedures outlined below.

3.1 Palmitoylation of Avidin

Particle surfaces are coated with avidin, a protein with four high-affinity binding sites for biotin, to enable surface display of a variety of biotinylated molecules such as pMHC and antibodies [12]. This method of surface modification is attractive because numerous proteins are commercially available with biotin modification, and avidin maintains picomolar affinity to biotin under a variety of in vitro and in vivo conditions [13] (*see* **Note 1** for further recommendations regarding biotin). Avidin is palmitoylated such that fatty acid chains partition into hydrophobic polymers that comprise aAPCs.

To conjugate palmitic acid to avidin:

1. Prepare 2 % (w/v) sodium deoxycholate solution by adding 16 g sodium deoxycholate to 700 mL sterile PBS and bringing the volume up to 800 mL.
2. Warm and stir sodium deoxycholate solution to 37 °C using a temperature-controlled magnetic stirrer platform.
3. In a 50 mL polypropylene tube with a tiny stir bar, prepare a 5 mg/mL solution of avidin by adding 100 mg avidin to 20 mL 2 % sodium deoxycholate.
4. Dissolve avidin by stirring in a 37 °C water bath.
5. After avidin is dissolved (brief incubation in a water sonication bath may be necessary), add 15-fold molar excess of NHS-palmitate, 8 mg NHS-palmitate to 100 mg avidin.
6. Sonicate this solution in a 37 °C water bath until no palmitate flakes remain.
7. Secure the vial in 37 °C water bath and allow reaction to continue for 3 h under stirring.
8. After reaction is complete, dialyze avidin-palmitate solution by transferring to Snakeskin 10,000 MWCO dialysis tubing and dialyzing against 2 % sodium deoxycholate at 37 °C overnight, stirring in a fume hood.
9. Use a BCA assay, following manufacturer instructions, to determine the protein content of avidin-palmitate solution.

3.2 Fabrication of Microparticles

Microparticles can be made using a single or double-emulsion technique, chosen depending on desired size range and type and degree of encapsulants. For instance, single emulsion techniques, also called oil/water (o/w) methods, are useful for encapsulating hydrophobic molecules like small molecule drugs and steroids. Because double emulsion, or water/oil/water (w/o/w), formulation strategies are best suited for encapsulation of hydrophilic molecules like proteins and peptides [1], we outline that procedure below:

1. Dissolve 100 mg 50:50 PLGA in 4 mL chloroform in glass test tube (Tube 1), creating a solution with a polymer/solvent ratio of 25 mg/mL.

2. Shake on plate shaker for 20 min to ensure homogenous dissolving in an eppendorf tube.
3. Prepare 100 μL of 100 μg/mL solution of IL-2 in sterile PBS in an Eppendorf tube.
4. Prepare a 400 mL beaker containing 100 mL of 0.3 % PVA, stirring gently in fume hood.
5. Prepare a test tube of 2 mL 2.5 % PVA and 2 mL 5 mg/mL avidin-palmitate (Tube 2).
6. While holding Tube 1 containing dissolved polymer on a benchtop vortex, use a Pasteur glass pipet to add 100 μL IL-2 solution dropwise to vortexing polymer/solvent solution, maximizing contact area between aqueous protein solution and organic polymer solution.
7. Continue vortexing for 30 s.
8. Using a benchtop vortex to mix Tube 2, containing PVA and avidin-palmitate, use a Pasteur glass pipet to add the contents of Tube 1 to Tube 2, continuing vortexing.
9. Add the contents of Tube 2 to the beaker containing 0.3 % PVA.
10. Allow solvent evaporation and polymer hardening to occur for 3 h at room temperature in fume hood.
11. Collect microparticles by centrifuging solution at 5600 RCF for 5 min.
12. Wash particles by dumping water, resuspending in 5 mL water by vortexing and bouts in water sonication bath, and centrifuging again at 5600 RCF for 5 min.
13. Dump water, resuspend in minimal water volume by vortex and water bath sonication, and transfer particle suspension to a preweighted scintillation vial.
14. Use liquid nitrogen to flash-freeze particle suspension.
15. Lyophilize for 48 h or until a dry powder is formed (*see* **Note 2** for further storage instructions).

3.3 Characterization of Microparticles

Microparticles can be sized in several ways depending on equipment availability. To collect particles in narrow size ranges, filters and centrifugation gradients may be used. Particle diameters may be quantified using free ImageJ software (NIH) to analyze images of particles coated in gold or carbon obtained by Scanning Electron Microscopy (SEM) (Fig. 4). Alternatively, hydrodynamic diameters of particles can be obtained by instruments like flow cytometers [14] or Beckman Coulter Counters [15]. To determine IL-2-protein loading of microparticles (*see* **Note 3**).

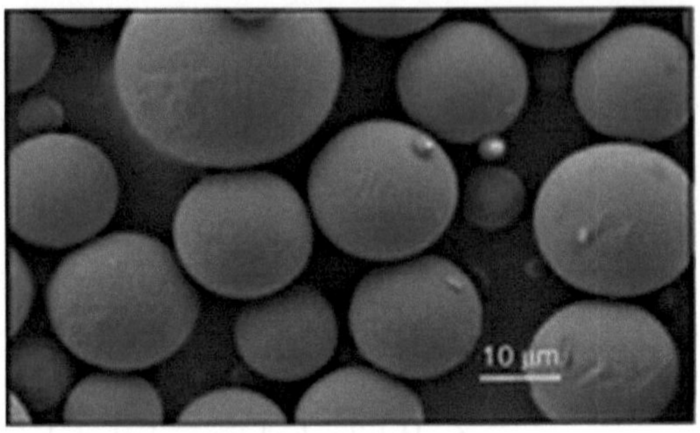

Fig. 4 Representative SEM image of microparticles. Adapted from [1]

3.4 BCA Assay to Detect Total IL-2 Loading

1. Mass out 2 mg of IL-2 loaded, avidin-coated microparticles into eppendorf tubes and wash once with DI water by adding 1 mL water and centrifuging at 2319.85 × *g* for 5 min and removing supernatant.
2. Dissolve particles by adding 500 μL 1 M NaOH with 1 % SDS, followed by mixing using a vortex and sonication in water bath. Allow particle degradation to occur for at least 30 min on a plate shaker or until solution is clear.
3. To create a standard, dissolve 2 mg empty, avidin-coated microparticles in 500 μL of the same NaOH/SDS solution, allowing to degrade for 30 min on plate shaker.
4. As not to interfere with BCA detection, the concentration of NaOH/SDS must be kept under 10 %. Therefore, dilute samples either 1:10 or 1:100, depending on how much protein you expect to be encapsulated (we recommend starting with both dilutions). For a 1:10 dilution, add 4.5 mL PBS to 0.5 mL particle/NaOH solution in a new eppendorf. For a 1:100 dilution, add 0.5 mL of 1:10 solution to 4.5 mL PBS in a new eppendorf.
5. Calculate how much BCA Working Reagent (WR vol) will be needed by multiplying the number of wells used (including standard wells) by 0.15 mL.
6. Mix WR following manufacturer instructions (adding 0.5*vol A, 0.48*vol B, 0.02*vol C).
7. Add 150 μL samples in triplicate to wells in a 96 well plate.
8. For standards, add 150 μL of 1:10 and/or 1:100 diluted blank particles to each well in a row, then serially dilute with protein of interest (or BSA standard from BCA kit if protein of interest is unavailable/expensive).
9. Add 150 μL WR to every well with protein solution in it.
10. Incubate at 37 °C for 2 h.

11. Read plate at absorbance 562 nm and follow the manufacturer's instructions to determine the protein concentrations.

3.5 Surface Modification with pMHC and Antibodies

Biotinylated ligands, such as pMHC and antibodies against CD28 and CD3, are added to avidin-coated aAPCs immediately before use, employing the following method:

1. Calculate the desired mass of aAPCs and ligand coating for experiments. In published reports, 1 μg ligand is added per mg of aAPC [7, 10], though it is advised to titrate surface ligand density for optimal T cell stimulation.
2. Create a 10 mg/mL solution of aAPC in sterile PBS in an eppendorf. In another eppendorf, create an equimolar solution of anti-CD28 and anti-CD3 or, if available, pMHC at 10 μg/mL.
3. Add desired amount of surface ligand cocktail to aAPC solution and allow to tumble on a rotisserie for 20 min at room temperature.
4. Wash particles by adding PBS with 1 % (v/v) Fetal Bovine Serum (FBS) to eppendorf tube, spinning down at 5600 RCF for 5 min, and removing supernatant.
5. Resuspend ligand-coupled aAPCs in complete RMPI-10 tissue culture medium for in vitro studies (*see* **Note 4** for instructions for in vivo experiments).

3.6 Antigen-Specific T Cell Expansion

Effective aAPCs will activate and expand antigen-specific T Cells. For clinical work, tumor-specific antigens or antigenic peptides are incorporated into aAPC platforms for incubation with autologous T cells. For proof-of-concept and murine studies, the antigenic peptide of model antigen ovalbumin (OVA) is loaded onto biotinylated pMHC complexes for incubation with OVA-specific T cells from transgenic mice. The spleens of OT-I mice (Jackson Lab) are transgenic mice bred to be enriched with OVA-specific CD8+ T cells. The following protocol stimulates and expands CD8+ T cells:

1. In a tissue culture hood, harvest T cells from the spleen of an OT-I mouse by using the back of a 5 mL syringe to mash the spleen through a cell strainer into a 50 mL Falcon tube, rinsing with sterile PBS.
   (a) Spin cells down at 1200 rpm for 5 min, discard supernatant, and add 5 mL ACK Lysing buffer to remove erythrocytes.
   (b) Incubate 5 min at room temperature.
   (c) Add 10 mL PBS, pellet cells, and discard supernatant.
2. Isolate CD8+ T cells using CD8+ negative selection kit, following manufacturer instructions.

3. Resuspend T cells in complete RPMI media (*see* **Note 5**).
4. Titrate surface-ligated aAPCs, suspended in media, in 96 well round-bottom plates, with a 100 μL volume per well. The highest aAPC concentration should not exceed a 1:1 molar ratio with T cells.
5. Add CD8+ T cells to each well for a final cell concentration of 5×10^5 cells/mL.
6. Allow aAPCs to stimulate CD8+ T cells for 3 days in tissue culture incubator set to 37 °C and 5.0 % CO_2.
7. Centrifuge plates at 208.7865 × *g* for 7 min and remove supernatant for ELISA analysis of proliferative cytokines IFN-γ and IL-2, following manufacturer instructions.

4 Notes

1. Experiments should use freshly hydrated and surface-modified aAPCs. It is not recommended to store aAPCs that have been coupled to biotinylated ligands.
2. Lyopholized aAPCs may be stored at −80 °C for up to 3 years.
3. To determine IL-2 protein loading of microparticles, a BCA protein detection assay may be used on either the supernatant of microparticles incubated in PBS at 37 °C for at least 1 week or on dissolved microparticles. The former method quantifies the amount of IL-2 released in physiologic conditions for a desired time range and is advised if researchers want to quantify the amount of IL-2 available to T cells. The latter method will yield the total amount of protein incorporated into particles, regardless of the amount released, and can only be used if empty particles, surface-modified with avidin, are used as a control, as the BCA will yield a positive signal for both avidin-palmitate and IL-2. Finally, while researchers may use an IL-2 Enzyme-Linked Immunosorbent Assay (ELISA) to quantify the amount of biologically active IL-2 released from or encapsulated in microparticles, we recommend using the more affordable BCA assay during particle optimization. Additionally, because of its conformational specificity, the IL-2 ELISA may only detect a fraction of IL-2 in particles.
4. For in vivo studies, suspend surface-modified aAPCs in sterile PBS before animal injections.
5. Tissue culture media may need to be supplemented with additional glutamine and changed frequently, as proliferating T cells exhibit high metabolism.

Acknowledgments

The authors thank past and present members of the Fahmy Lab, especially Dr. Erin Steenblock-Chia, for pioneering work in scalable adoptive immunotherapy.

References

1. Steenblock ER, Wrzesinski SH, Flavell RA et al (2009) Antigen presentation on artificial acellular substrates: modular systems for flexible, adaptable immunotherapy. Expert Opin Biol Ther 9(4):451–464
2. O'Hagan DT, Valiante NM (2003) Recent advances in the discovery and delivery of vaccine adjuvants. Nat Rev Drug Discov 2(9):727–735
3. Demento SL, Siefert AL, Bandyopadhyay A et al (2011) Pathogen-associated molecular patterns on biomaterials: a paradigm for engineering new vaccines. Trends Biotechnol 29 (6):294–306
4. Perica K, Bieler JG, Schutz C et al (2015) Enrichment and expansion with nanoscale artificial antigen presenting cells for adoptive immunotherapy. ACS Nano 9(7):6861–6871
5. Sunshine JC, Perica K, Schneck JP et al (2014) Particle shape dependence of CD8+ T cell activation by artificial antigen presenting cells. Biomaterials 35(1):269–277
6. Fadel TR, Sharp FA, Vudatu N et al (2014) A carbon nanotube–polymer composite for T-cell therapy. Nat Nanotechnol 9(8):639–647
7. Steenblock ER, Fahmy TM (2008) A comprehensive platform for ex vivo T-cell expansion based on biodegradable polymeric artificial antigen-presenting cells. Mol Ther 16 (4):765–772
8. Labowsky M, Fahmy TM (2012) Diffusive transfer between two intensely interacting cells with limited surface kinetics. Chem Eng Sci 74:114–123
9. Jain RA (2000) The manufacturing techniques of various drug loaded biodegradable poly(lactide-co-glycolide) (PLGA) devices. Biomaterials 21(23):2475–2490
10. Schneck JP, Slansky JE, O'Herrin SM et al (2001) Monitoring antigen-specific T cells using MHC-Ig dimers. Curr Protoc Immunol Chapter 17:Unit 17.2
11. Steenblock ER, Fadel T, Labowsky M et al (2011) An artificial antigen-presenting cell with paracrine delivery of IL-2 impacts the magnitude and direction of the T cell response. J Biol Chem 286(40):34883–34892
12. Lee SK, Siefert A, Beloor J et al (2012) Cell-specific siRNA delivery by peptides and antibodies. Methods Enzymol 502:91–122
13. Fahmy TM, Samstein RM, Harness CC et al (2005) Surface modification of biodegradable polyesters with fatty acid conjugates for improved drug targeting. Biomaterials 26 (28):5727–5736
14. Chandler WL, Yeung W, Tait JF (2011) A new microparticle size calibration standard for use in measuring smaller microparticles using a new flow cytometer. J Thromb Haemost 9 (6):1216–1224
15. van der Pol E, Coumans F, Varga Z et al (2013) Innovation in detection of microparticles and exosomes. J Thromb Haemost 11:36–45

Chapter 22

Exploiting Uptake of Nanoparticles by Phagocytes for Cancer Treatment

Mee Rie Sheen and Steven Fiering

Abstract

Many cancers including ovarian, pancreatic, colon, liver, and stomach cancers are largely confined to the peritoneal cavity. Peritoneal tumors are directly accessible by intraperitoneal injections. Previously we demonstrated that intraperitoneal injection of nanoparticles and subsequent ingestion by tumor-associated phagocytes can be used to either directly impact tumors or stimulate antitumor immune responses. Here we outline methods to specifically utilize iron oxide nanoparticles with the ID8-*Defb29/Vegf-A* murine ovarian cancer model and discuss the tendency of phagocytes to ingest nanoparticles and the potential of phagocytes to carry nanoparticles to tumors resulting in direct killing of tumor cells or stimulate antitumor immune responses in peritoneal cancers. This basic approach can be modified as needed for different types of tumors and nanoparticles.

Key words Peritoneal cavity, Peritoneal tumor, Intraperitoneal injection, Nanoparticles, Tumor-associated phagocytes, Antitumor immune responses, Iron oxide nanoparticles, ID8-*Defb29/Vegf-A*, Ovarian cancer

1 Introduction

It is now clear that the immune system plays a major role in the interaction between tumors and the patient carrying the tumors. The immune system recognizes tumors and moves to attack and eliminate tumors [1], but the tumors that become large enough to become a clinical issue (as opposed to those eliminated by the immune system before anyone ever knew they existed), invariably manifest local immunosuppression mechanisms that protect them. Rather than coexisting with the immune system, tumors manipulate both themselves and certain immune cells for protection from other immune cells [2]. Phagocytes of various sorts such as monocytes, macrophages, dendritic cells, and neutrophils play a major role in this interplay as the backbone of what is termed the innate immune system. This role in service of tumors is often as immunosuppressive cells that are recruited by the tumor and suppress attack

Reema Zeineldin (ed.), *Cancer Nanotechnology: Methods and Protocols*, Methods in Molecular Biology, vol. 1530, DOI 10.1007/978-1-4939-6646-2_22, © Springer Science+Business Media New York 2017

by other components of the immune system, a role attributed broadly to "myeloid derived suppressive cells" (MDSC) of various sorts [3]. This information is important in the context of immunotherapy and nanoparticle (NP)-mediated cancer treatment, because NP experimentalists generally go to great pains to avoid the ingestion of NPs by phagocytes [4]. Here we discuss ideas of how the tendency of phagocytes to ingest NPs can be exploited for cancer therapy using nanoparticles.

Most people, when considering immunology, focus on lymphocytes, (B and T cells), and their role in adaptive immunity. The vast majority of specialized immune cells are not lymphocytes, they are other leukocytes, referred to loosely as innate immune cells and they are very important in both starting and stopping the overall immune response, including the response against tumors. These innate cells can be either immunosuppressive and block immune responses, or immunostimulatory and support and generate immune responses [2]. As we consider how NPs can be utilized it is important to note that while most of us think about a direct effect on tumor cells when we consider NP-mediated cancer therapy, we should also consider that NPs can manipulate immune cells and support the antitumor immune response. This is particularly relevant for innate immune cells that actively ingest NPs they encounter. One idea to consider is that rather than trying to avoid ingestion of NPs by phagocytes, for example by coating them with polyethylene glycol [2, 5], there are ways to exploit the uptake of NPs by phagocytes to for example, eliminate immunosuppressive phagocytes or modify them to be immunostimulatory and thereby support the antitumor immune response [6, 7].

Mouse studies of cancer depend on various mouse cancer models and each model has unique strengths and weaknesses. Many common cancer types arise in the peritoneal cavity and metastasize there, at least initially. These include liver, colon, ovarian, stomach, pancreatic, and kidney cancers. It is important to consider that access to such cancers is through the blood stream, as with all cancers, but also through the peritoneal region itself, reagents injected into the peritoneum often have direct access to peritoneal tumor surfaces. In addition, phagocytes in the peritoneum are recruited to support the cancer and can be manipulated by intraperitoneal (IP) application of nanoparticles, as technically presented here.

Parental ID8 murine ovarian surface epithelial cancer cell line [8] and ID8 cell lines transduced either with vascular endothelial growth factor A (*Vegf-A*) (ID8-*Vegf-A*) or *Vegf-A* and β-defensin-29 (*Defb29*) (ID8-*Defb29/Vegf-A*) [9] are transplantable mouse models of ovarian cancer that establish tumors in syngeneic C57BL/6 mice. The models vary by aggressiveness and speed of cancer development with ID8 being the least aggressive and ID8-*Defb29/Vegf-A* much more aggressive with an end-stage of about

40 days. All three models accurately recapitulate characteristics of metastatic serous human ovarian cancer following IP inoculation, including tumor dissemination throughout the peritoneal cavity, development of ascites (excessive fluid in the abdomen), and recruitment and accumulation of great numbers of leukocytes such as tumor-associated immunosuppressive phagocytes in the peritoneal cavity [9–13]. These leukocytes are being recruited to the peritoneum by signals from the tumor and are subsequently entering the tumors themselves. Ovarian tumor cells and immune cells in the peritoneal cavity are easily accessible by IP injection, making it an excellent model for the study of NPs interaction with peritoneal cancers since the surface of the tumors and the leukocytes are both in direct contact with IP injected NPs [7].

Cancer nanotechnology includes the development and utilization of nanocarrier systems for therapeutic applications, which can be composed of bioactive entities, such as small-molecule drugs, peptides, proteins, and nucleic acids, and of nanosensor devices for detecting cancers, such as diagnostic devices, contrast agents, and analytical tools. This field is one of the most rapidly growing areas in cancer research with great potential [14]. NPs are broadly defined as particles with a diameter in the range of 10–200 nm. NPs have many potential uses for cancer therapy since they can be loaded with a variety of reagents in addition to manifesting the fundamental properties of the NP itself. NPs can be engineered with a wide range of functional surface/core properties, assembled and administered in vivo [14]. One metallic particle, iron oxide nanoparticles (IONPs) have attracted considerable interest due to features including magnetic properties, biocompatibility, solubility over time in vivo, stability, and non-toxicity [15].

As noted above, the tendency of NPs to be ingested by phagocytes can be utilized to manipulate the phagocytes and this can be immunostimulatory [14]. To illustrate this and related ideas concerning NPs and immunotherapy we outline and provide methods for the study of the ID8-*Defb29/Vegf-A* ovarian tumor model. NPs in this context are taken up by innate phagocytic cells traversing into the tumor and will carry those NPs and any NP they carry deep into the tumors themselves [7]. This is analogous to the Trojan horse that was brought by the Trojans into their city and led to their demise at the hands of the Greeks.

Isolation of peritoneal cells by collecting tumor ascites (peritoneal lavage supernatant) following IP injection of IONPs is an important technique for studying interactions between NPs and the peritoneal tumor and immune cells. The magnetic property of IONPs enables use of the MACS® column to gently separate magnetically labeled cells harboring IONPs. Subsequently the positively selected and magnetically labeled cell fraction from a heterogenous cell suspension can be spun onto the slides by use of cytospin technique and used for cytochemistry to visualize and evaluate the selected iron-containing cells. Prussian blue stain is a common way to detect the presence of iron in cells and tissues, which forms the purple Prussian blue dye in place and can be visualized as blue precipitate. Alternatively the positively selected and flow through cells (those not carrying IONPs) can be evaluated for cell types and effector function by flow cytometry and in vitro assays. In the following sections, with the example of IP injection of IONPs and ID8-*Defb29/Vegf-A* mouse ovarian cancer model, we describe methods to separate immune cells in the peritoneal cavity that ingests IONPs followed by IP injection and to visualize IONPs-harboring cells.

2 Materials

2.1 Injection of ID8-Defb29/Vegf-A Ovarian Tumor Cells and Bionized NanoFerrite (BNF)-Starch Coated IONPs

1. ID8-*Defb29/Vegf-A* ovarian tumor cells in culture.
2. Completed RPMI 1640 medium: RPMI 1640 medium supplemented with 10 % (v/v) fetal bovine serum (FBS), 2 mM L-glutamine, 1 mM sodium pyruvate, 0.1 mM MEM nonessential amino acids, 100 unit penicillin/streptomycin, and 0.05 mM 2-mercaptoethanol.
3. 0.25 % Trypsin/2.21 mM EDTA.
4. 1× phosphate-buffered saline (PBS).
5. BNF-starch coated IONPs (Micromod Partikeltechnologie GmbH, Germany).
6. 37 °C gassed (5 % CO_2) cell incubator.

2.2 Preparation of Peritoneal Lavage Supernatant

1. 70 % (v/v) ethanol.
2. Red blood cell lysis buffer: Weigh 4.1 g ammonium chloride (NH_4Cl), 0.5 g potassium bicarbonate ($KHCO_3$), and 0.1 g ethylenediamine tetraacetic acid (EDTA) and transfer to a glass beaker. Add about 900 mL ddH_2O and mix until the chemicals are completely dissolved. Add ddH_2O to bring the total volume of the solution to 1 L and filter the solution through a 0.22 μm membrane using a vaccum pump into a sterile container. Store at 2–8 °C.
3. Hemacytometer and microscope.
4. Styrofoam block and pins for mounting the mouse.

2.3 Separation of Magnetically Labeled Cells by MACS Columns

1. MACS column running buffer: Prepare a solution containing phosphate-buffered saline (PBS), pH 7.2, 0.5 % (w/v) bovine serum albumin (BSA), and 2 mM EDTA to equilibrate column. Degas buffer by applying vacuum at room temperature and keep buffer in the cold at 2–8 °C.
2. MACS LS columns (Miltenyi Biotec, San Diego, CA).

3. MACS MultiStand (Miltenyi Biotec, San Diego, CA).
4. MidiMACS separator (Miltenyi Biotec, San Diego, CA).

2.4 Cytospin of Separated Cells by MACS Columns

1. Ice cold 10 % FBS-containing media or PBS.
2. 0.1 % (w/v) poly-L-lysine solution in H_2O.
3. Cytocentrifuge (Shandon Inc., Shandon Cytospin 4, Pittsburgh, PA).
4. Cytospin sealed head (Shandon Inc., Pittsburgh, PA).
5. TPX single sample chambers and caps (Shandon Inc., Pittsburgh, PA).
6. Cytoclip stainless steel slide clip (Shandon Inc., Pittsburgh, PA).
7. Disposable white filter card (Shandon Inc., Pittsburgh, PA).

2.5 Prussian Blue Staining of Ferric Iron

1. 10 % (v/v) buffered formalin.
2. Iron Stain Kit Gomori Prussian Blue Reaction (Newcomer Supply, Middleton, WI).
3. Solution A: 20 % (v/v) hydrochloric acid aqueous solution.
4. Solution B: 10 % (w/v) potassium ferrocyanide aqueous solution.
5. Solution C: 1 % (w/v) nuclear fast red stain aqueous solution, (also known as Kernechtrot).
6. Permount solution (Fisher Scientific, Grand Island, NY).

3 Methods

3.1 Peritoneal Lavage to Retrieve Cells from Peritoneum that Have Ingested Iron Oxide Nanoparticles

1. Culture ID8-*Defb29/Vegf-A* cells and harvest when cells reach 80–85 % confluence. In such conditions cells should be more than 96 % viable (*see* **Note 1**).
2. Inoculate 1.5×10^6 ID8-*Defb29/Vegf-A* cells via intraperitoneal injection to establish tumor masses in the peritoneal cavity by disinfecting the injection site and injecting with a 25–27 gauge needle into the abdomen on the mouse's right side at about a 30° angle to avoid puncturing the cecum or other internal organs (*see* **Notes 2** and **3**).
3. At the desired time point after tumor inoculation (in this example, 4 weeks) administer BNF-starch coated IONPs (or nanoparticle of choice) intraperitoneally to mice bearing ID8-*Defb29/Vegf-A* tumor.
4. Next day, sacrifice the mouse by euthanasia with carbon dioxide gas inhalation.

5. After sacrifice of the mouse, spray the mouse and tools with 70 % (v/v) ethanol.
6. Insert a 23 gauge needle parallel to the peritoneal membrane in the lower right quadrant of the abdomen, slowly inject 5–10 mL of ice cold 1× phosphate-buffered saline (PBS) into the peritoneal cavity, and gently massage the mouse abdomen to incorporate free cells into the PBS (*see* **Note 4**).
7. After injection, collect the peritoneal fluid slowly with the same syringe avoiding blood contamination if possible (often the peritoneum itself is bloody from ID8-*Defb29/Vegf-A* tumors, but generally not before 4 weeks). If the needle gets clogged by fat tissue organs, gently move the tip of the needle around a little to enable collection of PBS wash.
8. Collect as much fluid as possible and deposit the collected fluid in a tube and place on ice.
9. To recover as much fluid as possible, cut through the skin and peritoneum with a scissors, and collect the remaining fluid from the peritoneal cavity using a 1 mL pipette while holding up the skin with a forceps, but again avoid blood as much as possible.
10. Centrifuge the peritoneal lavage fluid at 250 × *g* for 5 min (preferably at 4 °C), discard the supernatant and disperse the cell pellet by gently tapping (*see* **Note 5**).
11. If there is obvious blood, add 1 mL of red blood cell lysis buffer to the pellet for every 5 mL of the original peritoneal lavage fluid, completely resuspend the cells by pipetting up and down, and incubate on ice for 5 min with occasional shaking.
12. Stop red blood cell lysis by adding 10 mL of ice cold 1× PBS to the tube and then centrifuge at 250 × *g* for 5 min (preferably at 4 °C).
13. Discard the supernatant and disperse the cell pellet by gently tapping.
14. Repeat **steps 11–13** until the cell pellet appears white or light pink, indicating effective red blood cell lysis.
15. Resuspend the cell pellet in 1 mL of ice cold 1× PBS, pass the suspension through 40 μm cell strainer and rinse the tube and the cell strainer with an additional 1 mL of ice cold 1× PBS (*see* **Note 6**).
16. Discard the cell strainer and count cells using a hemocytometer.
17. Resuspend total cells in the appropriate final volume (up to 10^8 total cells in 500 μL of degassed column running buffer) to proceed with MACS column separation.

3.2 Magnetically Labeled Cells Separation by MACS LS Columns

Pick the optimal column based on the sample sizes and following applications.

1. Attach magnetic MidiMACS Separator to the MACS MultiStand.
2. Place LS column with the column wings to the front into MACS Separator and set up a labeled tube under the magnet and column to collect flow through (*see* **Note 7**). The MACS Column matrix provides a magnetic field strong enough to retain cells labeled with minimal amounts of magnetic material.
3. To prepare LS column, apply 3 mL of degassed column running buffer on top of the column and rinse the column by letting the column running buffer run through (*see* **Note 8**). MACS columns should not be allowed to run dry.
4. Discard effluent and change the collection tube. The LS column is now ready for magnetic separation (*see* **Note 9**).
5. Completely resuspend up to 10^8 total cells from the peritoneal lavage fluid in 500 μL of degassed column running buffer. (For higher total cell numbers, scale up the volume of running buffer accordingly.) (*see* **Note 10**).
6. Apply the cell suspension onto the prepared LS column and then collect the flow through, which contains the unlabeled negative cell fraction. IONPs-containing cells are retained on the column, while cells lacking IONPs flow through.
7. Wash the LS column with 3 mL degassed column running buffer three times by adding running buffer each times once the column reservoir is almost empty. Collect total effluent and this also contains the unlabeled cell fraction.
8. Remove the LS column from the MACS separator magnet and place the column on a new collection tube.
9. Pipette 5 mL of buffer onto the LS column then immediately flush out the retained cell fraction by firmly applying the plunger supplied with the column to elute the magnetically labeled cells that were retained on the column by the magnet. To increase the purity, the positive cell fraction can be passed over a new, freshly prepared LS column for separation of up to 1×10^8 magnetically labeled cells.

3.3 Cytospin of Separated Cells by MACS Column

1. Count separated cells using a hemocytometer and dilute a cell suspension to have a concentration of 1×10^5 cells per mL.
2. Wash cells twice with 1 mL ice cold 10 % (v/v) FBS-containing media or PBS and resuspend cells in 150 μL of ice cold 10 % (v/v) FBS-containing media or PBS. Be sure to keep cells on ice (*see* **Notes 11** and **12**).
3. Prepare glass microscope slides by coating with poly-L-lysine, which produces an adhesive surface, and pre-label the slides (*see* **Note 13**).

4. Remove the rotor from the Cytocentrifuge (*see* **Note 14**).
5. Prepare slide by placing a poly-L-lysine coated glass slide and one disposable white filter card with two holes on top of the slide into the slide Cytoclip. Next place the single sample chamber (Cytofunnel) onto the white filter card. Be sure that each filter card and slide pair are flush with each other and line up the holes in proper position so that the cells will be forced onto the slide.
6. Load 1×10^5 cells in a volume of 150 μL of ice cold 10 % (v/v) FBS-containing media or PBS into the sample chamber then mix well by pipetting up and down (*see* **Notes 15** and **16**).
7. Remove the cover of the rotor by pulling up on the silver lift tab in the center. Place each Cytoclip assembly (slide, white filter card, sample chamber, and Cytoclip) into the Cytospin head and balance them out.
8. Replace the rotor cover by pulling up on the silver lift tab, and pushing it down until it locks into place. Place the rotor into the Cytocentrifuge.
9. Adjust the setting on the Cytocentrifuge to get the correct setting for the protocol, in this case, spin at $120 \times g$ for 5 min. Push the start button to begin.
10. After cytocentrifugation, remove the rotor and the cover of the rotor, and remove each Cytoclip assembly without disarranging it.
11. Carefully detach the sample chamber and the white filter card without contacting the smears on the slide to avoid damaging the fresh cytospin.
12. Prepare a slide again by placing a poly-L-lysine coated glass slide and one disposable white filter card on top of the slide upside down into the slide Cytoclip to adhere cells to the second hole. Then place the single sample chamber (Cytofunnel) onto the white filter card.
13. Repeat **steps 6–11**.
14. Replace the rotor once empty. Wash the sample chamber in the sink. If infectious agents, such as bacteria, were used, wash the sample chamber with 10 % (v/v) bleach solution. Allow the sample chamber to completely dry.
15. Air dry the slides for a few minutes and examine each slide under the microscope to be sure that the cells are reasonably dispersed. The cells should appear to have normal morphology.
16. Dry the slides in a desiccation chamber or air dry overnight.
17. Proceed with immediate fixation or store the cytospun slides at −80 °C until ready for staining.

3.4 Visualization of Iron Oxide Nanoparticles-Harboring Cells by Iron Stain with Gomori Prussian Blue

This method is used to detect ferric iron in tissue sections. Use acid cleaned glassware for Prussian blue staining steps. If any residual iron solution remains on the staining glassware, then diffuse background staining will occur (*see* **Note 17**).

1. Fix the dried cytospun slides by immersion in precooled acetone (at −20 °C) or 10 % (v/v) buffered formalin for 10 min (*see* **Note 18**).
2. Pour off the fixative and allow fixative solution to evaporate from the slides for 20 min at room temperature.
3. Rinse fixed slides with two changes of 1× PBS for 10 min each.
4. Mark the area around the cytocentrifuged cells with a water repellent PAP pen, liquid blocker.
5. Hydrate the slides in distilled water for 5 min.
6. Mix equal parts of Solution A (20 % (v/v) Hydrochloric acid aqueous solution) and Solution B (10 % (w/v) Potassium ferrocyanide aqueous solution) before use to make a working solution.
7. Place slides (including positive and negative controls) in the working solution for 20 min.
8. Rinse the slides with distilled water 3–4 times.
9. Place slides in Solution C (1 % (w/v) nuclear fast red stain solution) for 5 min to counterstain cell nuclei (*see* **Note 19**).
10. Rinse the slides twice with distilled water.
11. Air dry the slides or dehydrate through graded ethyl alcohols (we recommend 10, 30, 50, 70 % (v/v) and finally two changes of 100 % ethanol) and xylene or xylene substitute, and place a coverslip on top with a mounting medium, Permount (*see* **Note 20**).
12. Examine the stained slide under the microscope. Ferric iron deposits will be dark blue, nucleus is dark red, and cytoplasm is light red or pink (Fig. 1).

4 Notes

1. Cells should be thawed 4–5 days prior to tumor challenge and quickly harvested when at 80–85 % confluence to ensure good viability.
2. Inserting the needle on the mouse's right side of the abdomen avoids puncturing the cecum, a large fluid-filled organ on the left side. The small intestines on the right side are less likely to be punctured by the needle. The needle should enter to a depth of about half a centimeter.

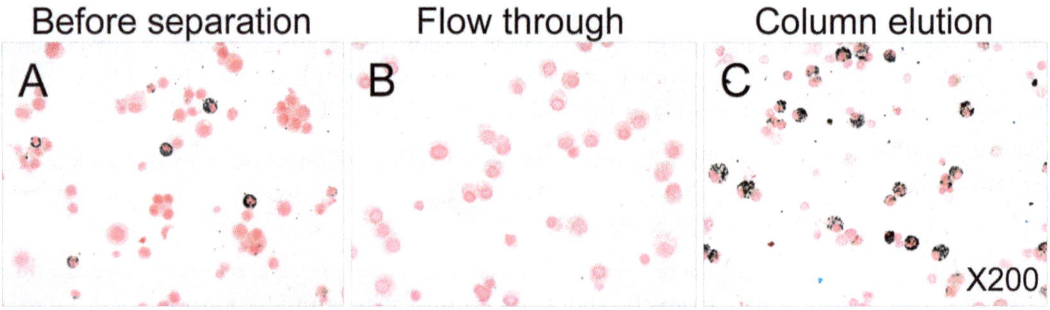

Fig. 1 Prussian blue staining of cytospin cells separated by MACS column. Representative histology pictures showing that Prussian blue staining of peritoneal lavage cells before separation (**a**), negative fraction of flow through (**b**), and magnetically labeled positively selected fraction (**c**). Pictures were taken with ×200 magnification

3. Aspirate once the needle has entered the abdomen to be sure that the needle has not penetrated the blood vessels or organs. For example, greenish brown aspirate indicates needle penetration into the intestines, and yellow aspirate indicates needle penetration into the urinary bladder. If any such fluid is aspirated into the needle, it indicates the solution is contaminated and must be discarded, and the injection procedure repeated with a new needle and syringe.
4. Insert the needle slowly and carefully into the peritoneum to avoid puncture of any organs or significant blood vessels.
5. After centrifugation, the cell pellet might be visible and tight, if not, remove about half of the supernatant and mix thoroughly.
6. Any visible chunks remaining in the cell suspension indicate the lysis/wash step is ineffective. Each time, the pellet must be completely dispersed and resolved.
7. MACS LS column capacity is 1×10^8 magnetically labeled cells from up to 2×10^9 total cells when manually separating. Column capacity may decrease when isolating larger cells than lymphocytes. Total enrichment rate is 50-fold to 1000-fold depending on the specificity and strength of the magnetic labeling. Typical flow rate of LS column for PBS is 1.3–2.0 mL/min.
8. Degas buffer before use by applying vacuum. Excessive gas in MACS column running buffer will form bubbles in the matrix inside of the column during cell separation and could block the column leading to clogging of the column and decreasing the quality of separation.
9. Do not store columns after rinsing, and use the column immediately to avoid formation of air bubbles.
10. Particles larger than 30 μm are not suitable for MACS separation with LS columns. To remove clumps and prevent

aggregates in the cell suspension, pass cells through 30 μm Pre-separation filter (Miltenyi Biotec, San Diego, CA).

11. Cells can be resuspended in 1 % BSA-containing media or PBS instead.
12. Fetal bovine serum provides nutrients to keep the cells healthy and alive throughout the cytospin procedure [16].
13. Glass slides should be clean before coating. Clean slides with 1 % (v/v) HCl in 70 % (v/v) ethanol (acid alcohol). Allow 0.1 % (w/v) poly-L-lysine solution to be room temperature before use. Place clean slides in 0.1 % (w/v) poly-L-lysine solution for 5 min. Dry slides in 60 °C oven for 1 h or overnight at room temperature [17–19].
14. The rotor must be removed from the cytocentrifuge before opening or closing the cover on the rotor. The rotor is very delicate and must be handled with care.
15. Load the sample in at least 100 μL and no more than 250 μL although the maximum sample volume for the white filter card is up to 500 μL.
16. When very few cells are available, load 100 μL of ice cold 1 % BSA-containing media or PBS (or 10 % FBS-containing media or PBS) without cells into the sample chamber and spin at 120 × *g* for 1–2 min. This will wet the filter card allowing more cells to reach the slide.
17. Clean glassware with acid alcohol, rinse thoroughly in distilled water, and dry.
18. Acetone fixative allows better antibody penetration but may wash out some antigen, especially in the case of cytosolic proteins. Avoid chromate fixatives when using glassware for staining.
19. Shake Solution C well before use. Do not filter.
20. The stained slides can be mounted with any compatible mounting medium.

Acknowledgment

We acknowledge the assistance of Dartmouth Transgenic and Genetic Constructs Shared Resource, and DartMouse Speed Congenics Shared Resource for animal maintenance. This study was supported by NIH grants: Dartmouth Immunology COBRE 5P30GM103415-03, NIH U54 CA151662-01, Norris Cotton Cancer Center Support Grant P30 CA023108-27, and R01CA157664.

References

1. Swann JB, Smyth MJ (2007) Immune surveillance of tumors. J Clin Invest 117 (5):1137–1146. doi:10.1172/JCI31405
2. Vatner RE, Cooper BT, Vanpouille-Box C, Demaria S, Formenti SC (2014) Combinations of immunotherapy and radiation in cancer therapy. Front Oncol 4:325. doi:10.3389/fonc.2014.00325
3. Fernandez A, Oliver L, Alvarez R, Fernandez LE, Lee KP, Mesa C (2014) Adjuvants and myeloid-derived suppressor cells: enemies or allies in therapeutic cancer vaccination. Hum Vaccin Immunother 10(11):3251–3260. doi:10.4161/hv.29847
4. Owens DE III, Peppas NA (2006) Opsonization, biodistribution, and pharmacokinetics of polymeric nanoparticles. Int J Pharm 307 (1):93–102. doi:10.1016/j.ijpharm.2005.10.010, S0378-5173(05)00668-X [pii]
5. Hong RL, Huang CJ, Tseng YL, Pang VF, Chen ST, Liu JJ, Chang FH (1999) Direct comparison of liposomal doxorubicin with or without polyethylene glycol coating in C-26 tumor-bearing mice: is surface coating with polyethylene glycol beneficial? Clin Cancer Res 5(11):3645–3652
6. Cubillos-Ruiz JR, Baird JR, Tesone AJ, Rutkowski MR, Scarlett UK, Camposeco-Jacobs AL, Anadon-Arnillas J, Harwood NM, Korc M, Fiering SN, Sempere LF, Conejo-Garcia JR (2012) Reprogramming tumor-associated dendritic cells in vivo using miRNA mimetics triggers protective immunity against ovarian cancer. Cancer Res 72(7):1683–1693. doi:10.1158/0008-5472.CAN-11-3160, 0008-5472.CAN-11-3160 [pii]
7. Toraya-Brown S, Sheen MR, Baird JR, Barry S, Demidenko E, Turk MJ, Hoopes PJ, Conejo-Garcia JR, Fiering S (2013) Phagocytes mediate targeting of iron oxide nanoparticles to tumors for cancer therapy. Integr Biol (Camb) 5 (1):159–171. doi:10.1039/c2ib20180a
8. Roby KF, Taylor CC, Sweetwood JP, Cheng Y, Pace JL, Tawfik O, Persons DL, Smith PG, Terranova PF (2000) Development of a syngeneic mouse model for events related to ovarian cancer. Carcinogenesis 21(4):585–591
9. Conejo-Garcia JR, Benencia F, Courreges MC, Kang E, Mohamed-Hadley A, Buckanovich RJ, Holtz DO, Jenkins A, Na H, Zhang L, Wagner DS, Katsaros D, Caroll R, Coukos G (2004) Tumor-infiltrating dendritic cell precursors recruited by a beta-defensin contribute to vasculogenesis under the influence of Vegf-A. Nat Med 10(9):950–958. doi:10.1038/nm1097, nm1097 [pii]
10. Cubillos-Ruiz JR, Engle X, Scarlett UK, Martinez D, Barber A, Elgueta R, Wang L, Nesbeth Y, Durant Y, Gewirtz AT, Sentman CL, Kedl R, Conejo-Garcia JR (2009) Polyethylenimine-based siRNA nanocomplexes reprogram tumor-associated dendritic cells via TLR5 to elicit therapeutic antitumor immunity. J Clin Invest 119(8):2231–2244. doi:10.1172/JCI37716, 37716 [pii]
11. Yang R, Cai Z, Zhang Y, Yutzy WH, Roby KF, Roden RB (2006) CD80 in immune suppression by mouse ovarian carcinoma-associated Gr-1 + CD11b + myeloid cells. Cancer Res 66(13):6807–6815. doi:10.1158/0008-5472.CAN-05-3755, 66/13/6807 [pii]
12. Kryczek I, Zou L, Rodriguez P, Zhu G, Wei S, Mottram P, Brumlik M, Cheng P, Curiel T, Myers L, Lackner A, Alvarez X, Ochoa A, Chen L, Zou W (2006) B7-H4 expression identifies a novel suppressive macrophage population in human ovarian carcinoma. J Exp Med 203(4):871–881. doi:10.1084/jem.20050930, jem.20050930 [pii]
13. Curiel TJ, Wei S, Dong H, Alvarez X, Cheng P, Mottram P, Krzysiek R, Knutson KL, Daniel B, Zimmermann MC, David O, Burow M, Gordon A, Dhurandhar N, Myers L, Berggren R, Hemminki A, Alvarez RD, Emilie D, Curiel DT, Chen L, Zou W (2003) Blockade of B7-H1 improves myeloid dendritic cell-mediated antitumor immunity. Nat Med 9 (5):562–567. doi:10.1038/nm863, nm863 [pii]
14. Sheen MR, Lizotte PH, Toraya-Brown S, Fiering S (2014) Stimulating antitumor immunity with nanoparticles. Wiley Interdiscip Rev Nanomed Nanobiotechnol 6(5):496–505. doi:10.1002/wnan.1274
15. Pankhurst QA, Thanh NTK, Jones SK, Dobson J (2009) Progress in applications of magnetic nanoparticles in biomedicine. J Phys D Appl Phys 42(22):224001–224015. doi:10.1088/0022-3727/42/22/224001
16. Ikeda K, Tate G, Suzuki T, Kitamura T, Mitsuya T (2010) Diagnostic usefulness of EMA, IMP3, and GLUT-1 for the immunocytochemical distinction of malignant cells from reactive mesothelial cells in effusion cytology using cytospin preparations. Diagn Cytopathol 39(6):395–401. doi:10.1002/dc.21398
17. Culling CFA, Allison RT, Bair WT (1985) Cellular pathology technique, 4th edn. Butterworth, Boston
18. Huang WM, Gibson SJ, Facer P, Gu J, Polak JM (1983) Improved section adhesion for

immunocytochemistry using high molecular weight polymers of L-lysine as a slide coating. Histochemistry 77(2):275–279

19. Mazia D, Schatten G, Sale W (1975) Adhesion of cells to surfaces coated with polylysine. Applications to electron microscopy. J Cell Biol 66(1):198–200

Chapter 23

Pulmonary Delivery of Magnetically Targeted Nano-in-Microparticles

Amber A. McBride*, Dominique N. Price*, and Pavan Muttil

Abstract

This chapter details the intratracheal delivery of dry powder microparticles termed nano-in-microparticles (NIMs) for the purpose of in vivo targeted pulmonary drug delivery. The dry powder NIMs technology improves on previous inhaled chemotherapy platforms designed as liquid formulations. Dry powder microparticles were created through the process of spray drying; a protocol detailing the formulation of NIMs dry powder is included as a separate chapter in this book. Dry powder NIMs containing fluorescent nanoparticles and magnetically-responsive superparamagnetic iron oxide nanoparticles are intratracheally delivered (insufflated) in the presence of a magnetic field and targeted to the left lung of mice. The targeting efficiency of dry powder NIMs is compared to the targeting efficiency of liquid NIMs to demonstrate the superiority of dry power targeting platforms. Targeting is assessed using fluorescence associated with NIMs detected in the mouse trachea, left lung, and right lung by an in vivo imaging system.

Key words Dry powder, Nano-in-microparticles, Intratracheal delivery, Insufflation, Superparamagnetism, Iron oxide nanoparticles, Pulmonary delivery, Targeted drug delivery

1 Introduction

1.1 Advantages of Pulmonary Drug Delivery Approach

Pulmonary administration of chemotherapeutics is a direct method of local delivery to the lung, as opposed to indirect methods such as parenteral and oral routes of delivery. Pulmonary drug delivery systems offer many advantages over traditional drug delivery systems [1]. First and foremost, drugs can be delivered regionally instead of systemically, directly to the disease site. Regional delivery allows for a lower drug dose to be used, often resulting in fewer systemic side effects. Also, barriers obstructing therapeutic efficacy are bypassed, such as poor gastrointestinal absorption and first-pass metabolism of drugs in the liver. In addition, pulmonary delivery is noninvasive and "needle-free" allowing for a wide range of

*These authors contributed equally to this work.

Reema Zeineldin (ed.), *Cancer Nanotechnology: Methods and Protocols*, Methods in Molecular Biology, vol. 1530, DOI 10.1007/978-1-4939-6646-2_23, © Springer Science+Business Media New York 2017

substances to be delivered, from small molecules to very large proteins [2]. The lungs have an enormous absorptive surface area (100 m^2) and a highly permeable membrane (0.2–0.7 μm thickness) in the alveolar region [3]. Large molecules with low gastrointestinal absorption rates can be absorbed in significant quantities due to the slow mucociliary clearance in the lung periphery resulting in prolonged residence in the lung [4].

Futhermore, inhalable drugs formulated as dry powders have many additional advantages. Dry powders have greater chemical and physical stability compared to aqueous dispersions for nebulization and thus often have increased product shelf lives and may not require refrigeration during storage. A nebulized suspension can prematurely release the drug payload, whereas we have shown that an inhaled dry powder can overcome this limitation in an in vitro setting [5]. Compared to a nebulizer, inhaler devices used to deliver dry powders are more efficient and less time-consuming. This reduces the overall treatment time and improves patient compliance.

1.2 History of Inhaled Chemotherapies

Although the development of inhalational agents for oncological use in humans has been limited [6], there is a large amount of published data regarding aerosol delivery of chemotherapy in preclinical studies. Futhermore feasibility of aerosol delivery has been shown using in vitro models [7, 8], animal models [9–15], and Phase I/II human trials for various cancers [16–20].

In 1968 the chemotherapeutic agent, 5-fluorouracil (5-FU), was investigated for inhalational therapy [21]. This study, published by Tatsumura and colleagues, treated patients with inhaled 5-FU preceded by surgery. Study results showed that 5-FU was found in higher concentrations in lung tumors than in the surrounding tissue. In a later study, Tatsumura et al. showed high 5-FU concentrations in the main bronchus and adjacent lymph nodes for nearly 4 h post-administration [18]. Furthermore, the formulation of 5-FU with lipid-coated nanoparticles showed sustained drug release and enhanced anticancer properties [22]. Similarly, Otterson and colleagues evaluated inhaled doxorubicin in a Phase I, and later in a Phase I/II, clinical study and demonstrated the promising efficacy of an aerosol treatment [16, 17]. However, the non-targeted aerosol delivery led to a moderate reduction of pulmonary function and pulmonary dose-limiting toxicity in some patients.

It is therefore critical to target inhaled chemotherapeutics, beyond local delivery, to tumors to protect healthy lung tissue. None of the studies described above used a targeting mechanism within the lung. To this end, Azarmi et al. formulated poly(butylcyanocrylate) nanoparticles with doxorubicin for inhaled, targeted drug delivery to the lung via encapsulation in lactose carrier particles made by spray-freeze drying [23]. This study showed successful in vitro uptake of the nanoparticles into H460 and A549 lung cancer lines through endocytosis rather than passive diffusion. Similarly, Dames et al. used a liquid suspension of magnetically-responsive superparamagnetic iron oxide nano-particles (SPIONs) and plasmid DNA (pDNA) (used as a drug surrogate) to target the different lobes of the lung in mice [11]. Unfortunately, while SPIONs were successful in tissue-targeting, pDNA was found to separate from the SPIONs during pulmonary administration. McBride and colleagues have formulated dry powder nano-in-microparticles (NIMs), incorporating SPIONs and chemotherapeutics in a dry powder lactose matrix that prevented pre-separation of SPIONs and therapeutic while maintaining the size and flow characteristics critical for lung delivery [5]. This formulation platform is detailed in another chapter of this book.

1.3 Micro- and Nanoparticles as Drug Delivery Vehicles

Delivery vehicles (nanoparticles (NPs), microparticles, or nanoparticles encapsulated within microparticles can range in size from several nanometers to a few micrometers. Microparticles intended for inhaled drug delivery should be 1–3 μm in size to achieve alveolar deposition [24]. Depending on the target delivery region, particles exhibit desirable particle size distribution ideally with aerodynamic diameters (d_a) of 5–10 μm for airways and 1–5 μm for deep lung delivery with a standard density of 1 g/cm^3. Particles less than 0.5 μm (NPs) are driven by diffusion and are likely to be exhaled, hence they are often encapsulated and delivered within microparticles.

This chapter describes targeted delivery of dry powder NIMs directly into the lungs of a mouse. NIMs are formulated to be magnetically-responsive, and can be used to target drug payloads to a particular lobe of the lung with the use of an external magnet [5]. NIMs dry powder matrixes have the benefit of physically binding the magnet-targeting SPIONs and drug payload (a fluorescent dye is used as a drug surrogate for visualization). Conversely, NIMs in a liquid suspension run the risk of SPION and drug separation, negating the targeting effect. To compare NIMs dry powder targeting efficiency to NIMs liquid suspension targeting, administration of a liquid suspension to mice using an intratracheal aerosolization device is also described below.

2 Materials

1. Balb/c mice (6–8 weeks old).
2. Intubation platform.
3. Nano-in-Microparticles (NIMs).
4. Penn Century dry powder Insufflator™.

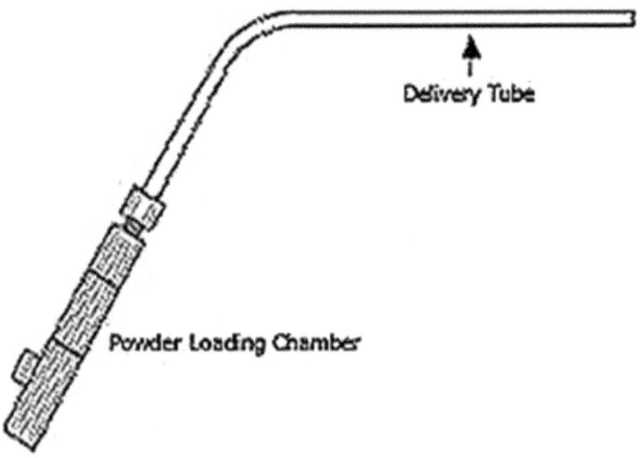

Fig. 1 A dry powder Insufflator™ for mouse (DP-4M). The device consists of a total of three pieces. The dry powder chamber is made up of two pieces; the chamber tube can be pulled apart and loaded with up to 2 mg of dry powder. To close the tube after the powder is loaded into the chamber, the two pieces are gently pressed together with pressure. The third piece of the device is the delivery tube and is attached by a screw thread to the delivery chamber tube. The delivery tube is 8″ in length from the bend angle to the tip of the tube. The insufflation device is fragile and extreme care must be taken to immediately clean the insufflator to prevent clogging. Photo of Dry Powder Insufflator™—Model DP-4 reprinted with permission of Penn-Century, Inc.

5. Neodymium-iron-boron (NdFeB) permanent cylindrical magnet (grade N52, 22 mm long × 20 mm in diameter).
6. Laryngoscope.
7. Mouse intratracheal aerosolizer.
8. In vivo fluorescence or bioluminescence animal imager.
9. The DP-4M Dry Powder Insufflator™ is specifically developed for pulmonary dry powder administration to mice, and variants suitable for rats, guinea pigs, and larger animals exist (*see* Fig. 1).

3 Methods

3.1 Intratracheal Administration of Dry Powder to Mice

1. Weigh mouse.
2. Administer anesthesia (*see* **Note 1**).
3. Weigh the clean insufflator, including the powder chamber and delivery tube. This initial weight will be used to calculate the final amount of powders delivered into the mouse lung.
4. Add 1–2 mg of dry powder NIMs to the insufflator chamber and close the chamber (*see* **Note 2**). Re-weigh the insufflator to ensure the proper powder amount has been loaded into the chamber.

5. Place the anesthetized mouse supine on the plexiglass intubation platform.
6. The platform should be situated at a 60° angle facing away from you. The operator will be facing the head of the mouse.
7. Using the incisor loop (plastic fishing line) hang the front incisors (teeth) of the mouse from the loop. A thin rubber band can then be placed over the mouse to secure the mouse on the intubation platform.
8. Using a cotton-tipped swab, gently roll the mouse tongue out of its mouth and to one side to expose the oropharynx.
9. Insert the laryngoscope into the mouth of the mouse. Using the light and blade features, depress the tongue to view the epiglottis. Adding a magnifying glass to the laryngoscope handle (using Velcro) will aid in the clear visualization of the small tracheal opening in a mouse. A white round opening, indicated by the opening and closing of the arytenoid cartilage around the tracheal opening should be visible (*see* **Note 3**).
10. The insufflator delivery tube (cannula) should be inserted down the trachea of the animal, gently proximal to the carina, until the curve of the cannula is positioned at the incisors. Attach the powder loaded chamber of the insufflator to the cannula. A 3 mL disposable plastic syringe is attached to the open end of the insufflator.
11. With the mouse situated on the plexiglass delivery platform, place the magnet over left lung as the mouse faces away from you, as shown in Fig. 2.
12. To insufflate the powders, depress the syringe attached to the insufflator with steady, forceful pressure using not more than 500 μL of air (*see* **Note 4**).
13. Note number of puffs given (*see* **Note 5**). Reweigh the insufflator after powder delivery (delivery tube and powder chamber) to quantify the amount of dry powder administered to the mouse lung.
14. If non-significant targeting exists (based on in vivo imaging), surgically open the animal and cut through the skin/ muscle to depth of the rib cage. Surgically expose the left lung by thoracotomy (*see* **Note 6**). Then re-place the magnet 1 mm above the incision, with the magnet's edge perpendicular to the upper section of the left lung. Follow **steps 8–13** again to deliver NIMs dry powder using the insufflator.
15. Sacrifice the mouse immediately. Remove lungs and trachea en bloc and separate (right lung, left lung, and trachea) into distinct tissues for evaluation of targeting efficiency of NIMs to the magnetized lobe. These tissues can be assessed for fluorescence and iron quantification.

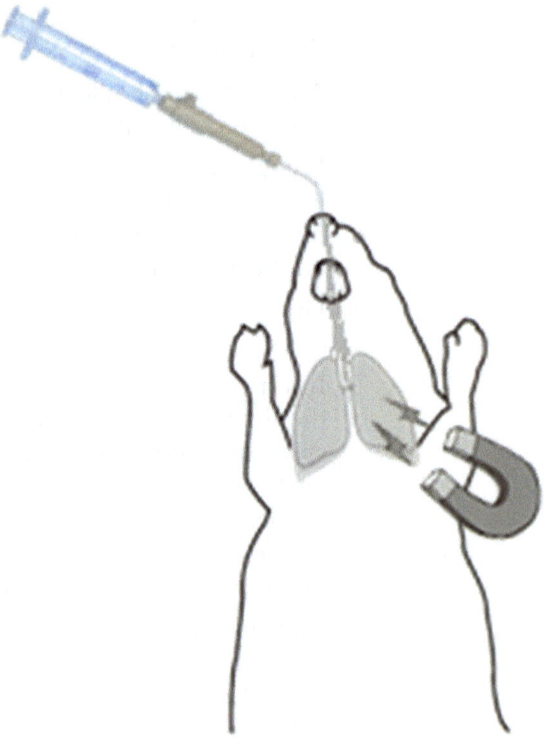

Fig. 2 Targeting NIMs to the left lung during insufflation using a permanent magnet. The mouse has been intubated with the insufflator. A magnet is held over the left lung lobe. NIMs will be dispersed into the lungs when the syringe plunger attached to the insufflator is depressed. NIMs will preferentially target the left lung compared to the right due to the magnetic field

3.2 Measurements to Be Noted

Weight of mouse: ________________________________ g

Theoretical amount of NIMs to be administered to mouse: ________________________________ mg

Insufflator weight loaded with 2 mg NIMs: ____________ mg

Insufflator weight post-NIMs administration: ____________ mg

Weight of NIMs administered: ____________ ________ mg

Number of insufflator "puffs" given to mouse: __________ puffs

3.3 Intratracheal Administration of Liquid Suspension to Mice

1. Weigh mouse.
2. Administer anesthesia (*see* **Note 1**).
3. Add 1.5 mg NIMs (*see* **Note 2**) to 0.5 mL saline and load into the aerosolization device.
4. With the mouse situated on the intubation platform, place the magnet over the left lung as mouse faces you (*see* **Note 3**).
5. Insert the laryngoscope into the mouth. Using the light and blade features, depress the tongue to view the epiglottis.

Adding a magnifying glass to the laryngoscope handle (using Velcro) will aid in the clear visualization of the small tracheal opening in a mouse. You should see a white round opening, indicated by the opening and closing of the arytenoid cartilage around the tracheal opening.

6. The liquid intratracheal aerosolization device should be inserted the trachea of the animal gently, proximal to the carina, until the curve of the cannula is positioned at the incisors.
7. To aerosolize the formulation, the plunger should be depressed firmly and with consistent force and speed (*see* **Note 7**). Once the plunger has been completely depressed, the liquid suspension will be administered into the mouse lung.
8. Carefully remove the aerosolizer delivery tube from the mouse trachea.
9. Sacrifice the mouse immediately. Remove lungs and trachea en bloc and separate (right lung, left lung and trachea) into distinct tissues for NIMs-targeting efficiency to the magnetized. These tissues can be assessed for fluorescence and iron quantification.

3.4 Comparison of Targeting Efficacy

1. Evaluate the presence of dye by measuring the fluorescence of each tissue (right lung, left lung, and trachea) (*see* **Notes 8** and **9**). Compare targeting efficiency of dye by first calculating NIM-associated fluorescence of each tissue over the total tissue fluorescence. This will tell you the percent of dye targeted to each tissue, and whether more dye was targeted to the left lung versus the right lung:

$$\%\text{Dye targeted to right lung} = \frac{\text{Fluorescene in right lung}}{\text{Total fluorescence (right lung + left lung + trachea)}}$$

$$\%\text{Dye targeted to left lung} = \frac{\text{Fluorescene in left lung}}{\text{Total fluorescence (right lung + left lung + trachea)}}$$

$$\%\text{Dye targeted to trachea} = \frac{\text{Fluorescene in trachea}}{\text{Total fluorescence (right lung + left lung + trachea)}}$$

2. Evaluate the presence of SPIONs by measuring iron content in each tissue (right lung, left lung, and trachea) (*see* **Note 10**). Compare targeting efficiency of SPIONs by first calculating the SPION-associated iron content of each tissue over the SPION-associated iron content of the total tissue. This will tell you the percent of SPIONs targeted to each tissue, and whether more SPIONs were targeted to the left lung versus the right lung:

$$\% \text{ SPIONs targeted to right lung} = \frac{\text{Iron in right lung}}{\text{Total iron (right lung + left lung + trachea)}}$$

$$\% \text{ SPIONs targeted to left lung} = \frac{\text{Iron in left lung}}{\text{Total iron (right lung + left lung + trachea)}}$$

$$\% \text{ SPIONs targeted to trachea} = \frac{\text{Iron in trachea}}{\text{Total iron (right lung + left lung + trachea)}}$$

3. Determine whether the SPIONs separated from the dye during targeting by comparing percentages (dye and SPIONs) for each tissue. The percentage deposited in each tissue will be significantly different if the SPIONs and dye separated during administration.

4 Notes

1. We used 100 mg/kg and 10 mg/kg body weight of ketamine and xylazine by intraperitoneal injection, respectively, for anaesthesia dosing.
2. Pre-weighing powders into a capsule speeds up the loading process and helps to ensure repeatability when loading similar amounts. For NIMs suspension (liquid) experiments we used the Penn Century Microsprayer® aerosolization device.
3. Morello et al. has published an excellent synopsis on the insufflation of dry powders into the lung of a mouse [25].
4. Hoppentocht et al. recently published data stating that 200 μL air volume, as recommended by the manufacturer, did not provide adequate dispersion of the NIMs in the insufflator leading to variable dry powder deposition in mouse lungs [26, 27]. We confirmed this observation and showed that a larger pulsed air volume of 500 μL was required for adequate NIMs dispersion in the lungs using the mouse insufflator. However, a higher air volume may have led to significant powder deposition in the trachea due to inertial impaction.
5. In our experience, ten puffs administered 25 % of the dry powder NIMs loaded in the insufflator. The remaining 75 % remained in the insufflator. Administering more than ten puffs did not dislodge the remaining NIMs from the insufflator.
6. A similar surgical protocol to expose the lungs for magnetic targeting is described by Dames et al. [11].
7. The force used to dispense the NIMs suspension from the liquid intratracheal aerosolization device was maintained at a constant rate.

8. Significantly more fluorescence (from the dye in the NIMs) was quantified in the trachea for dry powder NIMs than liquid suspension. We attribute this pitfall to the DP-4M insufflator delivery tool. The insufflator deposits the dry powder in the respiratory tract based on firm pushing of the syringe, which is necessary for the proper aerosolization and delivery of NIMs into the lung [25]. However, the high velocity air stream generated by the syringe (attached to the insufflator) leads to powder deposition in the upper conducting airways and the main tracheal bifurcation due to inertial impaction. Dry powder NIMs exiting the insufflator delivery tube had increased momentum and followed their trajectory until they collided with the tracheal wall [25]. NIMs that did not impact the upper respiratory tract were available for magnetic-targeting within the lung lobes. A passive dry powder inhaler that allows slow and deep inspiration may mitigate the upper respiratory tract deposition of NIMs.
9. For each tissue (right lung, left lung, and trachea), obtain total relative fluorescent units (rfu) as well as region of interest rfus (keeping the region of interest constant for each tissue).
10. We used Inductively Coupled Plasma–Atomic Emission Spectroscopy (ICP-AES) to determine tissue iron content. However, it is important to note that when using this method you must have a tissue control to subtract out the endogenous iron content of the tissues.

Acknowledgment

This research was supported by the University of New Mexico Health Science Center Research and Allocations Committee (RAC) grant. AAM was supported by NSF-IGERT Integrating Nanotechnology with Cell Biology and Neuroscience Fellowship (DGE-0549500) and the NCI Alliance for Nanotechnology in Cancer New Mexico CNTC Training Center. DNP was supported by Bill and Melinda Gates Grand Challenge Exploration (No OPP1061393) and UNM IDIP T32 training grant (T32-A1007538, P.I.– M. Ozbun).

References

1. Labiris NR, Dolovich MB (2003) Pulmonary drug delivery. Part I: Physiological factors affecting therapeutic effectiveness of aerosolized medications. Br J Clin Pharmacol 56:588–599
2. Wolff RK (1998) Safety of inhaled proteins for therapeutic use. J Aerosol Med 11:197–219. doi:10.1089/jam.1998.11.197
3. Patton JS, Byron PR (2007) Inhaling medicines: delivering drugs to the body through the lungs. Nat Rev Drug Discov 6:67–74. doi:10.1038/nrd2153
4. Agnew JE, Pavia D, Clarke SW (1981) Airways penetration of inhaled radioaerosol: an index to small airways function? Eur J Respir Dis 62:239–255

5. McBride AA, Price DN, Lamoureux LR et al (2013) Preparation and characterization of novel magnetic nano-in-microparticles for site-specific pulmonary drug delivery. Mol Pharm 10:3574–3581. doi:10.1021/mp3007264
6. Sharma S, White D, Imondi AR et al (2001) Development of inhalational agents for oncologic use. J Clin Oncol 19:1839–1847
7. Azarmi S, Tao X, Chen H et al (2006) Formulation and cytotoxicity of doxorubicin nanoparticles carried by dry powder aerosol particles. Int J Pharm 319:155–161. doi:10.1016/j.ijpharm.2006.03.052
8. Tseng C-L, Su W-Y, Yen K-C et al (2009) The use of biotinylated-EGF-modified gelatin nanoparticle carrier to enhance cisplatin accumulation in cancerous lungs via inhalation. Biomaterials 30:3476–3485. doi:10.1016/j.biomaterials.2009.03.010
9. Rao R, Markovic S, Anderson P (2003) Aerosol therapy for malignancy involving the lungs. Curr Cancer Drug Targets 3:239–250. doi:10.2174/1568009033481895
10. Hershey AE, Kurzman ID, Forrest LJ et al (1999) Inhalation chemotherapy for macroscopic primary or metastatic lung tumors: proof of principle using dogs with spontaneously occurring tumors as a model. Clin Cancer Res 5:2653–2659
11. Dames P, Gleich B, Flemmer A et al (2007) Targeted delivery of magnetic aerosol droplets to the lung. Nat Nanotechnol 2:495–499. doi:10.1038/nnano.2007.217
12. Hasenpusch G, Geiger J, Wagner K et al (2012) Magnetized aerosols comprising superparamagnetic iron oxide nanoparticles improve targeted drug and gene delivery to the lung. Pharm Res 29:1308–1318. doi:10.1007/s11095-012-0682-z
13. Gagnadoux F, Hureaux J, Vecellio L et al (2008) Aerosolized chemotherapy. J Aerosol Med Pulm Drug Deliv 21:61–70. doi:10.1089/jamp.2007.0656
14. Rodriguez CO, Crabbs TA, Wilson DW et al (2010) Aerosol gemcitabine: preclinical safety and in vivo antitumor activity in osteosarcoma-bearing dogs. J Aerosol Med Pulm Drug Deliv 23:197–206. doi:10.1089/jamp.2009.0773
15. Yi D, Wiedmann TS (2010) Inhalation adjuvant therapy for lung cancer. J Aerosol Med Pulm Drug Deliv 23:181–187. doi:10.1089/jamp.2009.0787
16. Otterson GA, Villalona-Calero MA, Sharma S et al (2007) Phase I study of inhaled Doxorubicin for patients with metastatic tumors to the lungs. Clin Cancer Res 13:1246–1252. doi:10.1158/1078-0432.CCR-06-1096
17. Otterson GA, Villalona-Calero MA, Hicks W et al (2010) Phase I/II study of inhaled doxorubicin combined with platinum-based therapy for advanced non-small cell lung cancer. Clin Cancer Res 16:2466–2473. doi:10.1158/1078-0432.CCR-09-3015
18. Tatsumura T, Koyama S, Tsujimoto M et al (1993) Further study of nebulisation chemotherapy, a new chemotherapeutic method in the treatment of lung carcinomas: fundamental and clinical. Br J Cancer 68:1146–1149
19. Zarogoulidis P, Darwiche K, Krauss L et al (2013) Inhaled cisplatin deposition and distribution in lymph nodes in stage II lung cancer patients. Future Oncol 9:1307–1313. doi:10.2217/fon.13.111
20. Lemarie E, Vecellio L, Hureaux J et al (2011) Aerosolized gemcitabine in patients with carcinoma of the lung: feasibility and safety study. J Aerosol Med Pulm Drug Deliv 24:261–270. doi:10.1089/jamp.2010.0872
21. Tatsumura T, Yamamoto K, Murakami A et al (1983) New chemotherapeutic method for the treatment of tracheal and bronchial cancers—nebulization chemotherapy. Gan No Rinsho 29:765–770
22. Hitzman CJ, Elmquist WF, Wattenberg LW, Wiedmann TS (2006) Development of a respirable, sustained release microcarrier for 5-fluorouracil I: in vitro assessment of liposomes, microspheres, and lipid coated nanoparticles. J Pharm Sci 95:1114–1126. doi:10.1002/jps.20591
23. Azarmi S, Lobenberg R, Roa WH et al (2008) Formulation and in vivo evaluation of effervescent inhalable carrier particles for pulmonary delivery of nanoparticles. Drug Dev Ind Pharm 34:943–947. doi:10.1080/03639040802149079
24. Gerrity TR, Lee PS, Hass FJ et al (1979) Calculated deposition of inhaled particles in the airway generations of normal subjects. J Appl Physiol 47:867–873
25. Morello M, Krone CL, Dickerson S et al (2009) Dry-powder pulmonary insufflation in the mouse for application to vaccine or drug studies. Tuberculosis (Edinb) 89:371–377. doi:10.1016/j.tube.2009.07.001
26. Hoppentocht M, Hoste C, Hagedoorn P et al (2014) In vitro evaluation of the DP-4M Penn-Century insufflator. Eur J Pharm Biopharm 88:153–159. doi:10.1016/j.ejpb.2014.06.014
27. Duret C, Wauthoz N, Sebti T et al (2012) Solid dispersions of itraconazole for inhalation with enhanced dissolution, solubility and dispersion properties. Int J Pharm 428:103–113. doi:10.1016/j.ijpharm.2012.03.002

Chapter 24

Neutron-Activatable Nanoparticles for Intraperitoneal Radiation Therapy

Derek Hargrove and Xiuling Lu

Abstract

Intraperitoneal internal radiation therapy is a cancer treatment option that is employed in situations where surgical resection, systemic chemotherapy, and external beam radiotherapy are not amenable for patients. However, exposure of noncancerous tissues to radiation continues to be a hindrance to safe and effective treatment of patients. In addition, reducing prolonged radiation exposure of personnel during preparation of internal radiation therapy agents makes their manufacture complicated and hazardous. Developments in nanotechnology have provided a platform for targeted treatments that combine dual imaging and treatment capabilities all in one package, while also being robust enough to withstand the intense stresses faced during neutron activation. Here, we describe a method for synthesizing neutron activatable mesoporous silica nanoparticles for use in radiotherapy of metastatic peritoneal cancers while limiting personal exposure to radioactive materials, limiting the leakage of radioactive isotopes caused by nanoparticle degradation during neutron activation, and increasing cancer tissue specificity of radiation.

Key words Nanotechnology, Neutron activation, Cancer, Radiation therapy, Intraperitoneal delivery

1 Introduction

The peritoneal cavity is a common site of metastatic disease [1, 2] from primary tumors found in the organs of the digestive tract and ovaries. Peritoneal metastatic disease is particularly characterized by poor patient outcomes and current treatment strategies include surgical resection in conjunction with intravenous chemotherapy [3–5]. In some cases, when patients fail to respond to these treatments, external beam radiation treatment is used. In general, these treatments are typically palliative in nature and are associated with high systemic toxicity [4]. In an effort to decrease the exposure of healthy tissues to harmful radiation and chemotherapeutics while also increasing local tumor exposure levels, intraperitoneal delivery of radiotherapeutics and chemotherapeutics has been employed [6–8].

Reema Zeineldin (ed.), *Cancer Nanotechnology: Methods and Protocols*, Methods in Molecular Biology, vol. 1530,
DOI 10.1007/978-1-4939-6646-2_24, © Springer Science+Business Media New York 2017

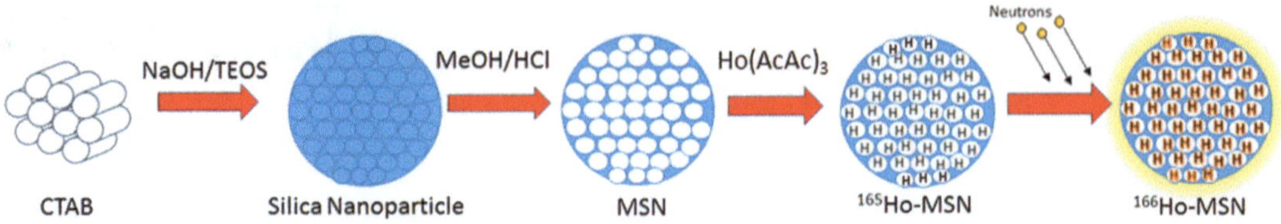

Fig. 1 Schematic of the synthesis pathway for Holmium-166 mesoporous silica nanoparticles. Under basic conditions the surfactant forms positively charged micelles that interact with the negatively charged TEOS forming a well ordered, hexagonal pore array covered in silica. After refluxing the particles in acidified methanol the surfactant is removed and all that is left are the hollow pores of the nanoparticles. Holmium acetylacetone ($Ho(AcAc)_3$) can then be added to the pores and the entire particle can be placed in a neutron flux to convert the stable Holmium-165 to the radioisotope Holmium-166

Nanomaterials provide a unique system that can increase the local concentration of radiotherapeutics with the ability to be tuned for specific tumor targeting through the use of targeting ligands [5, 9, 10]. If the particles have to be loaded with already radioactive materials, then the amount of exposure of the handlers during the synthesis of the nanoparticles may be high. These nanocarrier systems can be made radioactive after their manufacture using a neutron activation approach. However, in order for this to work, the particles have to be able to withstand the harsh environment of a nuclear reactor during neutron activation while still retaining its radioactive cargo and its targeting capabilities [11, 12].

In the mesoporous silica nanoparticle system (MSN) described in Fig. 1, we have demonstrated that the nanoparticles can be synthesized and loaded with a stable isotope of Holmium-165 in a well-studied 4-step process [13–17] without loss of cargo once it has been loaded [18]. The loaded nanoparticle can then be placed in a thermal neutron flux for conversion of Holmium-165 to its radioactive form of Holmium-166. Holmium-166 is useful in the treatment of cancer due to its emission of high-energy β-particles while also providing imaging capabilities with single-photon emission computed tomography due to the emission of γ- photons [19]. The relatively short half-life of 26.8 h also allows for limited radiation exposure of the patient and caregiver after intraperitoneal administration. The mesoporous silica nanoparticle structure is robust enough to withstand prolonged time in thermal neutron flux without the release of radioactive holmium [18]. The ability to make the particles radioactive post synthesis limits radiation exposure to the handlers and manufacturers of the particles, without sacrificing the integrity of the product. Upon intraperitoneal administration it has also been shown that these particles have the capability to selectively and passively accumulate in tumor tissues, thus limiting the exposure of healthy peritoneal tissues to radiation [18].

The following protocol details the preparation of monodisperse mesoporous silica nanoparticles loaded with Holmium-166. This includes the synthesis of particles with a well ordered hexagonal pore structure, Holmium-165 crystal preparation, loading the nanoparticles with the Holmium-165 crystals, and proper nanoparticle preparation for converting the entrapped Holmium-165 to the radioactive Holmium-166 isotope using neutron activation without nanoparticle degradation. Along with a detailed description of the preparation steps, multiple notes are introduced throughout the protocol in order to help bring attention to potential preparation pitfalls along with insight into potential protocol alterations for the optimization of the nanoparticles for more specific applications.

2 Materials

Prepare all solutions using type 1 (18.2 MΩ cm at 25 °C) ultrapure water and analytical grade reagents. Store all the stock reagents at room temperature and all prepared samples at 4 °C unless otherwise specified. It is best to freshly prepare all the necessary solutions before each synthesis to ensure highest product quality. Follow all waste disposal regulations when disposing waste materials.

1. Cetyltrimethylammonium bromide powder (CTAB). Store at room temperature.
2. 2 M sodium hydroxide (NaOH) solution, pH 14. Store at room temperature (*see* **Note 1**).
3. Acidified methanol: 1 % HCl solution in methanol. Add 1 mL of 37 % HCl to 100 mL of methanol and vortex until thoroughly mixed. Prepare fresh for each preparation.
4. Tetraethyl orthosilicate (TEOS) (Acros Organics, Pittsburgh, PA, USA). Store at room temperature.
5. 2,4-pentanedione (Acetylacetone, AcAc) (Acros Organics, Pittsburgh, PA,USA). Store at room temperature.
6. Holmium chloride (Acros Organics, Pittsburgh, PA, USA). Store at room temperature.

3 Methods

Perform all procedures at room temperature and in a certified fume hood unless otherwise specified.

3.1 Preparation of Mesoporous Silica Nanoparticles

1. Weigh out 0.2 g of CTAB powder in a weighing dish and transfer to a 250 mL Erlenmeyer flask. Add 100 mL of ultrapure water to the Erlenmeyer flask, add an appropriately sized

magnetic stir bar to the flask and cover the top with aluminum foil (*see* **Note 2**). Heat the solution using a water bath set to 80 °C and stir the solution at 200 rpm until the solution becomes clear.

2. Adjust the pH of the solution through the addition of 0.7 mL of 2 M NaOH. The pH of the solution should be 12. Maintain the CTAB solution at 80 °C and stirring at 200 rpm for 30 min (*see* **Note 3**).
3. After the 30 min have passed, increased the stirring rate from 200 rpm to 800 rpm. Using a 100 μL micropipette, add 1 mL of TEOS to the beaker in a dropwise fashion, making sure to drop one drop of TEOS every 30 s until the full volume is added (*see* **Note 4**). During this addition step the solution will become cloudy, indicating the formation of silica nanoparticles.
4. Keep heating and stirring at 80 °C and 800 rpm for 4 h. After this time, turn off the heat and allow the suspension to cool to room temperature while continually stirring for 12 additional hours.
5. Transfer the suspension to a 50 mL centrifuge tube and centrifuge at 12,000 × *g* for 5 min. Remove the supernatant and wash the pellet with methanol by resuspending the pellet in 30 mL of methanol and vortexing until a uniform suspension is created (*see* **Note 5**). Centrifuge the uniform suspension at 12,000 × *g* for 5 min and then remove the supernatant. Repeat this step two additional times with methanol and then three additional times using ultrapure water. This should remove the excess surfactant and TEOS that has not formed particles.
6. Following the last pellet wash with water, remove the supernatant and add 40 mL of the acidified methanol to the centrifuge tube containing the washed particle pellet and resuspend by sonicating the suspension in a bath sonicator at room temperature for 30 min (*see* **Note 6**).
7. Transfer the uniform suspension to a clean 125 mL Erlenmeyer flask and stir it with a magnetic stir bar at 800 rpm for 24 h in order to remove the surfactant from the particles. After the 24 h period, transfer the solution to a 50 mL centrifuge tube and centrifuge at 12,000 × *g* for 5 min. Discard the supernatant and then resuspend the pellet in another 40 mL of the acidified methanol using bath sonication, transfer the suspension back to the 125 mL Erlenmeyer flask and stir it again at 800 rpm for 24 h (*see* **Note 7**).
8. Transfer the suspension to a 50 mL centrifuge tube and centrifuge at 12,000 × *g* for 5 min. Remove the supernatant and wash the pellet with methanol by resuspending the pellet in 30 mL of methanol and vortexing until a uniform suspension is

created. Centrifuge the uniform suspension at 12,000 × *g* for 5 min and then remove the supernatant. Repeat this step two additional times with methanol and then three additional times using ultrapure water. This should remove the excess surfactant and methanol from the particles.

9. Following the last wash, place the centrifuge tube containing the washed nanoparticle pellet into a vacuum chamber and allow for the pellet to dry for 24 h (*see* **Note 8**). Store the dried pellet at 4 °C.

3.2 Holmium Acetylacetonate Crystal Preparation

1. Weigh out 18 g of acetylacetone in a 150 mL beaker. Add 100 mL of ultrapure water, cover with aluminum foil and mix with a magnetic stir bar at 150 rpm for 15 min. The pH for this solution should be between 3 and 4.
2. Slowly add ammonium hydroxide to the solution while it continues to stir at 150 rpm until the pH is 8.5. The solution should go from clear to yellow as the pH increases.
3. Weigh out 1 g of holmium chloride and dissolve in 15 mL of water. Slowly add this solution to the pH adjusted acetylacetonate solution while it is still stirring at 150 rpm. Cover the beaker with aluminum foil and allow to stir for 24 h at room temperature. The formation of crystals will become apparent as the solution will over time become cloudy.
4. Collect the holmium acetylacetonate crystals by pouring the suspension into Büchner funnel lined with coarse (particle retention >20 μm) filter paper that is connected to a 500 mL filtering flask. Use vacuum to increase the rate of filtration. The crystals should be pink in color.
5. Wash the crystals by pouring 300 mL of ultrapure water and pulling vacuum to remove excess water. After washing the crystals with ultrapure water, carefully transfer the wet crystals to a 20 mL glass vial. Cover the top of the vial with aluminum foil and poke some small holes in the aluminum foil (*see* **Note 9**). Transfer the vial to a vacuum chamber and dry the crystals for 48 h.

3.3 Loading Mesoporous Silica Nanoparticles with Holmium Acetylacetonate

1. Weigh out 10 mg of holmium acetylacetonate crystals and dissolve in 5 mL of anhydrous ethanol. Add the solution to a 10 mL glass vial. Weight out 10 mg of the previously prepared mesoporous silica nanoparticle powder and add to the holmium acetylacetonate and ethanol solution. Bath-sonicate the mixture for 1 h in order to create a uniform suspension of particles (*see* **Note 10**).
2. After the suspension is homogenous, add a magnetic stirrer to the vial and stir at 200 rpm and room temperature for 24 h.

3. Transfer the suspension to a 15 mL centrifuge tube and centrifuge at 12,000 × *g* for 5 min. Remove the supernatant and wash the pellet with ethanol by resuspending the pellet in 10 mL of ethanol and mixing using a vortex until a uniform suspension is created (*see* **Note 11**). Centrifuge the uniform suspension at 12,000 × *g* for 5 min and then remove the supernatant. Repeat this step two additional times with ethanol and then three additional times using ultrapure water. The remaining pellet is holmium loaded mesoporous silica nanoparticles (Ho-MSN).
4. Transfer the centrifuge tube to a vacuum chamber and dry the nanoparticle pellet for 24 h. Store at 4 °C until irradiation.

3.4 Neutron Activation of Holmium Loaded Mesoporous Silica Nanoparticles

1. Transfer around 1 mg of Ho-MSNs to the polypropylene sample vials in order to prepare for neutron activation (*see* **Note 12**).
2. Depending on the amount of radioactivity needed for the particular experiment, calculate the irradiation time by using Eq. 1 (*see* **Note 13**). Samples should be packaged in accordance with the proper radiation safety regulations.

$$A = nf\sigma\left(1 - e^{-\lambda T}\right)e^{-\lambda t} \tag{1}$$

Equation for determining the radioactivity produced in disintegrations per second, where n is the number of holmium atoms, f is the neutron flux density of the nuclear reactor being used (neutrons per cm^2 per second), σ is the thermal neutron capture cross section (cm^2), λ is the radiation decay constant, T is the irradiation time and t is the time between the end of irradiation and the count.

3. After irradiating the samples in the thermal neutron flux in a nuclear reactor facility for a specific time and returning to the lab following the radiation safety procedures, carefully remove the sample lids (*see* **Note 14**) and resuspend the particles in the appropriate amount of sterile phosphate buffered saline or sterile serum free media to make a nanoparticle concentration of 1 mg/mL (*see* **Note 15**).

4 Notes

1. The NaOH solution is usually not kept for more than 2 weeks and is preferably prepared fresh before each preparation. If stored, the pH is checked before every preparation to ensure no major changes have occurred.
2. The use aluminum foil helps to prevent the loss of water from the system during heating. This allows us to maintain the

concentration of surfactant well below the solubility point and also above the critical micelle concentration of 1 mM. It was found that aluminum foil worked best because of the necessity to constantly remove and replace the cover of the flask during nanoparticle preparation.

3. Adjusting the pH allows for the protonation of the surfactant and maintaining basic conditions is very important in order to properly form the hexagonal pore template upon which the silica source will form the particle.
4. We found it easier to work with the Erlenmeyer flask while it is stabilized in the water bath on a hot plate using a ring stand and adjustable clamp. Since the suspension will be spinning at a very high speed, it is imperative to keep the flask from moving due to some potential partial boiling in the water bath so that the magnetic stir bar can consistently spin without interruption. It is easiest to peel back a small part of the aluminum foil cover and quickly place the micropipette underneath the lid to drop TEOS into the flask. This will keep some of the water from evaporating. Slowly adding the TEOS drop by drop in 30 s intervals was found to form spherical particles of an even size distribution and prevent elliptical particles that do not fully form.
5. If large particles of silica are floating around in the tube after vortexing, bath-sonicate the sample in 30 min intervals until the sample is completely uniform before centrifuging the sample. If at all possible, avoid probe sonication of the sample. The coating on the probes has the potential to chip off into the sample. The extra microscopic metals can produce unwanted radioactive isotopes during irradiation.
6. Do not proceed to the day long stirring step until the suspension looks uniform. Continue bath sonication, checking every 30 min to see if the large particles have been separated. In the right image of Fig. 2 you can see some aggregation occurring even after sonication, so it is important to keep the particle suspension looking as uniform as possible to make sure all surfaces of the particle are exposed to the acidified methanol.
7. This step may need to be repeated multiple times in order to fully remove the surfactant. Without proper removal of the surfactant, the pores will not fully form and the amount of holmium loaded will be less. In the left image of Fig. 2 you can see the ordered pores of the MSN after successful removal of the surfactant.
8. The powder should be very fine. If the pellet forms a single block of silica, try breaking the pieces up with a spatula and then upon resuspension, use bath sonication to break it back up into individual particles.

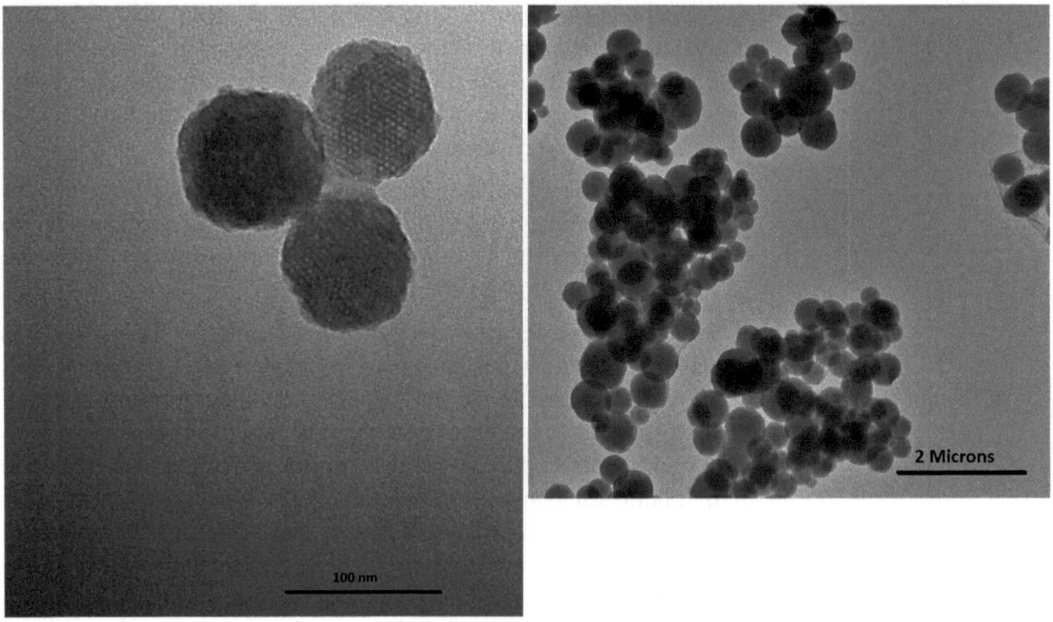

Fig. 2 TEM images of the prepared Holmium loaded mesoporous silica nanoparticles. (*Left*) At a high magnification the well-ordered pores become visible. The magnification is 250,000× with a scale bar of 100 nm. (*Right*) The particles have a high tendency to aggregate, so it is important to sonicate the sample well during the synthesis. The magnification is 18,500× with a scale bar of 2 μm. The average particle size is 120 nm using this preparation method

9. Make sure that the crystals are in a big enough container so that when vacuum is released the crystals are not sent airborne and out of your vessel completely.
10. The length of sonication can vary depending on how agglomerated the particles are. If resuspending the particles is a large issue, suspend the particles in the ethanol first and sonicate for extended periods of time before adding the holmium acetylacetonate crystals.
11. Use bath sonication if using a vortex is not enough to break up the large agglomerated particles.
12. 1 mg is used in order to easily resuspend the particles at a concentration of 1 mg/mL for cell and mouse experiments. This should decrease your radiation exposure time if everything is pre-weighed before irradiation.
13. In our experience we get about 20 % loading of elemental holmium to the nanoparticles. Therefore, our number of target atoms calculation is based on a holmium weight that is 20 % of the total weight of powder. The thermal neutron flux and neutron capture cross section is determined by the nuclear facility and was 1.8×10^{13} n/cm^2-s and 6.4×10^{-23} cm^2, respectively. The half-life of Holmium is 26.8 h and the decay

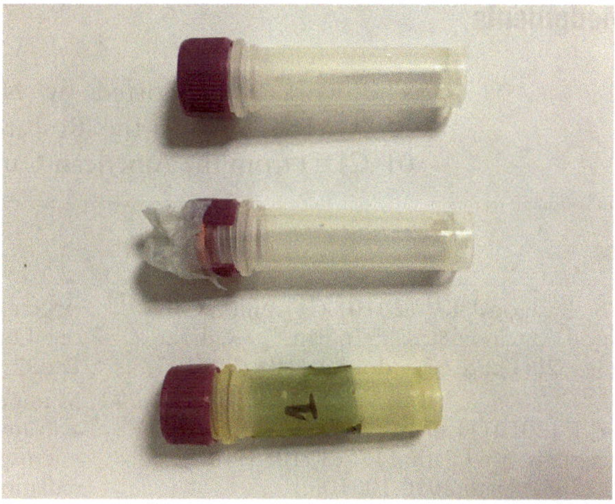

Fig. 3 Differences in the same lot of polypropylene sample vials after neutron activation of the Ho-MSN powders. (*Left vial*) 8 h in neutron flux caused extreme flimsiness in the vial and discoloration. (*Middle vial*) The cap was cracked while attempting to open it. (*Right vial*) Vial was carefully opened and did not present any noticeable breakage

constant is determined by calculating 0.693/half-life. Irradiation time up to 8 h has shown to have no determinable stability issues (holmium leaching from the pores, increased aggregation, and degraded nanoparticle structure). For our purposes, the irradiation time never exceeded 8 h. If the nuclear facility is not readily available, make sure to factor in the amount of time spent removing the samples from irradiation in the nuclear facility, packaging and shipping time, and experiment time in the amount of radioactivity needed for a particular experiment.

14. The vials will be quite flimsy and also have the tendency to break in some cases due to the long periods of time spent in the reactor (Fig. 3). Vials that are broken and compromised are not used in experiments in order to maintain accurate particle concentrations and to limit the need for having to weigh out certain amounts of powder for experiments. Resuspending directly in the vial saves time and limits radiation exposure. These specific vials are specially cleaned to remove sodium and other trace element contamination. Wear gloves when handling the vials in order to limit contamination. Follow radiation safety procedures diligently and make sure everything is set up in a way that limits personal exposure to the radioactive materials.

15. The sterile PBS is used in animal work and serum free media is used for cell work. Some of the powder may appear on the cap after irradiation and shipping. After carefully removing the cap to add the suspension media, make sure to carefully reattach the lid and shake the vial vigorously to try and recover the total mass of particles in the vial for accurate nanoparticle concentrations.

Acknowledgments

The work is supported by National Cancer Institute (NCI) R03CA184394 and the Research Scholar Grant, RSG-15-011-01-CDD from the American Cancer Society.

References

1. Smiti S, Rajagopal KV (2010) CT mimics of peritoneal carcinomatosis. Indian J Radiol Imaging 20(1):58–62. doi:10.4103/0971-3026.59757
2. Lengyel E (2010) Ovarian cancer development and metastasis. Am J Pathol 177(3):1053–1064. doi:10.2353/ajpath.2010.100105
3. Bajaj G, Yeo Y (2010) Drug delivery systems for intraperitoneal therapy. Pharm Res 27(5): 735–738. doi:10.1007/s11095-009-0031-z
4. Vicus D, Small Jr W, Covens A (2012) Chapter 59 - ovarian cancer A2. In: Gunderson L, Tepper JE (eds) Clinical radiation oncology, 3rd edn. Philadelphia, pp 1277–1297. doi:10.1016/B978-1-4377-1637-5.00059-6
5. Lu Z, Wang J, Wientjes MG, Au JLS (2010) Intraperitoneal therapy for peritoneal cancer. Future Oncol 6(10):1625–1641. doi:10.2217/fon.10.100
6. Bakri YN, Given FT Jr (1984) Radioactivity in blood and urine following intraperitoneal instillation of chromic phosphate in patients with and without ascites. Am J Obstet Gynecol 150(2):184–188
7. Spencer TR Jr, Marks RD Jr, Fenn JO, Jenrette JM 3rd, Lutz MH (1989) Intraperitoneal P-32 after negative second-look laparotomy in ovarian carcinoma. Cancer 63 (12):2434–2437
8. Wright AA, Cronin A, Milne DE, Bookman MA, Burger RA, Cohn DE, Cristea MC, Griggs JJ, Keating NL, Levenback CF, Mantia-Smaldone G, Matulonis UA, Meyer LA, Niland JC, Weeks JC, O'Malley DM (2015) Use and effectiveness of intraperitoneal chemotherapy for treatment of ovarian cancer. J Clin Oncol 33(26):2841–2847. doi:10.1200/jco.2015.61.4776
9. Kohane DS, Tse JY, Yeo Y, Padera R, Shubina M, Langer R (2006) Biodegradable polymeric microspheres and nanospheres for drug delivery in the peritoneum. J Biomed Mater Res A 77(2):351–361. doi:10.1002/jbm.a.30654
10. Wu CC, Yang YC, Hsu YT, Wu TC, Hung CF, Huang JT, Chang CL (2015) Nanoparticle-induced intraperitoneal hyperthermia and targeted photoablation in treating ovarian cancer. Oncotarget 6(29):26861–26875. doi:10.18632/oncotarget.4766
11. Mumper RJ, Ryo UY, Jay M (1991) Neutron-activated holmium-166-poly (L-lactic acid) microspheres: a potential agent for the internal radiation therapy of hepatic tumors. J Nucl Med 32(11):2139–2143
12. Hamoudeh M, Fessi H, Salim H, Barbos D (2008) Holmium-loaded PLLA nanoparticles for intratumoral radiotherapy via the TMT technique: preparation, characterization, and stability evaluation after neutron irradiation. Drug Dev Ind Pharm 34(8):796–806. doi:10.1080/03639040801918623
13. Bult W, Varkevisser R, Soulimani F, Seevinck PR, de Leeuw H, Bakker CJ, Luijten PR, van Het Schip AD, Hennink WE, Nijsen JF (2010) Holmium nanoparticles: preparation and in vitro characterization of a new device for radioablation of solid malignancies. Pharm Res 27 (10):2205–2212. doi:10.1007/s11095-010-0226-3
14. Slowing I, Trewyn BG, Lin VS (2006) Effect of surface functionalization of MCM-41-type mesoporous silica nanoparticles on the endocytosis by human cancer cells. J Am Chem Soc 128 (46):14792–14793. doi:10.1021/ja0645943
15. Slowing II, Vivero-Escoto JL, Wu CW, Lin VS (2008) Mesoporous silica nanoparticles as controlled release drug delivery and gene transfection carriers. Adv Drug Deliv Rev 60 (11):1278–1288. doi:10.1016/j.addr.2008.03.012
16. Lin Y-S, Tsai C-P, Huang H-Y, Kuo C-T, Hung Y, Huang D-M, Chen Y-C, Mou C-Y (2005) Well-ordered mesoporous silica nanoparticles as cell markers. Chem Mater 17 (18):4570–4573. doi:10.1021/cm051014c
17. Morelli C, Maris P, Sisci D, Perrotta E, Brunelli E, Perrotta I, Panno ML, Tagarelli A, Versace C, Casula MF, Testa F, Ando S, Nagy JB, Pasqua L (2011) PEG-templated mesoporous silica nanoparticles exclusively target cancer cells. Nanoscale 3(8):3198–3207. doi:10.1039/c1nr10253b
18. Di Pasqua AJ, Yuan H, Chung Y, Kim JK, Huckle JE, Li C, Sadgrove M, Tran TH, Jay M,

Lu X (2013) Neutron-activatable holmium-containing mesoporous silica nanoparticles as a potential radionuclide therapeutic agent for ovarian cancer. J Nucl Med 54(1):111–116. doi:10.2967/jnumed.112.106609

19. Munaweera I, Shi Y, Koneru B, Saez R, Aliev A, Di Pasqua AJ, Balkus KJ Jr (2015) Chemoradiotherapeutic magnetic nanoparticles for targeted treatment of nonsmall cell lung cancer. Mol Pharm 12(10):3588–3596. doi:10.1021/acs.molpharmaceut.5b00304

Chapter 25

Nanoparticle-Mediated X-Ray Radiation Enhancement for Cancer Therapy

Autumn D. Paro, Ilanchezhian Shanmugam, and Anne L. van de Ven

Abstract

Metallic nanoparticles with a high atomic number release Auger electrons in response to external beam X-ray radiation. When these nanoparticles are selectively delivered to tumors, they have the potential to locally enhance the effects of radiation therapy. Optimizing the therapeutic efficacy of these nanoparticles, however, remains a challenging and time-consuming task. Here we describe three different assays that can be used to experimentally quantify and optimize the in vitro therapeutic efficacy of nanoparticle-mediated X-ray radiation enhancement. These include an IC50 extended dose response curve, clonogenic cell survival assay, and immunoblotting. Collectively, these assays provide information about whether a given nanoparticle provides radiosensitization, the extent of the radiosensitization, and the potential mechanism of radiosensitization.

Key words Radiosensitization, Metallic nanoparticles, DNA damage, Clonogenic assay, IC50, Immunoblotting, Surviving fraction

1 Introduction

Cancer continues to be a major public health problem in the USA, with 595,690 new deaths anticipated in 2016, making it the second leading cause of death [1]. Radiation therapy, the use of ionizing radiation for cancer treatment, is currently administered to over half of all cancer patients to treat primary tumors, prevent recurrence, or relieve symptoms caused by cancer [2]. Radiation therapy can be used alone or in combination with chemotherapy or surgery, and is often selected for its ability to slow tumor growth and control energy deposition over time [3, 4]. Unfortunately, the use of high-intensity ionizing radiation poses significant risks to surrounding healthy tissue [5].

Several techniques have been used to minimize the radiation dose delivered to normal cells while maximizing that delivered to cancer cells. These methods include fractionating the radiation dose

Reema Zeineldin (ed.), *Cancer Nanotechnology: Methods and Protocols*, Methods in Molecular Biology, vol. 1530, DOI 10.1007/978-1-4939-6646-2_25,

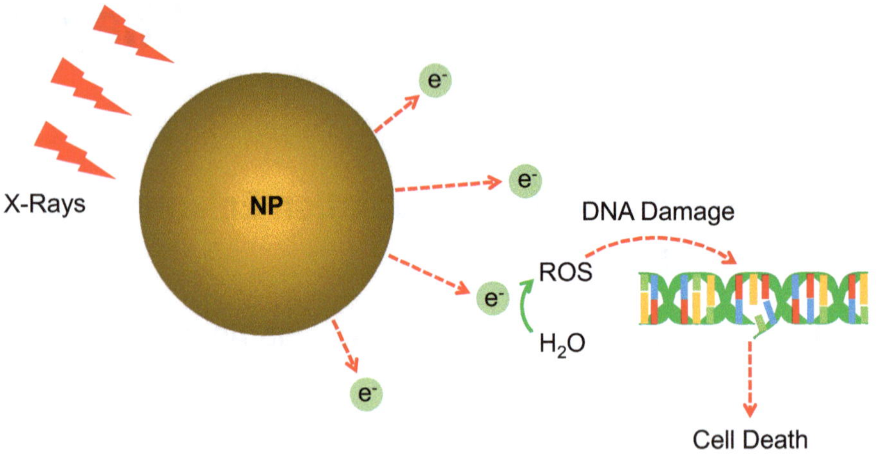

Fig. 1 The proposed mechanism by which metallic nanoparticles enhance radiation sensitivity in cells. Auger electrons released from the nanoparticle following X-ray radiation result in hydrolysis of water molecules within the cell, producing free radicals that interact with DNA to cause large numbers of single-stranded DNA breaks and eventual cell death. Adapted from [10]

over time, so that cancer cells can enter a more radiosensitive phase in the cell cycle before re-treatment, or fractioning over space by intersecting the tumor with lower-dose beams from multiple directions [6]. Other methods include systemic administration of radioprotective drugs to scavenge free radicals in healthy cells [7], radiosensitizers to selectively increase radiosensitivity of tumor cells [8], and metallic nanoparticles to locally enhance free radical production [9].

Designed to accumulate in tumors via the enhanced permeation and retention effect, metallic nanoparticles can selectively enhance the effect of X-rays in tumor cells via the localized release of Auger electrons (Fig. 1). Nanoparticles with a high atomic number absorb lower energy X-rays (30 keV–1 MeV), resulting in the displacement of an inner shell electron and its subsequent replacement by the fall of an electron from a higher level. The energy released during filling of the first electron vacancy can eject another electron from the atom, known as an Auger electron [9]. The released Auger electrons travel only very short distances, and thus tend to hydrolyze water molecules within the same cell, creating free radicals that induce DNA damage [11]. When paired with X-ray induced damage, the combination of single- and double-stranded DNA breaks makes DNA repair and replication more difficult, eventually resulting in cell death [10].

Several assays can be used to experimentally quantify and optimize the in vitro therapeutic efficacy of nanoparticle-mediated X-ray radiation enhancement. The IC50 extended nanoparticle dose response curve is used to determine relative toxicity of nanoparticles alone, in order to select a safe concentration range at which nanoparticles can be administered for radiation enhancement. In this assay, cell monolayers are treated with different concentrations of nanoparticles to identify the nanoparticle concentration that results in 50 % cell kill. Unlike conventional cytotoxicity studies, the IC50 assay described here is longer in duration in order to be sensitive to cell growth inhibition as a result of DNA damage [12]. The clonogenic cell survival assay is used to measure the fraction of surviving cells that retain proliferative capacity following X-ray irradiation [13, 14]. In this assay, cells are pretreated with nanoparticles, subjected to X-ray irradiation, and then re-plated at low seeding densities to enable the counting of individual cell colonies. Immunoblotting, or western blotting, is used to identify changes in protein expression following treatment. In this assay, protein expression is sampled at different time-points following X-ray irradiation, both the in presence and absence of nanoparticles, in order to determine how pretreatment with nanoparticles enhances radiation sensitivity [15]. Different primary antibodies can be selected based the putative mechanism of interest, such as DNA damage and repair, apoptosis, and ROS generation. Collectively, these assays provide information about whether a given nanoparticle provides radiosensitization, the extent of the radiosensitization, and the potential mechanism of radiosensitization.

2 Materials

2.1 Cell Culture Reagents for IC50 and Clonogenic Cell Survival Assay

1. Complete cell culture medium containing appropriate supplements for optimal cell growth. Store at 4 °C. Warm to 37 °C immediately before use.
2. Phosphate-buffered saline (PBS). Store at 4 °C.
3. 0.25 % trypsin with 1 mM EDTA. Store at −20 °C.
4. 0.4 % (w/v) trypan blue.
5. 10 % (v/v) neutral-buffered formalin.
6. 0.5 % (w/v) crystal violet solution.

2.2 Immunoblotting

1. Pierce BCA Protein Assay Kit (Thermo Fisher Scientific, Waltham, Massachusetts, USA) or equivalent commercially available protein quantification kit.
2. Mini Protean Tetra Cell with buffer tank, electrode assembly, lid, power cables, and buffer dam (Bio-Rad, Hercules, California, USA) or equivalent commercially available gel electrophoresis system.
3. Trans-Blot Turbo Transfer System (Bio-Rad, Hercules, California, USA) or equivalent commercially available gel transfer system.

4. Trans-Blot Turbo RTA Transfer Kit with transfer stacks and polyvinylidene difluoride (PVDF) membranes.
5. Lysis buffer: 1.0 % (v/v) Nonidet P-40 (NP-40), 50 mM Tris–HCl (pH 8.0), 150 mM NaCl in deionized water. Store at −20 °C.
6. 2× Laemmli sample buffer: 65.8 mM Tris–HCl (pH 6.8), 26.3 % (w/v) glycerol, 2.1 % SDS, 0.01 % bromophenol blue in deionized water. Store at room temperature.
7. 2× Sample buffer: (20 % (v/v) reducing agent (2-mercaptoethanol, dithiothreitol (DTT), or Cleland's reagent) in 2× Laemmli sample buffer. Prepare fresh.
8. Running buffer: 25 mM Tris–HCl (pH 8.3), 190 mM glycine, 0.1 % SDS in deionized water. Store at room temperature.
9. Washing buffer: 0.5 % (v/v) Tween 20, 50 mM Tris–HCl (pH 8.0), 150 mM NaCl in deionized water. Store at room temperature.
10. Blocking buffer: 3 % (w/v) bovine serum albumin (BSA) in washing buffer. Prepare fresh.
11. Transfer buffer: 25 mM Tris–HCl (pH 8.3), 190 mM glycine, 20 % (v/v) ethanol in deionized water. Store at 4 °C.
12. Western ECL Blotting Substrate Kit containing luminol enhancer and peroxide solution.
13. Precision Plus protein dual color standard (Bio-Rad, Hercules, California, USA). Store at −20 °C.
14. Precision Protein Strep Tactin-HRP conjugate (Bio-Rad, Hercules, California, USA). Store at 4 °C.
15. Primary antibody against the biomarker of interest. Store according to manufacturer's instructions. Potential biomarkers that may be examined are listed in Table 1.
16. ImageJ software, available from the NIH (http://imagej.nih.gov).

3 Methods

Carry out all procedures at room temperature unless otherwise noted.

3.1 IC50 Extended Nanoparticle Dose Response Curve

1. Seed cells (100,000/well) into 6-well cell culture plates and add 2 mL of complete cell culture medium. Prepare a sufficient number of plates to test multiple nanoparticle concentrations and controls in triplicate. Incubate plates at 37 °C in 5 % CO_2 for 24 h.

Table 1
Selected biomarkers for assessing X-ray radiation enhancement

Protein	Function	References
BAX	Pro-apoptotic regulator responsible for cell commitment to apoptosis	[16, 17]
BRCA1	DNA repair protein activated by double-stranded DNA breaks	[18]
BRCA2	DNA repair protein activated by single-stranded DNA breaks	[18]
Caspase-3	Protease activated during cell apoptosis	[19]
DNA polymerase theta	DNA repair protein activated by double-stranded DNA breaks	[18]
γH2AX	DNA damage marker activated by double-stranded DNA breaks	[18, 19]
KRas	Cell cycle regulator that can induce cell cycle arrest, apoptosis, or replicative senescence	[20]
Parp-1	DNA repair protein activated by single-stranded DNA breaks	[18, 19]
P53	Tumor suppressor protein activated by DNA damage	[17]
Rad51	DNA repair protein activated by double-stranded DNA breaks	[18]

2. Resuspend the nanoparticles of interest in a small volume of water or saline, and then sonicate or pipette to achieve a monodisperse suspension. To determine the concentration of nanoparticles that produces 50 % cell kill in the absence of radiation, nanoparticles are generally administered across the nM to mM dose range. Prepare several different dilutions of nanoparticles in complete media. Replace the cell supernant with 2 mL of cell culture medium with or without nanoparticles. Label the lid of each plate with the treatment conditions and incubate for at least 24 h.
3. 24 h after nanoparticle addition, harvest the cells for re-seeding at a lower cell density. Remove the media, wash each well once with PBS, and incubate with 0.5 mL pre-warmed 0.25 % trypsin–EDTA for 3 min or until the cells have detached. Neutralize the trypsin with 1 mL complete cell culture medium (or medium containing soybean trypsin inhibitor), pellet the cells in a 1.5 mL microcentrifuge tube, and resuspend cells in 1 mL media. Mix equal volumes of 0.4 % trypan blue and cells, and count the cells using an automated cell counter or hemocytometer.
4. Seed the cells in new 6-well plates at 500–5000 cells/well. Add 3 mL complete media and incubate for at least 1 week or until colonies form in the control wells.
5. After sufficient colonies have formed, remove the cell culture media, wash three times with 1 mL PBS, and add 500 μL of 10 % (v/v) neutral-buffered formalin (or 6 % (v/v)

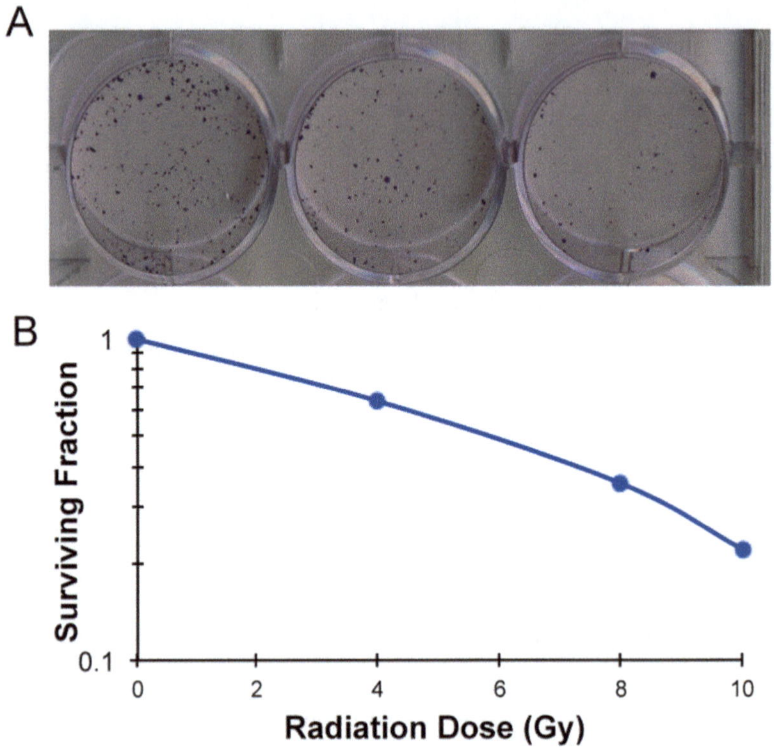

Fig. 2 Colonies of Capan-1 pancreatic cancer cells after 14 days of cell culture. (**a**) Cells were plated at a density of 2000, 1500, and 1000 cells/well (*left* to *right*) in 6-well plates 4 h after irradiation. (**b**) Colony counting following different doses of radiation yield a dose-dependent survival curve

glutaraldehyde) and 50 μL of crystal violet to each well for 30 min at room temperature. Remove formalin–crystal violet mixture with repeated washing using deionized water. Let the plates dry overnight. Example colonies of cells seeded at three different densities are shown in Fig. 2a.

6. Once the plates are dry, individual colonies can be counted manually using pen and paper or ImageJ software. The plating efficiency, PE, is calculated as

$$PE = \frac{\#\text{ colonies formed}}{\#\text{ cells seeded}}$$

using the number of colonies counted in the untreated controls. The surviving fraction, SF, for each treatment group is calculated as

$$SF = \frac{\#\text{ colonies formed}}{\#\text{ cells seeded} \times PE}$$

Once the survival fraction has been calculated for each dose, the survival curve can be plotted as shown in Fig. 2b.

3.2 Clonogenic Cell Survival Assay

1. Seed cells (100,000–300,000) into T25 cell culture flasks and add 3 mL of complete cell culture media. A minimum of two flasks is needed for each radiation dose: one with nanoparticle treatment and one without. Typical radiation doses include: 0, 2, 4, 6, 8, and 10 Gy. Incubate flasks at 37 °C in 5 % CO_2 until they reach ~70 % confluency, changing media as needed (*see* **Notes 1** and **2**).
2. Resuspend the nanoparticles of interest in a small volume of water or saline, and then sonicate or pipette to achieve a monodisperse suspension. Dilute the nanoparticle concentrate with a sufficient volume of complete media in order to fully replace that in the T25 flasks. Remove media from each T25 flask, add 3 mL of diluted nanoparticles or untreated media, and return the cells to the incubator for at least 24 h (*see* **Note 3**).
3. Twenty-four hours after nanoparticle treatment, irradiate the cells using a cabinet or small animal X-ray irradiator. For each radiation dose, you should have one plate treated with nanoparticles, and one without. Be sure to also bring the non-irradiated cells to the X-ray irradiator in order to subject the control cells to the same environmental conditions as the treated cells. After irradiation, return the cells to the incubator.
4. Four hours after irradiation, harvest the cells for replating in 6-well plates. One flask at a time, remove media, wash with 1 mL PBS, incubate with 1 mL pre-warmed 0.25 % trypsin-EDTA for 3 min or until the cells have detached. Neutralize the trypsin with 2–3 mL complete media (or media containing soybean trypsin inhibitor), pellet the cells in a 15 mL centrifuge tube, and resuspend cells in 2–3 mL media. Mix equal volumes of 0.4 % (w/v) trypan blue and cells, and count the cells using an automated cell counter or hemocytometer.
5. Seed the cells in triplicate in 6-well plates. The appropriate seeding density is usually on the order of 100–10,000 cells per well. This seeding density is deliberately low so that cells with proliferative capacity will appear as distinct, non-overlapping colonies following 2 weeks of culture. It may be necessary to plate the irradiated and/or nanoparticle-treated cells at a higher density than the untreated controls. Once the appropriate seeding density is determined (this may take several tries), dilute and seed the cells into 6-well plates, with each well containing 3 mL media. Incubate the colonies for at least 2 weeks, changing media only if needed.

6. After sufficient colonies have formed, label and count the cell colonies as described in **steps 5** and **6** under Subheading 3.1 above.

3.3 Immunoblotting

1. Prepare and treat cells seeded in 6-well plates with nanoparticles and radiation as desired. At the appropriate time-point following irradiation (as determined by the protein target of interest), prepare protein lysates as described in the Bio-Rad General Protocol for Western Blotting [21]. Generally, one confluent well yields sufficient protein for loading multiple gel lanes; however, it is recommended to prepare at least three replicates of each treatment condition when running multiple gels.
2. Determine the overall protein concentration of each cell lysate using the Pierce BCA Protein Assay. Protein lysates should be stored at −80 °C.
3. Preheat a hot plate to 100 °C. Place the lysis buffer, Precision Plus protein standards, reducing agent, and protein lysate on ice.
4. Prepare all reagents. The running, washing, and transfer buffers can be prepared in advance. The sample buffer and blocking buffer should be prepared fresh each time.
5. Place 1–4 gels on electrode assemblies, adding a buffer dam for odd numbers of gels. Fill the center of each electrode assembly with running buffer to verify the gasket is not leaking. Finish filling the buffer tank to the appropriate line, based on the number of gels being run. Using running buffer, wash each loading well by pipetting up and down several times (*see* **Notes 4** and **5**).
6. Aliquot the protein lysate into microcentrifuge tubes and dilute to ½ the final volume using with lysis buffer. Add 2× sample buffer, so that 50 % of the final volume is sample buffer and 50 % is protein lysate in lysis buffer (*see* **Note 6**).
7. Heat the protein samples at 100 °C for 5 min, and then centrifuge at 3000 rcf for 1 min, to collect the sample at the bottom of the tube.
8. Load each gel from left to right, placing 5–10 μL of Precision Plus Protein standard into the first well. Place the cover on the buffer tank and set the power supply to 150 V, 75 mA. Run the gel for desired amount of time to separate the protein band(s) of interest, generally 45–60 min, and then turn off power supply (*see* **Note 7**).
9. To prepare for gel transfer, soak two transfer stacks per gel in transfer solution. Soak PVDF or nitrocellulose transfer membranes in 95 % ethanol for 3 min, followed by 3 min in transfer

solution. In the meantime, open each gel, and place them into the transfer solution. For an even transfer, it is recommended to remove the tops of gels using a knife to create a straight top edge. If multiple gels are used with different protein concentrations, make note of which one is placed where for later reference when adding primary antibody.

10. Place a transfer stack into the transfer cassette, followed by the transfer membrane, then the gel, and finally another transfer stack. Make sure there are no air bubbles beneath each layer as it is placed down. Complete the assembly of the transfer cassette and place it into the transfer system. Set the power supply to 25 V, 1.0 A for 30 min. These time and power settings may vary based on the transfer method used.
11. When the transfer is finished, remove membranes from transfer cassette and place each into its own labeled plastic box. Add 15 mL of blocking buffer to each container and shake on an orbital shaker for 60 min to block non-specific binding (*see* **Notes 8** and **9**).
12. Remove the blocking buffer and add the primary antibody. If you plan to run multiple antibodies per membrane, cut the membrane and separate the pieces into new containers. Primary antibodies are diluted in blocking buffer as recommended by manufacturer. Place container in the fridge or on a refrigerated shaker overnight.
13. The next day, place the membranes on a shaker at room temperature for 2 h. Remove primary antibody, and wash four times with 10–15 mL TBST at 10-min intervals. Shake continuously (*see* **Note 10**).
14. Remove the TBST and replace with 15 mL of secondary antibody diluted in blocking buffer as per manufacturer's instructions. Make sure to use a secondary antibody that that is designed to bind the Fc domain of the primary antibody. For chemiluminescent detection, also add 1 μL of Strep Tactin HRP conjugate. Shake at room temperature for 1 h.
15. Remove the secondary antibody and wash four times with 10–15 mL TBST at 10-min intervals. Shake continuously.
16. Freshly prepare the chemiluminescent developer solution by combining Peroxide solution and Luminal Solution (1:1) from the Western ECL Substrate Kit. Prepare just enough to cover each membrane evenly. Remove one membrane at a time from the TBST, pat dry with a lint-free wipe, and place into developer solution for 5 min while shaking gently. After developing, pat the membrane dry, and cover in cling wrap, removing as many bubbles as possible. Image using a chemiluminescent imager (*see* **Note 11**).

17. Blots can be quantified using ImageJ software. More information can be found in Sect. 30.13 of the online ImageJ User Guide [22].

4 Notes

1. As an alternative to T25 flasks, cells can be seeded into 6-well plates.
2. Radiation doses are measured in Grey (Gy), where 1 Gy = 1 J/kg. The dose is calculated by the total exposure time multiplied by the energy of the X-ray beam.
3. Dilutions are calculated using the equation: $V_{np} = \frac{C_{want}}{C_{stock}} \times V_{total}$, where C_{want} is the concentration desired, C_{stock} is the concentration of the stock nanoparticle solution, V_{total} is the total volume to make, and V_{np} is the volume of nanoparticle stock needed.
4. Make sure to remove tape from bottom of gel before placing in the gel box. Make sure when placing electrode assemblies into the buffer tank, the correct electrodes are on the correct side.
5. When selecting or casting a gel, the size of the loading wells should be selected based on volume of protein to be loaded and the number of samples. Typically, as the well size increases, the number of available wells decreases.
6. The amount of protein prepared for a given gel is dependent on the concentration of the target protein and is generally determined experimentally when optimizing the use of each antibody.
7. For proteins of low molecular weight, a shorter running time is needed. If left too long proteins, will run off the bottom of the gel. For proteins of high molecular weight, or when using one membrane to sample multiple proteins, a longer running time is generally needed to separate the bands of interest.
8. In addition to labeling the protein loading concentration, it is helpful to record the primary antibody, antibody dilution, and the secondary antibody to be used.
9. This blocking step can also be performed using non-fat dry milk instead of BSA.
10. The primary antibody dilution can be saved and reused several times if stored at −20 °C.
11. For imaging, choose a standard exposure to start and then increase or decrease the exposure time based on the initial image. Take several images to verify that you have a good blot.

Acknowledgement

This work was supported in part by: NSF DGE-0965843, DOD W81XWH-09-2-0001, NCI 1R25CA174650-01A, and the Electronics Materials Research Institute at Northeastern University.

References

1. Siegal RL, Miller KD, Jemal A (2016) Cancer statistics, 2016. CA Cancer J Clin 66:7–30
2. Smith BD, Haffty BG et al (2010) The future of radiation oncology in the United States from 2010 to 2020: will supply keep pace with demand? J Clin Oncol 28(35):5160–5165
3. Terasawa T, Dvorak T et al (2009) Systematic review: charged-particle radiation therapy for cancer. Ann Intern Med 151(8):556–565
4. Elshaikh M, Ljungman M et al (2006) Advances in radiation oncology. Annu Rev Med 57:19–31
5. Kwatra D, Venugopal A, Anant S (2013) Nanoparticles in radiation therapy: a summary of various approaches to enhance radiosensitization in cancer. Transl Cancer Res 2 (4):330–342
6. Steel G (1997) Basic clinical radiobiology. Oxford University Press, London
7. Hosseinimehr S (2007) Trends in the development of radioprotective agents. Drug Discov Today 12:794–805
8. Wardman P (2007) Chemical radiosensitizers for use in radiotherapy. Clin Oncol 29:397–417
9. Bushberg J, Seibert J et al (2012) The essential of physics of medical imaging. Lippincott Williams & Wilkins, Philadelphia
10. Setua S, Ouberai M, Piccirillo SG et al (2014) Cisplatin-tethered gold nanospheres for multimodal chemo-radiotherapy of glioblastoma. Nanoscale 6:10865–10873
11. Adilakshmi T, Lease R, Woodson S (2006) Hydroxyl radical footprinting in vivo: mapping macromolecular structures with synchrotron radiation. Nucleic Acids Res 34(8):e64
12. Munshi A, Hobbs M, Meyn RE (2005) Clonogenic cell survival assay. Methods Mol Med 110:21–28
13. Shen Y, Rehman FL et al (2013) BMN 673, a novel and highly potent PARP1/2 inhibitor for the treatment of human cancers with DNA repair deficiency. Clin Cancer Res 19 (18):5003–5015
14. Franken N, Rodermond H et al (2006) Clonogenic assay of cells in vitro. Nat Protoc 1:2315–2319
15. Roa W, Zhang X et al (2009) Gold nanoparticle sensitize radiotherapy of prostate cancer cells by regulation of the cell cycle. Nanotechnology 20(37):375101
16. Hector S, Prehn J (2009) Apoptosis signaling proteins as prognostic biomarkers in colorectal cancer: a review. Biochim Biophys Acta 1795:117–129
17. Roos W, Kaina B (2006) DNA damage-induced cell death by apoptosis. Trends Mol Med 12(9):440–450
18. Wang H, Adhikari S et al (2014) A perspective on chromosomal double strand break markers in mammalian cells. Jacobs J Radiat Oncol 1 (1):1–8
19. Porter A, Janicke R (1999) Emerging roles of caspase-3 in apoptosis. Cell Death Differ 6 (2):99–104
20. Jancik S, Drabek J et al (2010) Clinical relevance of KRAS in human cancers. J Biomed Biotechnol 2010:1–13
21. Bio-Rad Laboratories, Inc. General protocol for western blotting (Bulletin 6376 RevA). www.bio-rad.com/webroot/web/pdf/lsr/literature/Bulletin_6376.pdf. Accessed 27 Jan 2016
22. Ferreira T, Rasband W (2012) ImageJ User guide. http://imagej.nih.gov/ij/docs/guide/146-30.html#infobox:Densitometry. Accessed 19 Dec 2015

Chapter 26

Radiosensitizing Silica Nanoparticles Encapsulating Docetaxel for Treatment of Prostate Cancer

Jodi Belz, Noelle Castilla-Ojo, Srinivas Sridhar, and Rajiv Kumar

Abstract

The applications of nanoparticles in oncology include enhanced drug delivery, efficient tumor targeting, treatment monitoring, and diagnostics. The "theranostic properties" associated with nanoparticles have shown enhanced delivery of chemotherapeutic drugs with superior imaging capabilities and minimal toxicities. In conventional chemotherapy, only a fraction of the administered drug reaches the tumor site or cancer cells. For successful translation of these formulations, it is imperative to evaluate the design and properties of these nanoparticles. Here, we describe the design of ultra-small silica nanoparticles to encapsulate a radiosensitizing drug for combined chemoradiation therapy. The small size of nanoparticles allows for better dispersion and uptake of the drug within the highly vascularized tumor tissue. Silica nanoparticles are synthesized using an oil-in-water microemulsion method. The microemulsion method provides a robust synthetic route in which the inner hydrophobic core is used to encapsulate chemotherapy drug, docetaxel while the outer hydrophilic region provides dispersibility of the synthesized nanoparticles in an aqueous environment. Docetaxel is commonly used for treatment of resistant or metastatic prostate cancer, and is known to have radiosensitizing properties. Here, we describe a systematic approach for synthesizing these theranostic nanoparticles for application in prostate cancer.

Key words Silica nanoparticles, Docetaxel, Drug delivery, Microemulsions, Prostate cancer, Bottom-up synthesis, Radiosensitization

1 Introduction

While chemotherapy is frequently used as a first line of treatment, adverse toxicities and low bioavailability associated with the non-specific systemic drugs often limit treatment timing and dosing in patients [1]. To overcome these toxicities and improve circulation time, many researchers are using nanoparticles as a means for delivery [2, 3]. Since radiation therapy is used in more than 50 % of the cancer patients, the development of nanoparticles formulations which can combine the two monotherapies, chemotherapy and radiation, will not only boost the therapeutic efficacy but also reduce the toxicities associated with monotherapies [4]. Currently, docetaxel is given systemically as Taxotere to patients via

Reema Zeineldin (ed.), *Cancer Nanotechnology: Methods and Protocols*, Methods in Molecular Biology, vol. 1530,
DOI 10.1007/978-1-4939-6646-2_26,

intravenous infusion once every 2–3 weeks to allow for recovery. Docetaxel is non-cell specific and acts on the microtubules of cells, preventing depolymerization. This traps the cell in G2/M phase, which also results in increased radiosensitizing properties [5]. As a result, co-delivery of docetaxel with radiation treatment can prove to be an effective dual treatment in the case of certain cancers. It is believed that this radiosensitization effect can lead to the use of lower doses to achieve synergistic therapeutic effects, while reducing the overall toxicity experienced during the treatment. Here, we propose the use of PEGylated (i.e., polyethylene glycol-functionalized) ultra-small silica nanoparticles to encapsulate docetaxel for combined chemoradiation therapy.

We describe a systematic protocol for synthesis of silica nanoparticles to encapsulate the hydrophobic drug in the core of nanoparticles. Silica nanoparticles can be formulated at various sizes, ranging from 10 to 250 nm in diameter [6, 7]. The core is nonpolar and can trap a variety of hydrophobic chemotherapeutics, small molecules, or dyes. The surface of the nanoparticles is modified with PEG and/or targeting ligands for long term circulation and targeted cellular uptake. The PEGylation of nanoparticles minimizes the opsonization process and allows for increased systemic circulation [8]. The functional groups on the surface of the nanoparticles can be used for conjugating targeting molecules like peptides, antibodies or aptamers [9]. Below, we describe the formulation of docetaxel-loaded ultra-small silica nanoparticles for radiosensitization in prostate cancer. We conjugate a near-infrared fluorophore, Cyanine 7.5, to the silica nanoparticles to track the nanoparticle in vitro and in vivo. First we describe the fabrication and purification of the nanoparticles, followed by characterization and quantification of drug loaded silica nanoparticles using various instrumentation techniques.

2 Materials

1. Aerosol-OT (AOT) or sodium bis (2-ethylhexyl) sulfosuccinate.
2. Hydrophobic drug or dye (*see* **Note 1**): Chemotherapeutic drug, docetaxel or fluorophore, cyanine 7.5 *N*-hydroxysuccinimide (NHS) ester.
3. Triethylamine.
4. Silane precursors vinyltriethoxysilane (VTES) and aminopropyl triethoxysilane (APTES).
5. 2-[METHOXY(POLYETHYLENEOXY)6-9PROPYL]TRIMETHOXYSILANE, tech-90.
6. HPLC grade solvents.

7. Dichloromethane.
8. Sterile spin filter tubes (100 kDa MWCO) (Pall Corporation).
9. Cellulose membrane 14 kDa cutoff pore size.

3 Methods

Carry out all procedures and keep all reagents at room temperature (25 °C) unless otherwise noted.

3.1 Modified Cy-7.5

1. Degas 1 mL dimethyl sulfoxide (DMSO) using argon to remove oxygen (~1 min) and add 1 mL of DMSO to 5 mg of Cy7.5 NHS ester to make 5 mg/mL concentration.
2. Add 20 μL of APTES to the dye solution (the color should now have a slight yellow tint) followed by addition of 20 μL of trimethylamine.
3. Add a small stir bar for stirring the reaction mixture gently and put a septum on the reaction vial. Purge the reaction mixture with argon gas overnight.
4. The final product, Cy 7.5 conjugated to APTES via the amine groups of APTES can be used without further purification. When added to the nanoparticles, the conjugate will polymerize along with VTES to form fluorescent nanoparticles (*see* **Note 2**).

3.2 Synthesis of Silica Nanoparticles

1. Prepare 2.2 % (w/v) AOT solution in deionized water (*see* **Note 3**). Weigh 220 mg of the surfactant AOT in a scintillation vial and add 10 mL of deionized water. To ensure accuracy in measurement and quick solvation, break AOT wax into small pieces before weighing.
2. Place a stir-bar in scintillation vial and stir on a magnetic stirrer at approximately 1200 rpm (*see* **Note 4**). The solution will be become cloudy in appearance as the AOT dissolves.
3. After 15–20 min of stirring, add 300 μL of 1-butanol (*see* **Note 4**). The solution should become clear upon addition.
4. After 5 min, add 75 μL of docetaxel (10 mg/mL in DMSO) and 50 μL modified Cy7.5 (5 mg/mL in DMSO) (*see* **Note 5**). Reaction mixture should be protected from light to avoid photo-bleaching using aluminum foil.
5. After 5 min of stirring, add 100 μL of silane precursor, vinyltriethoxysilane (VTES).
6. Stir the reaction mixture for 40 min and thereafter add 10 μL of ammonium hydroxide (*see* **Note 6**).

7. For PEGylation of the nanoparticles, add 10 μL 2-[methoxy (polyethyleneoxy)6-9propyl]trimethoxysilane 10 min after the addition of ammonium hydroxide.
8. Stir the solution overnight, or for at least 12 h to allow nanoparticle formation and Ostwald ripening (*see* **Note 7**).
9. Remove stir bar and store the nanoparticles at 4 °C if not immediately dialyzed.

3.3 Dialysis

The purpose of dialysis is to remove the surfactant, excess of reactants and any unencapsulated drug/fluorophore molecules from the nanoparticles solution.

1. Cut the dialysis tubing to approximately 5 in. and prepare the tubing as per manufacturer's recommended protocols.
2. Pipette as prepared nanoparticles solution into dialysis tubing while securing the end of the tubes with the dialysis clips.
3. Put the dialysis tubing with sample in a container with 4 L of deionized water.
4. Stir water at roughly 100 rpm. Caution: ensure that the dialysis tubing is stirring slowly and if required adjust speed accordingly.
5. Change deionized water (DI) every 30 min for 2 h, then again after 8 h. Change again at 24 and 36 h (*see* **Note 8**).
6. Remove the sample after 48 h of dialysis against DI water (*see* **Note 9**).

3.4 Preparation for High Performance Liquid Chromatography (HPLC) Analysis

Sonicate dialyzed nanoparticle solution for 1 min to allow for even dispersion of particles.

1. Pipette out 250 μL of the nanoparticles solution into a microcentrifuge tube. All samples must be taken in triplicate to ensure accuracy.
2. Add 250 μL of dichloromethane and 250 μL HPLC grade methanol to the tube.
3. Sonicate for 45 min.
4. Leave microcentrifuge tubes in fridge at 4 °C overnight.
5. Vortex for 10 s, then evaporate off the remaining dichloromethane with air.
6. Remove solution and transfer to spin filter centrifuge tubes. Centrifuge the tubes for 30 min at 16,128 rcf using a 100 mm rotor.
7. Remove filtrate from tubes and transfer to HPLC vials.
8. Add 250 μL of mobile phase (65:35 methanol in HPLC Water) and vortex briefly.
9. Run HPLC via standard protocol (*see* **Note 10**).

3.5 Dynamic Light Scattering (DLS)

1. Sonicate dialyzed nanoparticle solution for 1 min to allow for even dispersion of particles.
2. Place 1 mL of nanoparticles to clear 2 mL cuvette. Dilute if necessary.
3. Using 90Plus zeta sizer (Brookhaven) instrument perform measurements to determine hydrodynamic diameter of the nanoparticles (*see* **Note 11**).

3.6 Transmission Electron Microscopy

1. Sonicate dialyzed nanoparticle solution for 1 min to allow for even dispersion of particles.
2. The TEM grids were prepared by drop casting the sample (20 μL) dispersion onto an amorphous carbon coated 300 mesh copper grid.
3. Place copper grid on a filter paper to absorb the excess solvent and allow to dry before loading into chamber for TEM analysis using JEOL model JEM-100CX microscope at an acceleration voltage of 80 kV (*see* **Note 12**).

4 Notes

1. We have used a hydrophobic drug docetaxel to encapsulate inside silica nanoparticles. Similar synthetic strategies can be adopted to encapsulate other hydrophobic drugs.
2. The conjugation of Cy 7.5 to nanoparticles gives a purple color solution which can be due to the aggregation of dye molecules in the silica matrix whereas when the same fluorophore Cy 7.5 is encapsulated it gives a typical green color.
3. The surfactant AOT along with co-surfactant 1-butanol and DMSO when mixed together will create an oil-in-water microemulsion system. A surfactant like AOT highly reduces the interfacial tension at the water/oil interface. In this formulation, water is the bulk phase of the microemulsion, whereas DMSO forms the oil phase in the form nanosize droplets/reactors. The hydrophobic drugs/fluorophores will reside inside these droplets and exchange between the two microemulsion droplets will result in hydrolysis and polymerization of silane precursors (in basic pH) inside these nanosize droplets. This leads to entrapment of hydrophobic molecules in the silica matrix. Reverse micellar approach using a water-in-oil microemulsion system can also be used to synthesize silica nanoparticles. In such an instance, the polar groups are directed into the aqueous core, formulating nanoparticles which will entrap polar drugs/fluorophores [10, 11].

4. The size of the particles can be modulated by many variables including stirring speed of the reaction mixture. The amount of butanol (the oil phase) is a major factor in modulating the particle size. Addition of more butanol will increase the size of the nanoparticles. e.g., for synthesizing 200 nm silica, add 700 μL butanol to the AOT mixture, and for 30 nm silica add 300 μL butanol.
5. Docetaxel and Cy7.5 can be substituted by other hydrophobic drugs or dye. The quantity was determined by our loading efficiency of the drug. The HPLC protocol and mobile phase must be selected accordingly if the drug of choice is not Docetaxel.
6. Addition of ammonium hydroxide results in hydrolysis and polycondensation of vinyltriethoxysilane to vinylpolysiloxane inside the micellar core which leads to formation of small size nanoparticles.
7. Drug/dye encapsulated nanoparticles prepared as above will maintain a translucent appearance and be approximately 30 nm in size. The size of the particles can be checked with dynamic light scattering (DLS) and further confirmed with transmission electron microscopy (30 nm).
8. Dialysis must be done for 48 h with at least six water changes to ensure removal of excess reagents especially AOT which have known toxicities in both in vitro and in vivo systems.
9. Store nanoparticles in fridge at 4 °C. It is best to use a new batch of nanoparticles for experiments to limit the amount of drug/dye released from the particles.
10. Dispose of all waste for HPLC and after preparation according to hazardous waste management protocols.
11. Dynamic light scattering (DLS) measurements were performed by using 90Plus zeta sizer (Brookhaven Inc, NY). Zeta potential measurements can be acquired with the same instrument.
12. Transmission Electron Microscopy (TEM) images were obtained using a JEOL model JEM-100CX microscope at an acceleration voltage of 80 kV.

Acknowledgment

This work was supported by NSF-DGE- 0965843 and ARMY/W81XWH-12-1-0154.

References

1. Bissery MC, Nohynek G, Sanderink GJ, Lavelle F (1995) Docetaxel (Taxotere): a review of preclinical and clinical experience. Part I: Preclinical experience. Anticancer Drugs 6:339–355
2. Bolla M, Hannoun-Levi JM, Ferrero J-M et al (2010) Concurrent and adjuvant docetaxel with three-dimensional conformal radiation therapy plus androgen deprivation for high-risk prostate cancer: preliminary results of a multicentre phase II trial. Radiother Oncol 97:312–317. doi:10.1016/j.radonc.2010.08.012
3. Kumar R, Roy I, Ohulchanskyy TY et al (2008) Covalently dye-linked, surface-controlled, and bioconjugated organically modified silica nanoparticles as targeted probes for optical imaging. ACS Nano 2:449–456. doi:10.1021/nn700370b
4. Maitra A (1984) Determination of size parameters of water aerosol OT oil reverse micelles from their nuclear magnetic-resonance data. J Phys Chem 88:5122–5125. doi:10.1021/j150665a064
5. Najjar R (1970) Microemulsions—a brief introduction. Intech, Rijeka, Croatia
6. Peer D, Karp JM, Hong S et al (2007) Nanocarriers as an emerging platform for cancer therapy. Nat Nanotechnol 2:751–760. doi:10.1038/nnano.2007.387
7. Prasad PN (2012) Introduction to nanomedicine and nanobioengineering. Wiley, Hoboken, NJ
8. Roy I, Kumar P, Kumar R et al (2014) Ormosil nanoparticles as a sustained-release drug delivery vehicle. RSC Adv 4:53498–53504. doi:10.1039/C4RA10293B
9. Sharma RK, Das S, Maitra A (2004) Surface modified ormosil nanoparticles. J Colloid Interface Sci 277:342–346. doi:10.1016/j.jcis.2004.04.019
10. Szakács G, Paterson JK, Ludwig JA et al (2006) Targeting multidrug resistance in cancer. Nat Rev Drug Discov 5:219–234. doi:10.1038/nrd1984
11. Veronese FM, Mero A (2008) The impact of PEGylation on biological therapies. BioDrugs 22:315–329

Index

Reema Zeineldin (ed.), *Cancer Nanotechnology: Methods and Protocols*, Methods in Molecular Biology, vol. 1530, DOI 10.1007/978-1-4939-6646-2, © Springer Science+Business Media New York 2017